PHYSIOLOGY - LABORATORY AND CLINICAL RESEARCH

# AUDITORY CORTEX

## ANATOMY, FUNCTIONS AND DISORDERS

# PHYSIOLOGY - LABORATORY AND CLINICAL RESEARCH

Additional books in this series can be found on Nova's website under the Series tab.

Additional e-books in this series can be found on Nova's website under the e-books tab.

PHYSIOLOGY - LABORATORY AND CLINICAL RESEARCH

# AUDITORY CORTEX

## ANATOMY, FUNCTIONS AND DISORDERS

MOUNYA ELHILALI
EDITOR

NOVA BIOMEDICAL

*New York*

For permission to use material from this book please contact us:
Telephone 631-231-7269; Fax 631-231-8175
Web Site: http://www.novapublishers.com



Additional color graphics may be available in the e-book version of this book.

**Library of Congress Cataloging-in-Publication Data**

Auditory cortex : anatomy, functions, and disorders / editor, Mounya Elhilali.
p. ; cm.
Includes bibliographical references and index.
ISBN 978-1-62100-685-5 (hardcover)
I. Elhilali, Mounya.
[DNLM: 1. Auditory Cortex. 2. Auditory Diseases, Central. WL 307]

612.8'51--dc23

2011037403

*Published by Nova Science Publishers, Inc. † New York*

# Contents

# Preface

**There is no such thing as an empty space or an empty time.**
**There is always something to see, something to hear.**
**In fact, try as we may to make a silence, we cannot**
- John Cage

That auditory cortex interfaces sensory and cognitive processes to guide perception is pretty much established. It is the most central stage along the auditory pathway and a gateway to projections onto multimodal association areas. What is less clear however is its exact role in mediating this sensory/cognitive interaction? What is its exact function in sensory perception? Does it play any role in learning and memory? Is it truly a unimodal unit? Is it a homogenous unit? What are its cyto- and chemo-architectures? Suffices to say that we have more questions about auditory cortex than we have answers…

The current volume attempts to elucidate some of these questions through a series of overviews and research studies. The chapters highlight recent technological advances that begin opening the door to address questions about auditory cortex, and canvass findings obtained from intracellular and extracellular electrophysiology, optical imaging, and quantitative electroencephalography in addition to reviews of molecular techniques, functional imaging approaches and histological anatomy.

Drs Hong, Lee and Yeo start with a general overview of the complex structure that is auditory cortex. In this first chapter, they review the known anatomy, function and disorders of auditory cortex. One the intriguing contributions of this chapter is that it highlights some of the unknown and sometimes paradoxical facts about auditory cortex. E.g. (i) Auditory cortex represents acoustic information via highly sparse and synchronized volleys of activity; yet, neurons can respond vigorously and in sustained fashion to acoustic features that drive them best. (ii) Stimulus-locked cortical responses are sluggish and undergo a temporal-to-rate transformation; yet, cortical temporal firing patterns can be highly precise and able to trace fine details of the temporal structure of sounds. (iii) Auditory cortex is a multisensory nucleus and inputs from multiple modalities modulate the cortical representation of sounds; yet, multisensory stimulation is not ‘effective’ with the same degree depending on its dynamics relative to the auditory stimulus. Overall, the chapter is an excellent stage setter for the complex system that is auditory cortex.

Building on the review from chapter I, Dr. Ojima puts the spotlight on the complex ascending and descending pathways at the level of auditory cortex. The second chapter presents a holistic view of auditory cortex, specifically primary auditory cortex A1, in the context of its entire network of subcortical pathways, extrinsic and intrinsic connections and cortical modules. It fuels the debate about the role of A1 as a "whiteboard" of acoustic information. Instead, the author underscores the cognitive role of primary auditory cortex; and argues that the community should contemplate its function as an association cortex rather than a primary one.

In chapter III, Drs Filippov, Hudoerkov, Krebs and Pugachev review recent results exploring infraslow brain potentials and their role in cortical information processing. The study shows evidence implicating slow oscillatory activity with cortical neural processing. Particularly, the authors disambiguate the role of infraslow activity (at the subHertz level) in providing bilateral thalamo-cortical modulation of cortical processing; while multisecond potentials implicate interactions between primary auditory cortex and brainstem and basal forebrain nuclei. These findings complement results presented in the previous chapter and paint a picture of auditory cortex as a dynamical structure where a systems-view is the only way to integrate the complex recurrent projections from and to it.

Chapter IV by Drs Song, Nishimura and Saitoh reviews the anatomical and functional structure of auditory cortex. They employ new techniques using in vivo optical imaging combined with acoustic and electrical stimulation to provide a detailed parceling of the guinea pig auditory cortex. The analysis reveals a total of nine subfields within auditory cortex, some of them lacking a tonotopic organization. The findings also suggest possible disparate functional roles of each subfield in processing auditory information.

In chapter V, Drs Depireux and Shechter provide a different flavor of studies of cortical function, one based on characterizing receptive fields of cortical neurons. The authors expand on the traditional linear system approaches classically adopted with receptive field techniques and look into the neural coding of acoustic features operating at different time-scales. The study highlights the differences in tuning dynamics of cortical neurons over short, medium and long time scales. The authors argue that these variable coding schemes operate synergistically in generating stable and invariant time-frequency representations of complex acoustic signals. They also discuss their potential role in guiding noise-robust processing of auditory scenes, such as cocktail party effects.

Next, Drs Sakai and Sato continue along the same lines as the previous chapter and explore functional roles of cortical responses in mediating perception. This chapter focuses particularly on category perception, and uses the commonly studied example of voice-onset-time (VOT) intervals in plosive consonant-vowels. The authors present evidence linking the perceptual phenomenon of categorical perception to an interplay between excitatory and inhibitory post-synaptic potentials in A1 neurons along with plastic modulation of thalamo-cortical projections. Such findings argue that VOT-based categorization is a general non-speech-specific phenomenon. In such as view, the temporal interplay between synchronized neural responses in A1 plays a major role in guiding the dynamics of cortical responses and hence the emergence of categorical VOT perception.

Last but not least, Drs Pirini, Mancini and Chiari review cortical activity during postural audio-biofeedback. Using quantitative EEG, the authors show how audio biofeedback complements other sensory information for postural control. Though not exclusively focusing on auditory cortex alone, this chapter explores the interaction between audition, vision and proprioception. It shows modulation of auditory cortical responses possibly to generate spatial cues that provide a feedback for the control of postural sway. Such activation is only observed in asbence of visual inputs. The results highlight the complex and possibly multi-level interaction of multisensory information, likely via a re-weighting process. Such view alters the classic beliefs of multisensory interaction that shield primary sensory cortices from such interactions.

*Mounya Elhilali, Ph.D.*
*Johns Hopkins University*

In: Auditory Cortex: Anatomy, Functions and Disorders
Editor: Mounya Elhilali
ISBN 978-1-62100-685-5


*Chapter I*

# The Anatomy, Physiology and Disorders of the Auditory Cortex

***Seok Min Hong,[1] So Yoon Lee[2] and Seung Geun Yeo[2]***
[1]Department of Otorhinolaryngology-Head and Neck Surgery,
College of Medicine, Hallym University, Korea
[2]Department of Otorhinolaryngology-Head and Neck Surgery,
School of Medicine, Kyung Hee University, Korea

## Abstract

The auditory cortex occupies a large proportion of the ventral bank of the lateral sulcus and superior temporal gyrus in humans and primates. In humans, this area includes the transverse temporal gyri of Heschl and the planum temporale, roughly corresponding to Brodmann's areas 41, 42, 52, and 22. One interesting structural feature of the cortex is that a central primary or core region lies adjacent to a number of secondary areas that forms a belt around the core. Many brain areas receive inputs from the cortex. These auditory-related regions are located in the temporal, parietal, and frontal lobes, and tend to feature multisensory convergence. Among species, the auditory cortex differs in relative position, arrangement, connections with other regional subdivisions, and tonotopic organization.

The cortex is important in the processing of sounds used for communication. The human auditory cortex processes both elementary speech sounds and other temporally complex acoustic signals. Multisensory integration occurs in the cortex. Apart from auditory stimuli, accompanying visual and somatosensory signals assist in auditory perception. Cross-modal plasticity has been observed; the auditory area may be activated by visual or sign language in congenitally deaf adults

Damage to the auditory cortex causes cortical deafness, pure word and auditory sound agnosia, and sensory amusia, depending on the extent of the auditory system lesion and other clinical characteristics. In patients with auditory hallucinations or subjective chronic tinnitus, functional magnetic resonance imaging has shown that the auditory cortex is active.

# Introduction

This chapter outlines the anatomy, function and disorders of the auditory cortex and is intended for medical students, general otologists, neurologists, and psychiatrists, as well as anyone else interested in the auditory cortex. To date, most books on these subjects have focused on the cochlea and cochlear nerve, mainly discussing patients with lesions in these organs. Lesions in the auditory cortex itself are rare, and few studies have been performed especially in humans. Moreover, most studies on the auditory cortex have been performed postmortem or by noninvasive physiology. To overcome these limitations, recent studies have incorporated quantitative methods, functional imaging, and measurements of the expression levels of enzymes, proteins and neurotransmitters. Therefore, the first two parts of this chapter describe the basic anatomy and function of the auditory cortex, while the third part presents a general overview of disorders in the auditory cortex. We hope to provide new insights of human auditory organization, as well as the function and disorders of the auditory cortex.

# Anatomy of the Auditory Cortex

## Development

The brain cortex develops through two different phases. The first phase involves the intrinsic development of central neural pathways; during this phase, development of the brain cortex is not related to external input signals and development proceeds according to biological programs, regardless of external signals. For example, axonal growth cones in the central nervous system seem to have predetermined destinations for synaptic termination. During this period, thalamic afferents reach the brain cortex. In the second or late phase, sensory signal inputs direct development; during this time, the tonotopic organization of the auditory cortex can be affected by over-exposure to a narrow range of stimuli. In humans, thalamic afferents pass through the cerebral cortex in the middle of intrauterine life, whereas, in rats and cats, these afferents pass through the cerebral cortex around 3.5 and 5 days, respectively, before birth [1]. Herein, we will describe the development of the human auditory cortex in utero and after birth.

### *First Trimester*

The peripheral auditory organs (i.e. the cochlea and cochlear nerve) form during this period, and auditory centers and pathways can be identified in the brainstem [2]. Axons of the trapezoid body in the auditory nucleus pass through the brainstem and innervate the superior olivary complex [3], and the medial geniculate body can be identified [4]. At 8 weeks, axons arising from the inferior colliculus reach the thalamic center and cells accumulate around the external surface of the cerebral cortex, forming a dense layer (i.e. the cortical plate) in the forebrain. The marginal layer includes large and early maturing cells. The auditory cortex consists of a dense cellular cortical plate and a clear marginal laryer [5] (Figure 1).

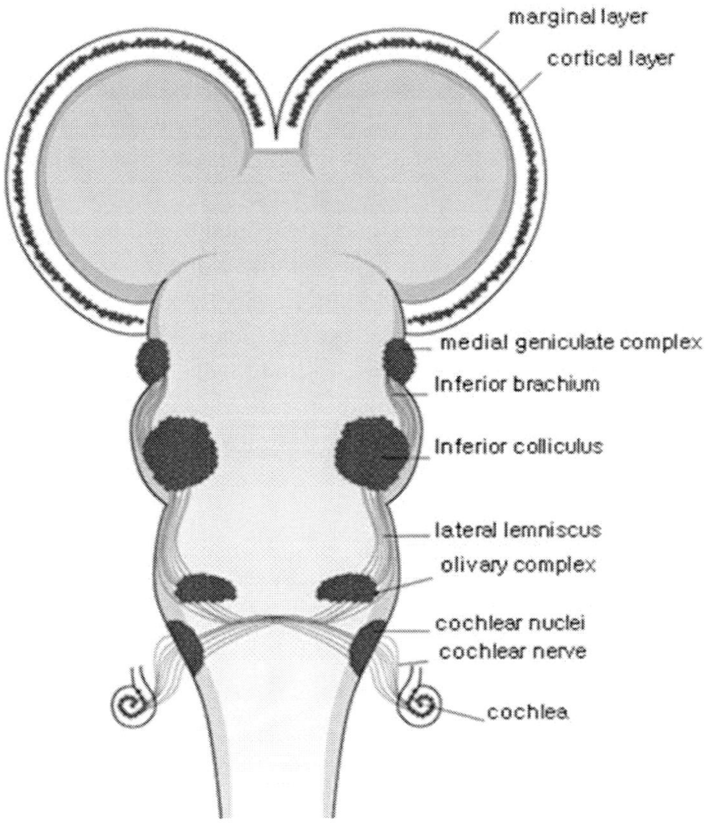


Figure 1. Schematic diagram of the human auditory system during the first trimester. The inferior colliculus projects to the medial geniculate nucleus of the thalamus and medial geniculate complex also projects the auditory cortex. The cortex consists of a densely cellular cortical plate and a clear marginal layer.

### *Second Trimester*

The cortical plate, which consists of narrow vertical columns of cells, doubles in thickness during this period [6]. Large intrinsic neurons produce thick axons running horizontally in the deepest portion of the layer, passing through many apical dendritic tufts of cortical plate neurons in the marginal layer [7]. These intrinsic neurons express neurochemicals (e.g. reelin, acetylcholinesterase, and calcium-binding proteins). They play an important role in attracting migrating neuroblasts and guiding them to exact locations on the cortical plate. These neurochemicals may also act as attractants to the afferent axons of the thalamus, which first enter the cortical plate during 22nd week of gestation [8, 9]. At this time, the upper portion of the marginal layer probably receives many axons, which enter the cortex from the reticular formation [10].

A distinct temporal lobe forms during 27th week of gestation. A group of axons arising in the lower level continue to increase in the marginal layer [11]. These axons are capable of directing cortical arousal, as premature infants born during gestational weeks of 25 to 27 show cortical evoked potential (CEP) [12].

### *Perinatal Period (Third Trimester to Sixth Postnatal Month)*

As the temporal lobe expands, there is a division between the transverse temporal gyrus and the secondary auditory cortex of the superior temporal gyrus. The marginal layer is prominent during the perinatal period [10]. Axons of intrinsic neurons that traverse the dendrites thicken due to the development of the marginal layer. In addition, a dense lower tier of fiber forms and the upper layers of the thin afferent axons become thickened. Despite of their long course and passage through large numbers of dendrites, these axons are expected to direct cortical arousal. In animal experiments, stimulation of the marginal layer caused potential shifts in the deeper-lying cortical neurons [13]. Axons in the marginal layer are considered the only source of long latency evoked potentials, such as $N_2$ and mismatch negativity (MMN), found in infants. Therefore, $N_2$ and MMN are generated by marginal layer afferents in the deeper cortical layer, although mature axons are absent and the very long latencies of potentials reflect the slow conduction of thin and lightly myelinated axons [14].

### *Early Childhood*

In children aged 6 months to 1 year, the prominence of the marginal layer decreases markedly and thalamic input matures. The deeper tier of the intrinsic neurons completely disappears, and cortical neurons are mature in appearance. In 1-year-olds, the auditory radiation of the core of the temporal lobe and the deeper layer of the cortex contain filament-filled axons. There is a distinctively restricted distribution of the projection from the ventral division of the medial geniculate complex [10, 15].

The arrival of the thalamic input to the cortex changes the pattern of infants' responses to language stimuli. Six-month-old infants show differential responses to phonemes of their native tongue and foreign languages, and pay attention to features of ambient language [16]. Similar findings were observed in studies of MMN. For example, the MMN of 6–12-month-old Finnish infants showed increased responses to vocalized sounds in Finnish, but decreased responses to vocalized sounds in Estonian [17].

The primary change observed at 3 years is the maturation of axons in the deeper layer. Filament-stained axons form an open meshwork in layers 4, 5 and 6. By the of age 5 years, axons run perpendicularly through the narrow column of the cortex, with a density similar to that in adults, in the process of projection from the ventral medial geniculate complex.

### *Later Childhood*

The final phase of structural development of the auditory cortex occurs during later childhood, at ages 6 to 12 years. During this period, the axons mature in superficial layers, and the upper cortical layers also mature. These two processes enhance the ability of an individual to distinguish language under difficult conditions. The perception of language in a noisy background improves from late childhood to adolescence. Moreover, 5–12-year-old children show steady improvement in the ability to distinguish masked and degraded speech [18, 19]. The increased abilities to discriminate language reflect a capacity for more complex auditory processing, resulting from the increased interactions between auditory cortices in the left and right brain hemispheres, as well as the broader interaction of cortices within the same hemisphere [10].

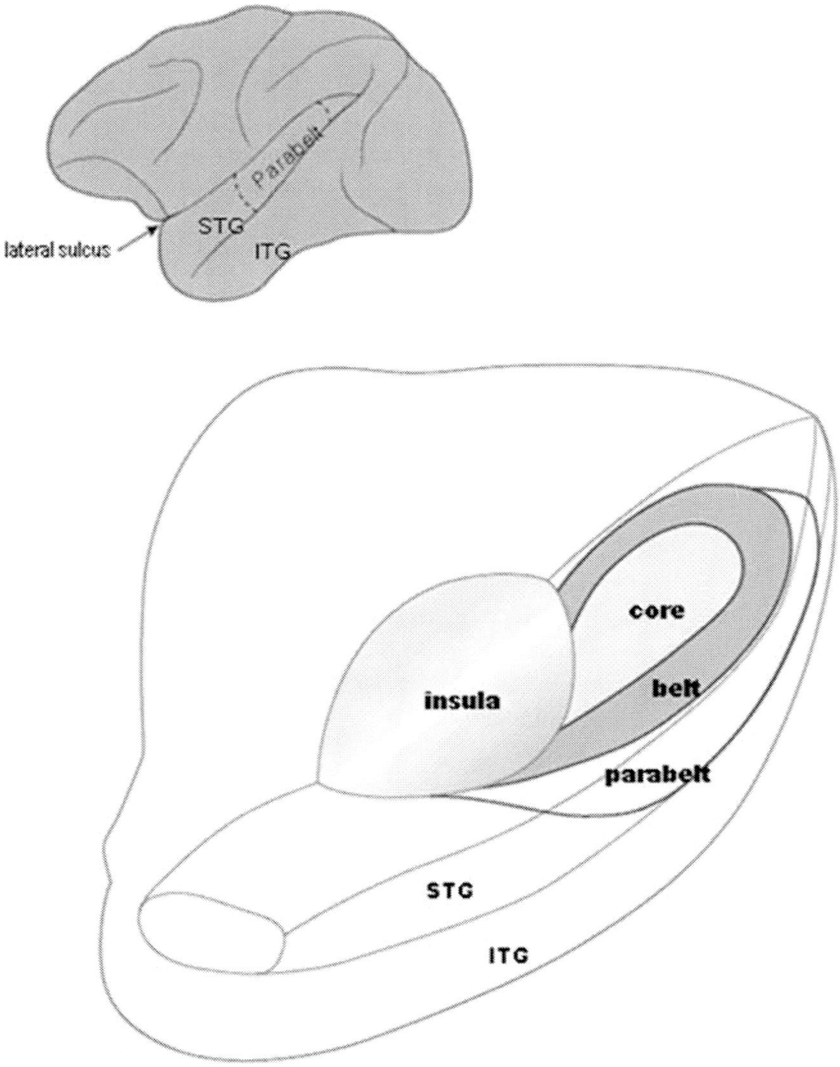


Figure 2. Schematic diagram of the left hemisphere of the macaque monkey, Top, left hemisphere showing the location of the parabelt region of the auditory cortex on the superior temporal gyrus (STG). Bottom, dorsolateral view of the lateral sulcus (LS). Abbreviations: ITG, inferior temporal gyrus.

## Localization

The auditory cortex is the area of the cerebral cortices that is the main receiver of signals from the ventral and dorsal portions of the medial geniculate complex of the thalamus. Thus, the auditory cortex of human and nonhuman primates occupies many areas within the ventral portion of the lateral sulcus and superior temporal gyrus. In humans, these correspond to areas 41, 42, 52, and 22 of Brodmann [20] and enclose the transverse temporal gyri of Heschl and the planum temporal [21].

The auditory cortex consists of a central primary, or core, region, containing several areas with one or more subareas, and a belt region. The core region receives signals from the ventral division of the medial geniculate complex, to which the core region is connected, and has cellular characteristics of the primary sensory cortex. Belt regions around the primary auditory cortex receive signals from the dorsal division of the medial geniculate complex, and have the cellular structure of an associated cortex [22]. In primates, this model has been expanded to a third region known as the parabelt region [23, 24]. Like the belt region, the parabelt region receives signals from the dorsal division of the medial geniculate complex. Unlike the belt region, however, the parabelt region is not directly connected to the core. The belt region is thought to be a mediator of signals from the core to the parabelt region [25] (Figure 2).

Structural models of the auditory cortex have been formulated in several species (e.g. bats, cats, ferrets, rats, monkeys). These auditory cortices show species-specific characteristics, including differences in the number of areas, their relative location and arrangement, their connection to surrounding areas, and their tonotopic organization. Brain size is usually associated with the number of auditory areas. Although hemispheric imbalances in the function and structure of each area have been observed, the number of areas is thought to be the same.

Each of the three main regions (i.e. the core, belt and parabelt regions) contains areas interconnected to the other two regions. Monkeys have three subdivisions, seven belt regions and two subdivisions of the parabelt region. Each region has a unique set of connections to the thalamus and other areas of the cortices, with some information processed in parallel by two or more areas, whereas other information is not. These connecting patterns indicate both serial and parallel processes within the network of the auditory cortex [26].

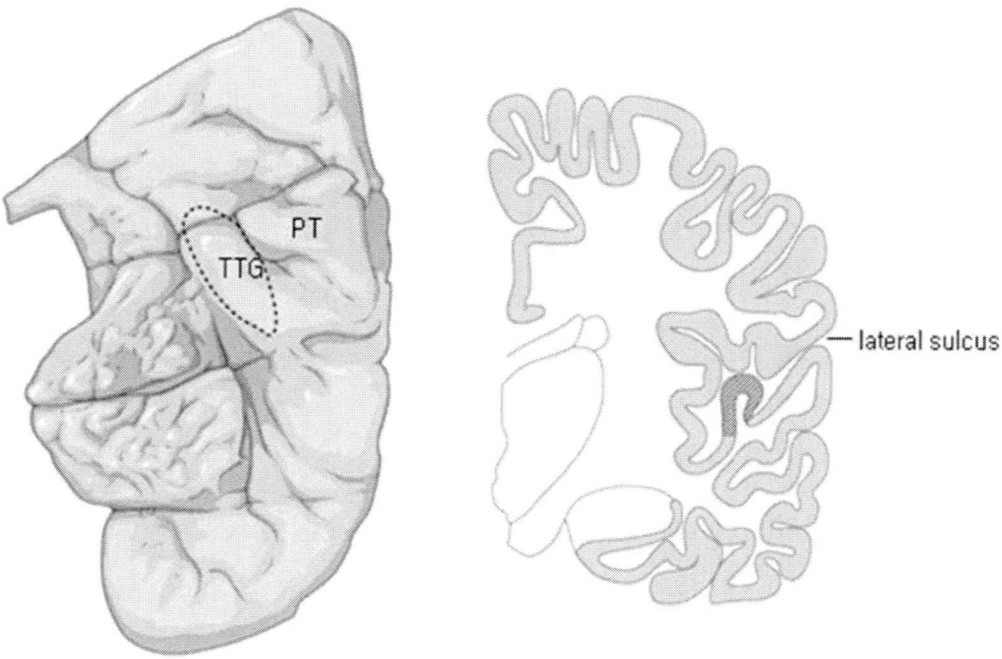


Right, Coronal sections of the auditory cortex. The stripe indicates the location of the core region.

Figure 3.Human auditory cortex. Left, dorsal views of the superior temporal plane. Transverse temporal gyrus(TTG) and planum temporale (PT) are indicated.

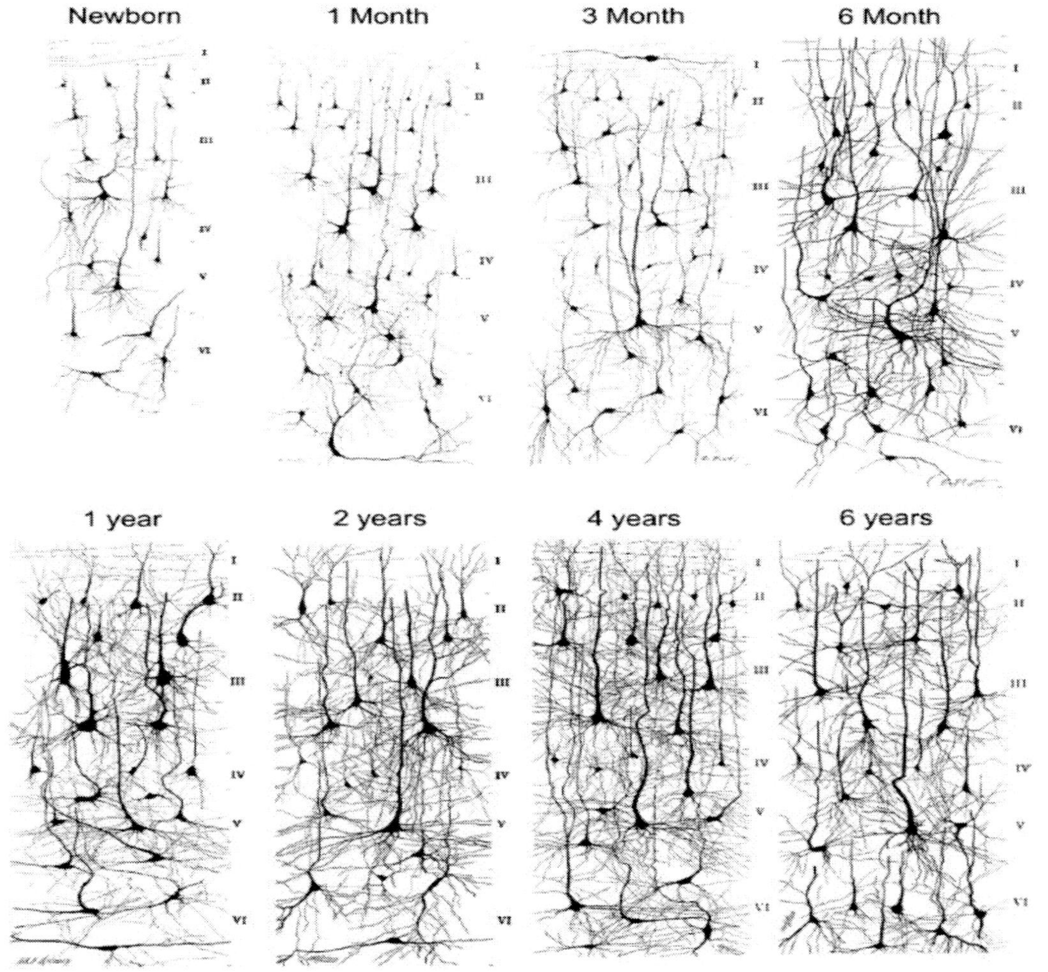




Figure 4. Development of the human primary auditory cortex, Conel (1939–1967). Dendritic complexity increases during postnatal development, as the synaptic densities increases.

In contrast to other species, information is available on the organization of the auditory centers in humans. Most of these studies involve biopsies taken from cadavers or noninvasive physiological examinations. At present, however, the functional characteristics of these areas are being assessed by measurements of the expression of enzymes, proteins, and neurotransmitters, studies that may provide knowledge about their functional properties [21].

Closer examination of the organization of the human auditory center shows that the core occupies two thirds of the posteromedial area of the transverse temporal gyrus, corresponding almost to Brodmann area 41 [20]. The transverse temporal gyrus is single in some individuals and paired in others and may be located between the cerebral hemispheres. Thus, the exact location of the core varies according to the number of transverse temporal gyri. The core occupies most single transverse temporal gyri. Not exceeding the boundaries of the sulcus, either in front or in the rear. In individuals with paired transverse temporal gyri, the core occupies the sulcus between the two gyri [21] (Figure 3).

The belt region borders the core at the anteromedial and posterolateral sides of the transverse temporal gyrus. The front portion of the belt region is located between the core region and the circular sulcus of insula, corresponding to Brodmann area 52; whereas the rear portion of the belt region occupies part of the planum temporale, corresponding to Brodmann area 42 [27]. Brodmann area 22, part of which extends toward the planum temporale from the superior temporal gyrus to the lateral side of Brodmann area 42, is thought to correspond to some or most of the parabelt region [21].

## Histology

The human auditory cortex is divided into six layers. These six layers have been observed in immature brains, leading to a recently updated, computer-generated model [28]. Layer I, a molecular or plexiform layer, has few or no nerve cells and is composed of horizontal or diagonal axons; it receives unspecific input signals from the thalamus. Layer II contains small pyramidal cells and is rich in small double-bouquet cells; this layer is connected to other layers or areas of other cortices on the same side. Layer III is composed of large pyramidal cells and double-bouquet cells; this layer sends output signals to areas of other cortices and is connected to neurons located in layer IV, in areas of cortices on the opposite side. Layer IV, which contains primarily non-pyramidal or stellate cells, is the area that receives most input signals projected from the ventral portion of the thalamus. Layer V consists primarily of large pyramidal cells and has a long axon that extends to subcortical structures. Layer VI contains pyramidal and fusiform cells and receives input signals from other layers. In addition, layer 6 may project signals into the thalamus and peripheral nuclei of ascending sensory pathways.

A study of the histological distribution of the auditory cortex showed that pyramidal cells are present in laminae layers II–VI and are particularly dense in laminae layers II, III, and V [29]. All dendrites of pyramidal cells are covered with spines. Smooth stellate cells are observed in layers II and V, whereas spiny stellate cells are rare in layers II, III, IV and VI. Giant cells are observed in all layers except layer I and are particularly rich in layers V and VI [30] (Figure 4).

## Descending Auditory Pathways

The descending projection from the auditory cortex consists of mutually connected auditory pathways. The descending pathways form a feedback loop, which supplies circuit modulating information processed by the peripheral apparatus to the cortex. There are two descending pathways, the corticofugal system and the cortico-cochlear system. The corticofugal system is a projection pathway from the auditory cortex to the thalamus, whereas the cortico-cochlear system is a projection pathway from the auditory cortex to the cochlear nucleus and the cochlea. The two pathways cross and also have individual, non-crossing pathways. In particular, there are many corticofugal pathways, through which descending signals are transmitted to the lower structure [31].

Signals projected into the medial geniculate complex and the inferior colliculus are structured as projections into the periolivary nuclei and send olivocochlear efferents toward the cochlea [31]. This structure was identified in owl monkeys by injecting radioactive proline into the primary auditory cortex and rostral field, resulting in strong labeling in the ventral portion, corresponding to the principal and dorsal nuclei of the medial geniculate complex, as well as labeling in the inferior colliculus [32].

Although descending pathways in peripheral organs such as the cochlea have been previously identified in humans, less is known about higher peripheral apparatus. Descending pathways in humans may be identical to those of other species. At lower levels, descending pathways are thought to be related to the sensitivity of the cochlea and its frequency selectivity because its connection to hair cells of the inner ear, located, in the olivocochlear bundle, affects the mechanics of the cochlea [33].

# Function of the Auditory Cortex

## Cortical Mechanism in Hearing

To determine the cortical mechanism associated with hearing, it is necessary to understand the structurally and functionally distributed pathway as a type of information processing. The thalamocortical auditory projection in monkeys provides a basis of hierarchical transformation in which auditory signals are sequentially processed in the core, the belt and the parabelt regions. These auditory signals are subsequently transmitted to various parts of the temporal, parietal, and frontal areas. Information transmitted from the core to other parts of the brain is thought to pass through the belt region. During this process, responses in the belt areas can be considered transformations of the property of the core to some extent. Within this framework, there is also a basis for parallel processing. That is, the pathway of parallel processing begins with the parallel projection from the primary thalamus to several core cortical fields and ends with parabelt projections within the temporal and parietal areas. The concept of parallel processing suggests that different areas at the same level perform partial and parallel information processing with specialization. Several fields (e.g. the primary auditory cortex, rostral fields, and other belt fields) are thought to perform parallel information processing, with some degree of specialization [34].

Two principal streams are thought to be present in the cortex, the 'where (dorsal)' and 'what (ventral)' pathways. The 'where' pathway connects, through the caudomedial area of the belt, the primary auditory cortex to the frontal eye field and the parietal area, related to the spatial processing, where is important in recognizing a sound source. The 'what pathway' is an information stream, in which information originating from the anterior core and belt areas affect the target within the temporal lobe. These hypotheses are supported by the results of recent human imaging analyses. That is, more posterior region, that is, the posterior temporal area, the parietal cortex, and the superior frontal sulcus portion are activated during spatial processing, whereas the auditory cortex and the inferior prefrontal lobe are activated during the processing of auditory stimuli of pitch, working memory and phonemes [35, 36].

## Properties of Auditory Cortical Responses

Physiological studies on the functional topography of the auditory cortex have shown that neurons tuned to narrow frequency ranges are organized tonotopically in the core regions of many species. Functional magnetic resonance imaging (fMRI) has shown that the core region in macaques has a mirror-symmetric tonotopic organization. That is, the primary auditory cortex has a high-to-low frequency representation, whereas the rostral core field has a low-to-high frequency representation. Moreover, many belts have a tonotopic organization that parallels that of the neighboring core areas [37].

Many studies of the human auditory cortex have found that high frequency sound activates not only the small lateral area in front of the intersection of Heschl's gyrus and the superior temporal gyrus but also the wide medial area at the rear of the tip of Heschl's gyrus. Furthermore, low frequency sound activates the lateral area in the middle of Heschl's gyrus and the posterior portion of the superior temporal gyrus [38-40].

The method by which the auditory cortex represents auditory stimuli has been assessed experimentally. For example, the neuronal population of the auditory cortex can be represented by a structure in which a handful of selective nerve cells are activated at a given moment, rather than being represented by a high density structure composed of many nerves activated simultaneously in a wide area. The sparseness of representation of the auditory cortex in rats was recently revealed by measuring nerve activity using the method of cell-attached record. These findings indicate that the sparseness of auditory activation is associated with advantages in processing some information. For example, it is easier to recognize one person shouting in a quiet crowd than many people shouting simultaneously because only very small nerves are activated [41].

In addition, the response of the auditory cortex is precise. Whereas the visual cortex jitters within 5 milliseconds in reaction to its most reliable stimulatory spike, the auditory cortex jitters within 1 millisecond [42]. This precise spike timing is considered important in tracing the minute temporal structure of complex sounds or in distinguishing among animal sounds [43]. Moreover, during trial-to-trial stimulation, nerves of the visual cortex show a very high variability in spike count, whereas counts of neurons of the auditory cortex control vary within narrow limits. This finding also indicates that the auditory cortex is more precise [44].

Repetitive transient and temporal modulation of tone and noise has been used to assess the functions of the auditory complex. The firing rate of nerve cells in the auditory complex represents amplitude modulation at high frequency, and synchrony coding of nerve cells is related to amplitude modulation at low frequency. Despite differences in reactivity to various stimuli, their temporal transfer functions can be quite similar [45], suggesting that the responses of the auditory cortex to various ranges of time-varying auditory signals are shaped by a common temporal filtering process, probably synaptic depression and facilitation [46].

Studies of cortical processing of complex sounds in humans have yielded results similar to those in animals. Neuroimaging has shown that activation of the auditory cortex increases as the stimulation becomes more spectro-temporally complex [47]. In addition, the subregions of the auditory cortex may differ based on their spectro-temporal sensitivity. For example, the core region is mainly affected by temporal changes, whereas the belt area is stimulated more efficiently by spectral manipulation [48].

## Coding of Intensity

The firing rates of neurons in the auditory cortex of primates vary according to intensity, with two types of neurons, monotonic and nonmonotonic, present in the auditory cortex [49]. Many neurons of the primary auditory cortex have similar rate-intensity functions as the auditory nerve, with a monotonic firing rate showing an increase of 10–40 dB. In contrast, other neurons are sharply nonmonotonic and may be reduced to a spontaneous level in some cases. Wide band noise has been found to raise the threshold of neurons of the cortex; thus, above a certain level of sensitivity to noise, the firing rate increases in a manner similar to an unmasking condition, with the intensity profile remaining largely unchanged [50]. In addition, a continuous rise in the level of masking noise alters the intensity profile gradually toward higher sound pressure levels, resulting in an increased signal to noise ratio and allowing individuals to hear better in noisy environments. Animal experiments have shown that some cortical neurons are intensity selective. These cells respond only to a given range of intensity, but, collectively, the neurons generally cover a wide range of intensity.

## Neural Coding of Temporal Information

Neural representation of time-varying signals in the auditory cortex is particularly important in understanding the concept of speech processing. The time-varying signal is a fundamental component of sound for communication, including human speech and animal vocalization. Both humans and animals recognize information included in temporally modulated sounds across a wide range of time intervals, from several to several hundred milliseconds. Therefore, time is an essential variable of the input signal [51]. Temporal information on auditory signals can be represented as the temporal pattern of neuronal activity throughout the early phase of the auditory nervous system. That is, auditory nerve fibers at the auditory periphery represent the fine structure of complex sound in a temporal discharge pattern. As the signal is subsequently processed along the ascending auditory pathways, the upper limit of this stimulus-synchronized temporal representation gradually decreases. When this signal encoding acoustic information reaches the auditory cortex, a temporal firing pattern alone is inadequate to represent the entire range of sounds that vary over time and are recognized by humans and animals. Therefore, these modifications of neural coding occur in the auditory cortex.

Many studies have stressed the role of spike timing for information coding in the auditory cortex. Spike timing is a form of neural spike onset latency, a tool to distinguish animal vocalization and a guideline to understanding the fine temporal structure of complex sounds [51]. Observations on the primary auditory cortex of awakened marmosets have shown that some neurons in the auditory cortex have a time-locked response to sound stimuli, whereas other neurons do not. These latter neurons respond only to sounds at short interclick intervals. Two types of cortical responses to periodic click stimuli were eventually identified, one exhibiting a stimulus-synchronized response to sounds with long interclick intervals (i.e. slow sounds), and the second type showing monotonically changing discharge rates at short interclick intervals (i.e. quick sounds).

By the time an auditory signal reaches the auditory cortex, there has already been a considerable temporal-to-rate transformation. Unsynchronized neural responses are important in the transformation of temporal coding because they represent processed rather than preserved temporal information. Complex integration at this auditory cortical level is necessary because a higher level of processing requires temporal integration over a time window preceding and following a particular time of interest. A reduction in the temporal limit of stimulus-synchronized discharges in the auditory cortex is necessary for multi-sensory integration in the cerebral cortex. Auditory information is encoded at the periphery at a much higher temporal modulation rate than is visual or tactile information at the periphery, but discharge synchrony rates are similar across primary sensory cortical areas. The slowing of the temporal response rate along the ascending auditory pathway and the accompanying temporal-to-rate transformation are necessary for the cerebral cortex to rapidly integrate auditory signals with information from other sensory organs [52].

## Multisensory Interaction in the Auditory Cortex

Human speech represents a multisensory behavior involving both auditory and non-auditory factors. Multisensory integration in the auditory cortex offers many advantages to the perception and behavior of sounds, including for language comprehension and sound localization; input signals from multiple modalities increase the representation of sounds. Multisensory language perception is found at an early level [53], with visual-auditory integration at the neural level in particular taking place during early levels of cortical processing [54]. Auditory processing in both animals and humans is influenced by various multimodal stimuli, with the auditory cortex not being the sole domain of the cochlea receptor [55, 56].

Input of visual signals has been found to evoke responses in the auditory cortex, as shown by electroencephalography (EEG) and functional magnetic resonance imaging (fMRI), causing higher amplitude responses and higher firing rates than responses to a single auditory stimulation. The interaction of auditory with sense and somatosensory stimuli has attracted less attention than auditory-visual interaction, but somatosensory signals have been shown to have a considerable influence on sound perception. A well-combined auditory-tactile stimulation increases the strength of the perceived signal [57].

Research on neural mechanisms may explain the temporal principle of interactions in the auditory cortex. The dynamics of auditory-somatosensory interactions in the primary auditory cortex were evaluated by comparing neural responses to unimodal versus bimodal stimuli, with asynchrony varying between 0 ms (synchronous auditory and somatosensory stimuli) and 976 ms (somatosensory stimuli 976 ms after auditory stimuli). Synchronous stimulation and three asynchronous bimodal stimulations (at 27 ms, 140 ms and 781 ms, respectively) enhanced multisensory interactions. In contrast, neural responses to three other asynchronous bimodal stimulations (at 14 ms, 67 ms, and 320 ms) showed a greater decrease than observed with single mode stimulations. These findings indicate that neural responses to multisensory stimulations increase in a non-linear manner and that non-auditory signals can enhance the activity of accompanying auditory input when they arrive within several temporal "windows" [58].

To achieve multisensory integration in the auditory cortex, the visual or somatosensory stimulus must have a pathway that transmits a signal to the auditory cortex. Non-auditory signals may be sent to the auditory cortex as a feedforward source, via the posterior and postero-medial areas of the thalamus and the magnocellular divisions of the medial geniculate body, and also as a cortical feedback and lateral source, via the caudomedial area of the auditory association cortex, superior temporal polysensory area, intraparietal sulcus, and pre-frontal cortex (Figure 5).

## Lateralization of Function

Unilateral lesions in the cerebral hemisphere have been shown to lead to decreases in function of the contralateral ear. This may be explained by findings showing that the ears send more auditory signals to the auditory cortex on the opposite than on the same side. Stimulating the auditory cortex on the opposite side requires a 5–20 dB lower auditory threshold than stimulating the cortex on the same side [59]. Measurements of field potential in the auditory cortex during neurosurgery showed that stimulation of the opposite side had a higher potential [60]. Measurements of late auditory evoked potentials in human temporal and parietal lobes differed when the same or opposite side was stimulated.

## Reorganization of the Auditory Cortex Following Deafness

Because sensory pathways in the auditory cortex are influenced by internal development of the nervous system and external stimulations, the normal growth and connectivity necessary for a functional auditory system are interrupted when, as in deafness, there is no stimulation by external input signals. The development of a normal central nervous system is a prerequisite for the development of conversation and language skills; hence, for a child who has difficulty hearing, normal development of these skills is impossible.

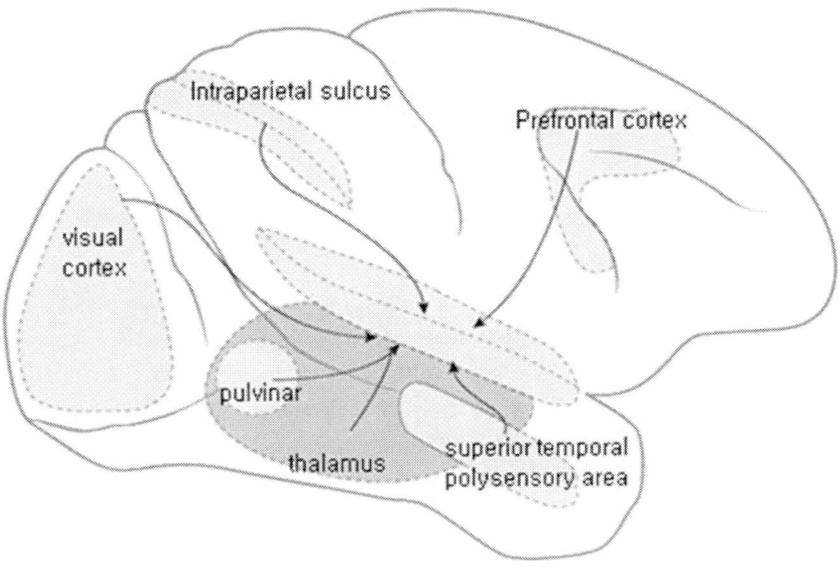


Figure 5. Schematic diagram of multisensory input to the auditory cortex. The diagram shows the macaque brain with established non-auditory sources and their pathways to the auditory cortex.

The congenitally deaf white cat is a good model for research on cortical organization. These cats have a restricted activation pattern in the layer of the primary auditory cortex and unsynchronized activity among different cortical layers. Electrical stimulation after the sensitive period of central auditory development results in delayed activation of the supragranular layer and non-activation of the infragranular layer in the cortex. The non-activation of the infragranular layer may affect a feedback projection to the subcortical auditory structure and suggests the functional decoupling of a higher order auditory cortex and the primary auditory cortex [61].

Cortical development after stimulus deprivation has been assessed in humans primarily by measuring cortical evoked potential (CAEP). Cochlear implant surgery resolves the harmful aspects of stimulation deprivation by bypassing damage to the cochlea and directly stimulating the spiral ganglion, making it a good method for assessing the reorganization of the auditory cortex following re-input to the auditory cortex after stimulation deprivation. The magnitude of CAEP change after cochlear implantation was dependent on the duration of deafness prior to implant surgery. That is, implant surgery performed during early childhood shows small changes, whereas later implant surgery results in greater changes in the normal development of CAEP. According to Sharma et al. [62], Congenitally deaf patients receiving cochlear implants at than 3.5 years, at 3.5–7 years, and 7 years of age showed normal P1 latencies, abnormal cortical response latencies, and variable cortical response latencies, respectively. The N1 component showed a normal response in patients who received implants before age 3.5 years. These findings indicate that congenitally deaf children who receive implants at an early age experience normal auditory stimulation and are expected to achieve normal language development and behavioral outcomes after childhood.

Following auditory deprivation, there is cross-modal plasticity and reorganization between auditory and non-auditory areas. Auditory stimulation in children who undergo cochlear implant surgery does not activate the auditory association area, which is involved in processing input signals from other modalities [63]. Moreover, when brain activity was assessed by fMRI in congenitally deaf adults who were shown visual stimuli, there was significant activity in the temporal cortex, in particular in the area of the auditory cortex [51]. Similar results have been observed in response to stimulations such as sign language, lip movement, and somatosensory stimuli [52].

## Imaging of the Auditory Cortex

The development of various imaging techniques, including positron emission tomography (PET) and fMRI, has engendered many studies on the auditory cortex. PET uses a scanning device that detects photons emitted by a radioactive tracer injected into the body. Brain activity can be determined by measuring local blood flow and glucose metabolism. PET and fMRI have revealed physiological and anatomic structures of humans, such as anatomic location and tonotopic arrangement. Studies are currently ongoing assessing the activity of the auditory cortex during the processing of acoustic features (including sound intensity, pitch and location) and auditory attention.

The middle portion of the auditory cortex around Heschl's gyrus is activated by sound intensity, with the spatial distribution of activation varying by sound intensity and being identical to ampliotopic organization [64]. fMRI demonstrated sound lateralization, in that to the auditory cortex of each cerebral hemisphere responded more to sound stimulation of the ear on the opposite than on the same side [65]. Studies in primates showed that the posterior region of the auditory cortex is more narrowly tuned in sound location than the anterior region, whereas the anterior region of auditory cortex is more narrowly tuned into spectral feature. This result is consistent with the 'what' and 'where' auditory pathways of the human auditory cortex [66] (Figure 6).

## Disorders of the Auditory Cortex

Among the lesions that can occur in the unilateral temporal lobe containing the auditory cortex are tumors, cerebral hemorrhage, trauma and cerebral infarction. These lesions can affect the auditory cortex. Symptoms are generally diffuse and auditory hallucinations may occur, but changes in auditory threshold levels are not very large. Damage to the primary auditory cortex usually does not result in a high degree of hearing threshold elevation even for sound stimulation contralateral to the side of the lesion. Most patients show normal speech discrimination, in contrast to patients with lesions of the auditory system. Lesions in the auditory cortex may be detected by the low redundancy speech test [67], which assesses speech discrimination using interrupted or very rapid speech, unlike general speech discrimination tests.

Pure tone audiometry tests have shown normal results in patients with astrocytomas of the left temporal lobe affecting the auditory cortex. However these patients show greatly decreased speech discrimination when their right ears are exposed to distorted speech [68] (Figure 7).

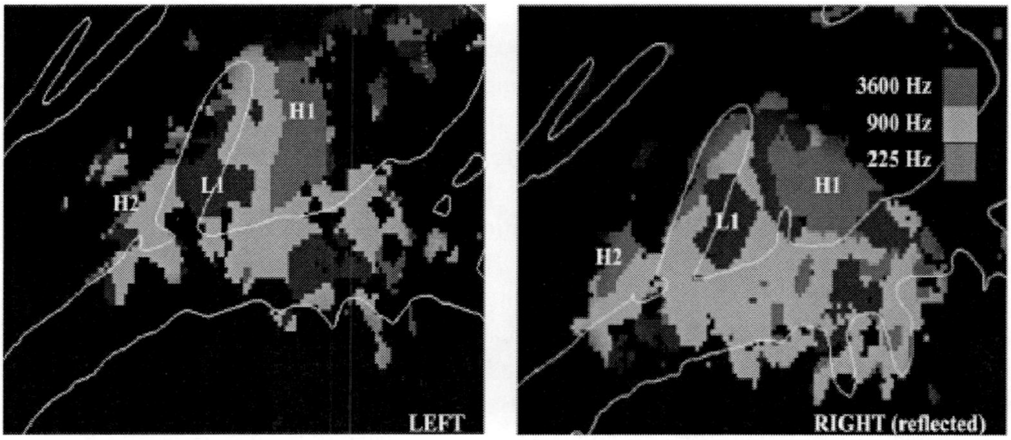


Figure 6. Mirror-image tonotopic organization of the auditory cortex in the left and right hemispheres. Plots show regions with significant activations coded by the frequency that produced maximal activation at that point. Red = 3600 Hz, Green = 900 Hz, Blue = 225 Hz. All values were averaged over subjects, continuous and sparse sampling, sound spatial position, and sound intensity. Activation maps are shown on the average gyral structure (white lines) of the left and right hemispheres. z-score threshold = 4.0. H1 and H2 indicate the posterior and anterior foci, respectively, driven by high-frequency tones, whereas L1 indicates the central region driven by low-frequency tones.

**Table 1. Clinical features of disorders in the auditory cortex**

| Disorder | Impairments | Lesion |
|---|---|---|
| Cortical deafness | Audiometric sensitivity. Speech comprehension and repetition. Recognition of familiar sounds. Musical perception | Bilateral PAC or auditory radiations |
| Cortical auditory disorder | Speech comprehension and repetition. Recognition of familial sound. Musical perception. | Bilateral AAC |
| Pure word deafness | Speech comprehension and repetition, Musical perception. | Bilateral AAC or left auditory radiations and callosal fibers from right AAC |
| Auditory sound agnosia | Recognition of familiar sounds, Musical perception | Right or bilateral AAC |
| Sensory amusia | Musical perception+/- | Unilateral AAC |

PAC, primary auditory cortex; AAC, auditory association cortex.

Bilateral lesions in the auditory cortex include cortical deafness, pure word deafness, auditory sound agnosia, and sensory amusia, depending on the types of sound sources that cannot be recognized and the location of the lesion (Table 1). These patients are unable to recognize language and/or non-linguistic sounds.

## Cortical Deafness

Cortical deafness is rare; persons with this condition cannot recognize sounds and cannot discriminate among sounds. The most common cause of the disorder is two sequential unilateral strokes. Because individuals with this condition have profound impairment in processing auditory stimuli, they are unable to perceive, discriminate among, or recognize verbal and nonverbal sounds. This disorder is also accompanied by impairments in temporal auditory analysis and/or the spatial localization of sound. However, few have signs of aphasia, which, if present, is mild.

Cortical deafness should be distinguished from ‘cortical auditory disorder’ [69]. Although the two conditions are similar, cortical auditory disorder is the associative form of cortical deafness. Both conditions show most functional impairments in sound perception, when tests of auditory abilities are sufficiently comprehensive. Some patients with cortical deafness may progress to cortical auditory disorder. Bilateral destruction of the cortex, including the primary auditory cortex, in animals has been shown to lead to complete hearing loss [70]. Patients presenting with complete destruction of the primary cortex, however, do not show permanent loss of audiometric sensitivity [71]. These findings indicate that auditory disorders that include impairments in detecting and discriminating among sounds occur in a much more complex and selective manner. Behavioral research has shown that patients with cortical deafness who pay attention to hearing sounds have an enhanced ability to detect and localize sounds, despite their impairment [72].

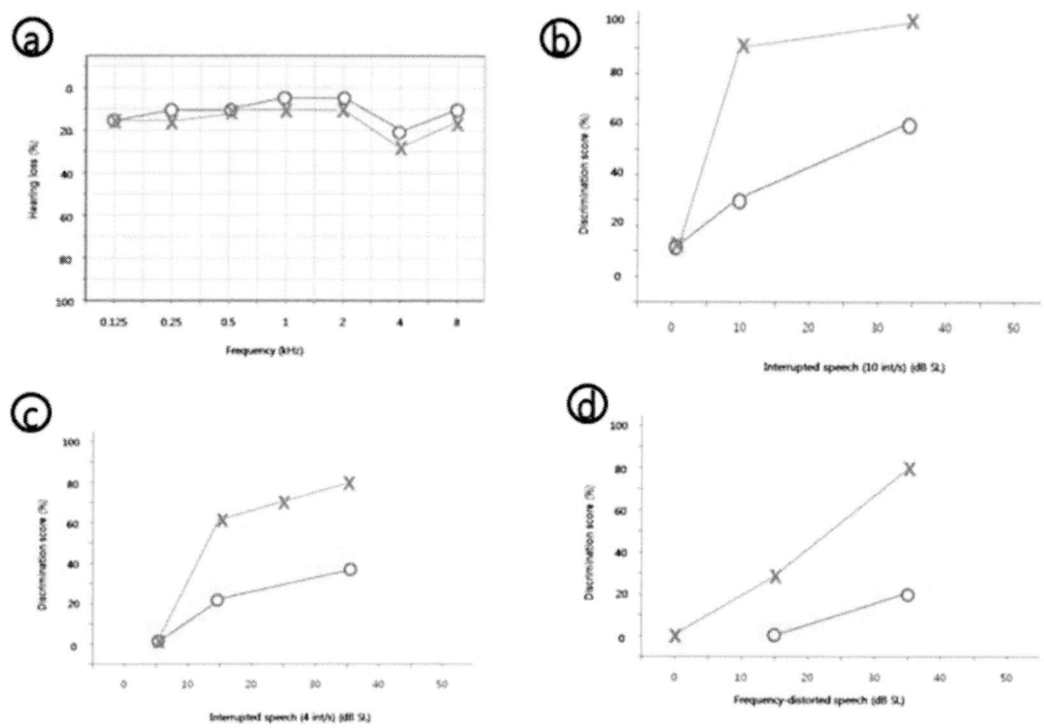


Figure 7. (a) Pure tone audiogram in a patient with a tumor (astrocytoma) in the left temporal lobe. (b) Speech discrimination for interrupted speech (10 interruptions per sec) (c) Speech discrimination of frequency filtered speech. (d) Speech discrimination of time-compressed speech.

Cortical deafness can also be caused by Moyamoya disease. The development of this disease is frequently biphasic, with the first phase of aphasia and hemiparesis caused by unilateral damage, followed by a secondary phase of sudden total hearing loss caused by damage to the opposite side [72]. Cortical deafness is thought to be caused by bilateral damage to either auditory radiations or the primary auditory cortex. Although damage to the bilateral temporal lobes most commonly affects the primary cortex, part or all of this area can be spared. The major cause of cortical deafness may be the disconnection of pathways toward the bilateral auditory cortices, not just isolated lesions of the cortex itself [73]. Pathophysiologically, however, the correlation between the cortex and subcortical region is still unclear. Cortical auditory disorder may be caused by bilateral lesions of the uninvolved auditory cortex. That is, cortical auditory disorder may be caused by injury to the auditory association cortex itself. Alternatively, it can be caused by the disconnection of pathways involving the auditory association cortex, while sparing the primary auditory cortex [74].

## Pure Word Deafness

Auditory agnosia is a condition in which an individual cannot understand the meaning of sounds regardless of their normal pure tone recognition. There are two types of auditory agnosia. In the first, verbal auditory agnosia or 'pure word deafness', an individual is unable to understand spoken language. In the second, nonverbal auditory agnosia or 'auditory sound agnosia', an individual is unable to recognize nonlinguistic sounds such as a siren or a barking dog. Patients with pure word deafness have unimpaired reading and writing abilities, and can recognize nonverbal sounds, yet they cannot understand spoken language. They can voluntarily write, but cannot take dictation.

This disorder is thought to be caused by disruption of the ascending auditory pathway towards the left auditory word center from the bilateral subcortical area [75]. Most patients with pure word deafness show bilateral, cortical-subcortical lesions in the anterior portion of the superior temporal gyri while the left Heschl's gyrus is preserved. Some patients, however, have subcortical lesions only in the dominant temporal lobe, presumably destroying not only callosal fibers from the opposite auditory region but also the ipsilateral auditory radiations.

In general, damaged areas in patients with pure word deafness result in the disconnection of Werniche's area from auditory input signals. Lesions restricted to this area usually result in destruction of this area, thus explaining the low prevalence of pure word deafness [76]. One study reported that pure word deafness in 30 of 37 patients was caused by cerebrovascular disease [77], although it can also be caused by encephalitis or neoplasm [76]. During childhood, pure word deafness may be associated with Landau-Kleffner syndrome. Patients with Landau-Kleffner syndrome often show a successive process of verbal disability, starting with sensory aphasia and followed by generalized auditory agnosia and, ultimately, by pure tone deafness [78].

Pure word deafness can also occur during recovery from Wernicke's aphasia [79]. As paraphasia disappears, along with the inability to read and write, patients are able to communicate by writing, even if they cannot understand spoken language. These patients are not deaf because their pure tone audiometric findings are normal. Patients with Wernicke's aphasia may have auditory hallucination or symptoms of temporary euphoria or paranoia [69]. Although they do not understand verbal speech, they have various responses to speech. For example, they may say, "the words sound like a foreign language", "I can hear the sound, but not the words", or "the words seems to be spoken really fast" [69].

Many studies have emphasized the role of auditory-perceptual processing in the occurrence of pure word deafness, with disabilities in temporal resolution and phonemic discrimination being of particular importance. For example, one study reported that the primary problem in pure word deafness is the temporal resolution of auditory stimulation rather than unique phonemic discrimination [79]. In addition, a patient with a lesion of the cortex and subcortical white matter on the left temporal lobe was found to be unable to process dynamic auditory changes in a short period of time, suggesting an explanation for the impaired temporal processing observed in this disorder [80].

Pure word deafness may be caused by two types of disease mechanism [81]. The first is a disturbance in prephonemic temporal auditory acuity caused by bilateral damage to the temporal lobe. The second is phonemic discrimination due to the damage from left temporal lesions associated with Wernicke's aphasia, regardless of temporal auditory acuity [81].

However, electrophysiological abnormalities have been observed in six patients with pure word deafness related to Landau-Kleffner syndrome [82]. These patients showed a delay in N1 in cortical evoked potential (CEP) to tone and speech sounds compared with controls. This delay in N1 was consistently found over the lateral temporal cortex. Thus, in these patients, the processing of auditory stimuli in the secondary auditory cortex of the lateral temporal lobe was slow for both speech and tone, suggesting that the perceptual impairment associated with pure word deafness is not speech-specific.

## Auditory Sound Agnosia

Auditory sound agnosia is a rare condition with a lower prevalence than pure word deafness. Patients with this condition have no problem understanding language and have normal test scores on pure tone audiometry, but they cannot recognize non-verbal sounds such as the ringing of a telephone. Most of these patients do not show symptoms of aphasia. The low prevalence of this disorder may be due in part to its low rate of detection. Because these individuals appear normal on pure tone audiometry and speech discrimination tests, and have fewer complaints than patients who have problems understanding verbal language, they may go unrecognized.

Auditory sound agnosia can develop from generalized agnosia, in which individuals cannot recognize verbal and non-verbal sounds, or it may progress to other conditions, in which patients cannot recognize speech sounds and other auditory stimuli. A recent case study described a typical patient with auditory sound agnosia [83]. The patient, a 65-year-old man who had experienced hemiplegia 3 years earlier, visited the healthcare unit with major complaints of anxiety and headache. Audiologic tests showed moderate hearing loss on both sides at high frequencies, but the patient could not recognize common sounds. He did not show signs of aphasia nor other agnosia deficits, and his sound localization was normal. Matching to sample tests showed that his inability to recognize sounds was not due to an acoustic disability. Postmortem examination showed old, sharply demarcated infarcts around the right center of the parietal lobe, the superior temporal or angular gyrus, the insula, and the inferior parietal and frontal gyri of this patient. In addition, several studies have described patients with auditory sound agnosia who had unilateral lesions [84].

Taken together, these reports indicate that the inability to recognize environmental sounds may be due to damage in the right unilateral hemisphere. These findings also suggest that the acoustic processor of the right hemisphere is responsible for processing non-linguistic sounds, whereas the acoustic processor of the left hemisphere is responsible for processing linguistic sounds. Auditory sound agnosia has also been reported in patients with bilateral subcortical lesions and bilateral ventricular enlargement without cortical lesions. Thalamic hemorrhages in patients with generalized auditory agnosia were shown to result in auditory sound agnosia. Auditory sound agnosia may also be caused by a head injury. Although abnormalities in the cortex and subcortical area were not observed on CT or MRI scans of this patient, intraventricular hemorrhage and enlargement were observed on CT scans only [74,85].

Comprehensive evaluation can reveal the pathophysiological localization of this disease. Recent neuroimaging research suggests that the right primary auditory cortex and the auditory association cortex (AAC) are necessary to integrate environmental sounds, and that the left temporal and frontal lobes are associated with the analysis of language information [86]. In human dialogue, verbal language cannot only impart the meaning of words, but can also show a speaker's emotional state by the volume, timbre, or pitch of speech. One case study [87] described a patient with a lesion in the right temporal-parietal lobes who could not understand serious speech in which no emotion was involved. This subtype of auditory sound agnosia is called "auditory affective agnosia."

## Sensory Amusia

Patients with sensory amusia have the ability to detect normal pure tone but are unable to appreciate the diverse characteristics of music. Most patients with amusia do not consider the disorder a serious one, and even medical doctors regard it as a marginal symptom. Thus, few patients are diagnosed with sensory amusia. These patients usually have lesions on the right temporal lobe or the insula. Patients who experience cerebral infarctions in the right cerebral hemisphere, especially infarctions that involve the insula, may have difficulty recognizing music, but retain the ability to understand language and to detect environmental noise [88]. In addition, patients with sensory amusia lack the ability to analyze a rapid temporal sequence of notes or to sense movements of sound sources [89]. Recognition of music, however, may be a multifactorial process involving the cooperation of both bilateral cerebral hemispheres. For example, a dichotic listening study found that the right cerebral hemisphere is important in processing music and non-verbal sounds, whereas the left cerebral hemisphere is important in sequential processing [90].

A comprehensive non-verbal auditory test on two patients with lesions in the bilateral auditory cortex showed that both could recognize environmental and speech sounds, but they could not recognize tune, prosody and voice [91]. This behavioral dissociation suggested that, although the processing of music differs from the processing of speech or environmental noise, the two share common processing of distinct classes of auditory material such as voice, melody and prosody. For example, recognition of a specific voice or musical instruments depends on timbre, and recognition of tunes depends on pitch. Therefore, although the anatomical system of processing speech and environmental sounds overlaps with that of processing music, their compartments differ.

## Other Diseases Involving the Auditory Cortex

### *Auditory Hallucinations*

Auditory hallucinations can occur following injury to all portions of the central and peripheral auditory pathways. These hallucinations may consist of 'unformed' sounds, such as ringing, clicking, buzzing and humming sounds, or 'formed' sound, such as voice or music. Both unformed and formed auditory hallucinations can occur in various disorders (e.g. deafness, psychotic depression, drug intoxication, seizure). Examination of disorders in relation to the auditory cortex has shown that electric stimulation of Heschl's gyrus resulted in unformed auditory hallucinations in the opposite ear. Peripheral lesions give rise to auditory hallucinations on the ipsilateral side, whereas cortical lesions give rise to either contralateral or bilateral auditory hallucinations. Cortical lesions on the posterior superior temporal gyrus, including the primary auditory cortex and the planum temporal, are associated with this disorder. People with schizophrenia often complain of prolonged, formed auditory hallucinations [92]. Moreover, fMRI analysis has shown that schizophrenic patients with auditory hallucinations have smaller volumes of gray matter in the superior gyrus of both temporal lobes [93, 94].

### *Transcranial Magnetic Stimulation in Tinnitus Patients*

Subjective tinnitus is a disorder in which an individual can recognize sound in the absence of an intrinsic or extrinsic sound stimulus. Although its biologic mechanism is not yet fully understood, subjective chronic tinnitus may result from a reorganization process in the central nervous system induced by changed peripheral auditory and somatosensory input signals [95]. That is, deafferentiation of peripheral organs may cause an imbalance between the functions of excitatory and inhibitory signals, resulting in maladaptive plastic changes in structural and functional organization at certain levels of the central auditory nervous system. fMRI analysis has shown structural and functional changes in the central auditory pathway of patients with tinnitus [96].

## Conclusion

In this Chapter, we have described the development, organization, mechanism of hearing, imaging, and diseases, of the auditory cortex. Auditory cortical researches have proceeded on the basis that hearing mechanisms of the cortices of human and non-human primates are very similar or even identical. However, the physiology of the human auditory cortex has yet to be explored in detail. Future studies utilizing novel methods will yield definitive information on the anatomy and physiology of the auditory cortex; such knowledge will assist in the understanding of diseases of the cortex.



## References

[1] Kral, A. Unimodal and cross-modal plasticity in the 'deaf' auditory cortex. *Int. J. Audiol*, 2007, 46, 479-93.

[2] Cooper, ERA. The development of the human auditory pathway from the cochlear ganglion to the medial geniculate body. *Acta Anat*, 1948, 5, 99-122.

[3] Moore, JK. Organization of the human superior olivary complex. *Microsc. Res. Tech*, 2000, 51, 403-12.

[4] O'Rahilly, R; Gardner, E. The timing and sequence of events in the development of the human nervous system during the embryonic period proper. *Z. Anat. Entwickl-Gesch*, 1971, 134, 1-12.

[5] Meyer, G; Gonza´lez-Herna´ndez, T. Developmental changes in layer I of the human neocortex during prenatal life: A DiI-tracing, AChE and NADPH-d histochemistry study. *J. Comp. Neurol*, 1993, 338, 317-36.

[6] Krmpotic-Nemanic, J; Kostovic, I; Nemanic, D. Prenatal and perinatal development of radial cell columns in the human auditory cortex. *Acta Otolaryngol*, 1984, 97, 489-95.

[7] Marin-Padilla, M; Marin-Padilla, TM. Origin, prenatal development and structural organization of layer I of the human cerebral (motor) cortex: A Golgi study. *Anat. Embryol*, 1982, 164, 161-206.

[8] Meyer, G; Goffinet, AM. Prenatal development of reelinimmunoreactive neurons in the human neocortex. *J. Comp. Neurol*, 1998, 397, 29-41.

[9] Spreafico, R; Arcelli, P; Frassoni, C; Canetti, P; Giaccone, G; et al. Development of layer I of the human cerebral cortex after midgestation: Architectonic findings, immunocytochemical identification of neurons and glia, and in situ labeling of apoptotic cells. *J. Comp. Neurol*, 1999, 410, 126-42.

[10] Moore JK; Linthicum FH Jr. The human auditory system: A timeline of development. *Int. J. Audiol*, 2007, 46, 460-78.

[11] Marin-Padilla, M; Marin-Padilla, TM. Origin, prenatal development and structural organization of layer I of the human cerebral (motor) cortex: A Golgi study. *Anat. Embryol*, 1982, 164, 161-206.

[12] Starr, A; Amlie, RN; Martin, WH; Sanders, S. Development of auditory function in newborn infants revealed by auditory brainstem potentials. *Pediatrics*, 1977, 60, 831-9.

[13] Cauller, LJ; Connors, BW. Synaptic physiology of horizontal afferents to layer I in slices of rat S1 neocortex. *J. Neurosci*, 1994, 14, 751-62.

[14] Moore, JK; Linthicum, FH Jr. The human auditory system: a timeline of development. *Int. J. Audiol*, 2007, 46, 460-78.

[15] Hashikawa, T; Molinari, M; Rausell, E; Jones, EG. Patchy and laminar termination of medial geniculate axons in monkey auditory cortex. *J. Comp. Neurol*, 1995, 362, 195-208.

[16] Kuhl, PK; Williams, KA; Lacerda, F; Stevens, KN; Lindblom, B. Linguistic experience alters phonetic perception in infants by 6 months of age. *Science*, 1992, 255, 606-8.

[17] Cheour, M; Ceponiene, R; Lehtokoski, A; Luuk, A; Alho, K; et al. Development of language-specific phoneme representations in the infant brain. *Nature Neurosci*, 1998, 1, 351-3.

[18] Elliott, LL. Performance of children aged 9 to 17 years on a test of speech intelligibility in noise using sentence material with controlled word predictability. *JASA*, 1979, 66, 12-21.

[19] Eisenberg, LS; Shannon, RV; Martinez, AS; Wygonski, J; Boothroyd, A. Speech recognition with reduced spectral cues as a function of age. *JASA*, 2000, 107, 2704-10.

[20] Brodmann, K. Vergleichende Lokalisationslehre der Grosshirnrinde.Leipzig: Barth, 1909.

[21] Hackett, TA. Anatomical Organization of the Auditory cortex. *J. Am. Acad. Audiol*, 2008, 19, 774-9.

[22] Kaas, JH; Hackett, TA; Tramo, MJ. Auditory processing in primate cerebral cortex. *Curr. Opin. Neurobiol*, 1999, 9, 164–70.

[23] Morel, A; Kaas, JH. Subdivisions and connections of auditory cortex in owl monkeys. *J. Comp. Neurol*, 1992, 318, 27–63.

[24] Hackett, TA; Stepniewska, I; Kaas, JH. Subdivisions of auditory cortex and ipsilateral cortical connections of the parabelt auditory cortex in macaque monkeys. *J. Comp. Neurol*, 1998, 394, 475–95.

[25] Kaas, JH; Hackett, TA. Subdivisions of auditory cortex and levels of processing in primates. *Audiol. Neurootol*, 1998, 3, 73–85.

[26] Rauschecker, JP; Tian, B; Pons, T; Mishkin, M. Serial and parallel processing in rhesus monkey auditory cortex. *J. Comp. Neurol*, 1997, 382, 89–103.
[27] Hackett, TA. The comparative anatomy of the primate auditory cortex. In: Ghazanfar A, ed. Primate Audition: Behavior and Neurobiology. Boca Raton: CRC Press, 2003, 199–226.
[28] Conel, JL. The Post-natal Development of Human Cerebral Cortex. Vol. I-VIII Cambridge MA: Harvard University Press, 1939-67.
[29] Seldon, HL. Structure of human auditory cortex I. Cytoarhcitectonics and dendritic distributions. *Brain Res*, 1981, 229, 277-94.
[30] Conel, JL. The Postnatal Development of the Human Cerebral Cortex, Vols I–VIII, Cambridge, London, Harvard University Press, 1939.
[31] Harrison, JM; Howe, ME. Anatomy of the descending auditory system. In "handbook of Senosry physiology:"(Keidel WD and Neff WD, ed.) Vol 5, Part 1, Springer-Verlag, Berlin and New York, 1974, 363-88.
[32] FitzPatrick, KA; Imig, TJ. Organization of auditory connections: The primate auditory cortex. In "cortical sensory organization"(C.N. Woolsey, ed.), Vol 3, Clifton, New Jersey. Human Press, 71-109.
[33] Haines, DE. Fundamental Neuroscienece for basic and clinical applications. Elsevier Inc. Philadelphia, PA, USA, 2006.
[34] Semple, MN; Scott, BH. Cortical mechanisms in hearing. *Curr. Opin. Neurobiol.* 2003, 13, 167-73.
[35] Maeder, PP; Meuli, RA; Adriani, M; Bellmann, A; Fornari, E; Thiran, JP; Pittet, A; Clarke, S. Distinct pathways involved in sound recognition and localization: a human fMRI study. *Neuroimage*, 2001, 14, 802-16.
[36] Clarke, S; Bellmann Thiran, A; Maeder, P; Adriani, M; Vernet, O; Regli, L; Cuisenaire, O; Thiran, JP. What and where in human audition: selective deficits following focal hemispheric lesions *Exp. Brain Res.* 2002 ,147,8-15.
[37] Petkov, CI; Kayser, C; Augath, M; et al. Functional imaging reveals numerous fields in the monkey auditory cortex. *PLoS Biol*, 2006, 4, 215.
[38] Bilecen, D; Scheffler, K; Schmid, N; et al. Tonotopic organization of the human auditory cortex as detected by BOLD-FMRI. *Hear Res*, 1998, 126, 19–27.
[39] Engelien, A; Yang, Y; Engelien, W; et al. Physiological mapping of human auditory cortices with a silent event-related fMRI technique. *Neuroimage*, 2002, 16, 944–53.
[40] Wessinger, CM; Buonocore, MH; Kussmaul, CL; et al. Tonotopy in human auditory cortex examined with functional magnetic resonance imaging. *Human Brain Mapp*, 1997, 5, 18–25.
[41] Hroma´ dka, T; Deweese, MR; Zador, AM. Sparse representation of sounds in the unanesthetized auditory cortex. *PLoS Biol*, 2008, 6, 16.
[42] DeWeese, MR; Wehr, M; Zador, AM. Binary spiking in auditory cortex. *J. Neurosci*, 2003, 23, 7940-9.
[43] Elhilali, M; Fritz, JB; Klein, DJ; Simon, JZ; Shamma, SA. Dynamics of precise spike timing in primary auditory cortex. *J. Neurosci*, 2004, 24, 1159-72.
[44] Barbour, DL; Wang, X. Auditory cortical responses elicited in awake primates by random spectrum stimuli. *J. Neurosci*, 2003, 23, 7194-206.

[45] Liang, L; Lu, T; Wang, X. Neural representations of sinusoidal amplitude and frequency modulations in the primary auditory cortex of awake primates. *J. Neurophysiol*, 2002, 87, 2237-61.

[46] Malone, BJ; Scott, BH; Semple, MN. Context-dependent adaptive coding of interaural phase disparity in the auditory cortex of awake macaques. *J. Neurosci*, 2002, 22, 4625-38.

[47] Hall, DA; Johnsrude, IS; Haggard, MP; Palmer, AR; Akeroyd, MA; Summerfield, AQ. Spectral and temporal processing in human auditory cortex. *Cereb. Cortex*. 2002, 12, 140-9.

[48] Seifritz, E; Esposito, F; Hennel, F; Mustovic, H; Neuhoff, JG; Bilecen, D; Tedeschi, G; Scheffler, K; Di Salle, F. Spatiotemporal pattern of neural processing in the human auditory cortex. *Science*, 2002, 297, 1706-8.

[49] Pfingst, BE; O'Connor, TA. Characteristics of neurons in auditory cortex of monkeys performing a simple auditory task. *J. Neurophysiol*. 1981, 45, 16-34.

[50] Phillips, DP. Neural representation of sound amplitude in the auditory cortex: effects of noise masking. *Behav. Brain Res,* 1990, 37, 197-214.

[51] Schnupp, JW; Hall, TM; Kokelaar, RF; Ahmed, B. Plasticity of temporal pattern codes for vocalization stimuli in primary auditory cortex. *J. Neurosci*, 2006, 26, 4785–95.

[52] Wang, X; Lu, T; Bendor, D; Bartlett, E. Neural coding of temporal information in auditory thalamus and cortex. *Neuroscience*, 2008, 157, 484-94.

[53] Gogate, LJ; Walker-Andrews, AS; Bahrick, LE; The intersensory origins of word comprehension: an ecological-dynamic systems view. *Developmental Science*, 2001, 4, 1–18.

[54] Ghazanfar, AA; Nielsen, K; Logothetis, NK. Eye movements of monkeys viewing vocalizing conspecifics. *Cognition*, 2006, 101, 515–29.

[55] Sams, M; Aulanko, R; Hamalainen, M; Hari, R; Lounasmaa, OV; Lu, ST; Simola, J. Seeing speech: visual information from lip movements modifies activity in the human auditory cortex. *Neurosci. Lett*, 1991, 127, 141–5.

[56] Schroeder, CE; Foxe, J. 2005. Multisensory contributions to low-level, 'unisensory' processing. *Curr. Opin. Neurobiol*. 15, 454–458.

[57] Schurmann, M; Caetano, G; Jousmaki, V; Hari, R. Hands help hearing: facilitatory audiotactile interaction at low sound-intensity levels. *J. Acoust. Soc. Am*, 2004, 115, 830–2.

[58] Musacchia, G; Schroeder, CE. Neuronal mechanisms, response dynamics and perceptual functions of multisensory interactions in auditory cortex. *Hear Res*, 2009, 258, 72-9.

[59] Mountcastle, V. Central neural mechanisms in hearing. In V. Mountcastle ed. Medical physiology (vol.2) St.Louis; CV Mosby

[60] Celesia, GG. Auditory cortical areas in man. *Brain*, 1976, 99, 403-14.

[61] Kral, A; Heid, S; Tillein, J; Hartmann, R; Klinke, R. Postnatal cortical development in congenital auditory deprivation. *Cereb. Cortex*, 2005, 15, 552-62.

[62] Sharma, A; Dorman, MF; Spahr, AJ. A sensitive period for the development of the central auditory system in children with cochlear implants: implications for age of implantation. *Ear Hear*, 2002, 23, 532-9.

[63] Rosen, S. Temporal information in speech: acoustic, auditory and linguistic aspects. *Philos. Trans. R. Soc. Lond. B. Biol. Sci*, 1992, 336, 367–73.

[64] Woods, DL; Stecker, GC; Rinne, T; et al. Functional maps of human auditory cortex: effects of acoustic features and attention. *PLoS ONE*, 2009, 4, 183.

[65] Petkov, CI; Kang, X; Alho, K; et al. Attentional modulation of human auditory cortex. *Nat. Neurosci*, 2004, 7, 658–63.

[66] Rauschecker, JP; Tian, B. Mechanisms and streams for processing of 'what' and 'where' in auditory cortex. *Proc. Natl. Acad. Sci. U S A*, 2000, 97, 11800–6.

[67] Bocca, E; Calearo, C; Cassinari, V. A new method for testing hearing in temporal lobe tumours. *Acta otolaryngol (Stockh),* 44, 219, 1954.

[68] Moller, AR. Hearing: Anatomy, Physiology, and Disorders of the Auditory System. 2nd ed. U.S.A, Academic Press, 2006, 245
"This article was published in Hearing: Anatomy, Physiology, and Disorders of the Auditory System, 2nd ed, Moller, AR, pg 245, Copyright Elsevier (2006)."

[69] Bauer, RM; McDonald, CR. Behavioral neurology and neuropsychology. 2nd Ed. Edited by Feinberg TE, Farah MJ. USA: McGraw-Hill companies Inc. 2003, 257-67.

[70] Massopoust, LC; Wolin, LR. Changes in auditory frequency discrimination thresholds after temporal cortex ablation. *Exp. Neurol*, 1967, 19, 245-51.

[71] Wohlfart, G; Lindgren, A; Jernelius, B. Clinical picture and morbid anatomy in a case of "pure word deafness". *J. Nerv. Ment. Dis*, 1952, 116, 818-27.

[72] Grade, MM; Cowey, A. "Deaf hearing": Unacknowledged detection of auditory stimuli in a patient with cerebral deafness. *Cortex*, 2000, 36, 71-80.

[73] Tanaka, Y; Kamo, T; Yoshida, M; Yamadori, A. "So-called" cortical deafness. Clinical, neurophysiological, and radiological observation. *Brain*, 1991, 114, 2385-401.

[74] Motomura, N; Yamador, A; Mori, E; Tamaru, F. Auditory agnosia: Analysis of a case with bilateral subcortical lesions. *Brain*, 1986, 29, 379-91.

[75] Lichteim, L. On aphasia. *Brain*, 1885, 7, 433-84.

[76] Kanter, SL; Day, AL; Heilman, KM; Gonzalez-Rothi, LJ. Pure word deafness: A possible explanation of transient-deterioration after extracranial-intracranial bypass grafting. *Neurosurgery*, 1986, 18, 186-9.

[77] Buchman, AS; Garron, DC; Trost-Cardamone, JE. Word deafness: One hundreds years later. *J. Neurol. Neurosurg. Psychiatry*, 1986, 49, 489-99.

[78] Kaga, M. Language disorders in Landau-Kleffner syndrome. *J. Child Neurol*, 1999, 14, 118-22.

[79] Albert, ML; Bear, D. A case study of word deafness with reference to the role of time in auditory comprehension. *Brain*, 1974, 97, 373-84.

[80] Wang, E; Peach, RK; Xu, Y. Reception of dynamic acoustic patterns by an indivisual with unilateral verbal auditory agnosia. *Brain Lang*, 2000, 73, 442-55.

[81] Auerbach, SH; Allard, T; Naeser, M. Analysis of a case with bilateral lesions and a defect at the prephonemic level. *Brain*, 1982, 105, 271-300.

[82] Klein, SK; Kurtzberg, D; Brattson, A. Electrophysiologic manifestation of impaired temporal lobel auditory processing in verbal auditory agnosia. *Brain Lang*, 1995, 51, 383-405.

[83] Spreen, O; Benton, AL; Fincham, R. Auditory agnosia without aphasia. *Arch. Neurol*, 1965, 13, 84-92.

[84] Clarke, S; Bellmann, A; Meuli, RA; Assal, G; Steck, AJ. Auditory agnosia and auditory spatial deficit following left hemispheric lesions. *Neuropsychologia*, 2000, 38, 797-807.

[85] Lambert, J; Eustache, F; Lechevalier, B. Auditory agnosia with relative sparing of speech perception. *Cortex*, 1989, 25, 71-82.

[86] Engelien, A; Stern, E; Silbersweig, DA. Functional neuroimaging of human central auditory processing in normal subjects and patients with neurological and neuropsychiatric disorders. *J. clin. Exp. Neuropsychol*, 2001, 23, 94-120.

[87] Heilman, KM; Scholes, R; Watson, RT. Auditory affective agnosia. *J. Neurol. Neurosurg. Psychiatry*, 1975, 38, 69-72.

[88] Griffiths TD, Rees A, Witton C, Cross PM, Shakir RA, Green GG. Spatial and temporal auditory processing deficits following right hemisphere infarction. A psychological study. *Brain* 1997, 120, 785-794.

[89] Griffiths TD, Bench CJ, Frackowiak RS. Human cortical areas selectively activated by apparent sound movement. *Curr. Biol.* 1994, 4, 892-895.

[90] Blumstein, S; Cooper, W. Hemispheric processing of intonation contours. *Cortex*, 1974, 10, 146-58.

[91] Perez, I; Kolinsky, R; Tramo, M; et al. Functional dissociations following bilateral lesions of auditory cortex. *Brain*, 1994, 117, 1283-1301.

[92] Devinsky, O; D'esposito, M. Neurology of cognitive and Behavioral disorders. Oxford university Press Inc. New York USA. 1st ed. 2004.

[93] Cachia, A; Paillère-Martinot, ML; Galinowski, A; Januel, D; de Beaurepaire, R; Bellivier, F; Artiges, E; Andoh, J; Bartrés-Faz, D; Duchesnay, E; Rivière, D; Plaze, M; Mangin, JF; Martinot, JL. Cortical folding abnormalities in schizophrenia patients with resistant auditory hallucinations. *Neuroimage*, 2008, 39, 927-35.

[94] Marti-Bonmati, L; Lull, JJ; Carcia-Marti, G; Aquilar, EJ; Moratal-Peres, D; Poyatos, C; et el. Chronic auditory hallucinations in schizophrenic patients: MR analysis of the coincidence between functional and morphologic abnormalities. *Radiology*, 2007 Aug, 244(2), 549-56.

[95] Shulman, A; Goldstein, B; Strashun, AM. Final common pathway for tinnitus: Theoretical and clinical implications of neuroanatomical substrates. *Int. Tinnitus J*, 2009, 15, 5-50.

[96] Lanting, CP; de Klein, E; van Dijk, P. Neural activity underlying tinnitus generation: result from PET and fMRI. *Hear Res*, 2009, 255, 1-13.

In: Auditory Cortex: Anatomy, Functions and Disorders
Editor: Mounya Elhilali
ISBN 978-1-62100-685-5


*Chapter II*

# Primary Auditory Cortex as a Node of the Ascending, Descending, and Local Connectivity

***Hisayuki Ojima****
Cognitive Neurobiology, Graduate School of Medical and Dental Sciences,
Tokyo Medical and Dental University, Tokyo, Japan

## Abstract

Auditory cortex (AC) of mammals has long been studied with the aim at understanding how neuronal responses to acoustic parameters decoded in cochlea are integrated for perception of natural sounds. Of several hierarchical fields in the AC, the primary auditory field (A1) has been intensively investigated for anatomical network and response properties. Connectivity of AI has been schemed by revealing subcortical pathways, extrinsic and local intrinsic connections, cortical modules, and architectures based on imaging techniques. Functional evaluation of A1 has also clarified response properties to basic acoustic parameters, response modulation by activation of non-auditory fields, and state-dependent shift of response pattern. These lines of evidence cast light on each piece of a jigsaw puzzle in detail but seem to be far away from showing the full extent of the puzzle. Each piece may correspond to a cortical module. Indeed, it will be noticed that in most textbooks virtually no links has been described between individual modules' functions such as frequency selectivity and perception of natural sounds such as vocalization. As a prerequisite for this holistic interpretation, in this short chapter, a certain attempt has been made to degrade presumed cortical modules into constituent neurons from the point of view of their connectivity at the single cell level and response properties at the synaptic level. Such degradation will help readers grasp a hint to integrate information of module's functions into the function of A1, and ultimately the AC.

* Phone: 81-3-5803-5446, Fax: 81-3-5803-0186. E-mail: yojima.cnb@tmd.ac.jp.

# Introduction

Cerebral cortex in general receives projections from subcortical structures and other cortical areas, and project efferent to them. Unitary architecture receiving or projecting these connections is thought to be column-like and extend throughout the cortical depth, referred to as cortical module or column.

Auditory cortex (AC) receives three major ascending systems designated as lemniscal (tonotopic), nonlemniscal (diffuse) and multimodal (polysensory). These pathways are well segregated while ascending from the cochlear nucleus (CN) through the inferior colliculus (IC) to the medial geniculate body (MGB) [1]. Thalamocortical (TC) connectivity is principally divergent in the sense of projection to multiple cortical fields from one thalamic nucleus, though individual neurons may project dominantly to single fields [2]. Conversely, TC connectivity is convergent in the sense of projection to one cortical field from multiple thalamic nuclei. Fields in the AC are delineated on the basis of topography to sulci and overall representation of the cochlear basilar membrane, tonotopy. Well-defined tonotopic fields, for example, such as primary, anterior, posterior and ventroposterior auditory fields in cats, or 2 to 3 fields including primary auditory field (A1) within core region in monkeys, contain neurons with distinct frequency selectivity reflecting the lemniscal ascending system, while ill-defined fields, such as secondary auditory field in cats (e.g., connectivity between cat AC and MGB in Figure 1) or several fields within belt region in monkeys, contain neurons with less distinct frequency selectivity reflecting the nonlemniscal ascending system. Anatomically, however, tonotopic fields are targets of projections via both lemniscal and nonlemniscal pathways, but probably so with different proportions of their contribution. In addition, each field receives projection via multimodal pathway. For example, A1 receives a major lemniscal projection from the anterior part of the ventral MGB nucleus (vMGB) and a minor one from the lateral nucleus of the posterior complex, together with a weak but substantial input from the multimodal medial MGB nucleus (mMGB) and a slight contribution possibly from parts of the dorsal MGB nucleus (dMGB) belonging to the nonlemniscal system. Note that this field is said to be tonotopic, since it contains a set of modules that represents a systematic gradient in the frequency selectivity derived from the dominant lemniscal projections, despite of the contribution of the multimodal and non-lemniscal systems. Thus, each AC field could potentially be influenced by lemniscal, nonlemniscal and multimodal input. Similarly, the descending systems from AC comprise segregated divergent pathways to distinct thalamic [3, 4, 5] and subcortical [6] stations.

Evidence for interactions of the AC including A1 with areas of other sensory modalities through corticocortical (CC) connections [7, 8, 9] and with higher order and multisensory cortical areas through feedback projection system [10, 11] has been accumulating. It is assumed that such connectivity is mediated by module-to-module connections. Anatomical findings of related connections raise the possibilities that A1 neurons may respond to non-auditory stimuli or that their responses to acoustic stimuli are modulated by non-auditory stimuli. Indeed, recent studies showed the modulation of response properties of AI neurons by visual [9, 12], and somatosensory [9, 13] stimuli. Far prior to these, it had been reported that the responsiveness of single AC neurons, some in a region corresponding to the current A1 of the cat, could be modulated by higher cognitive functions such as attention [14].

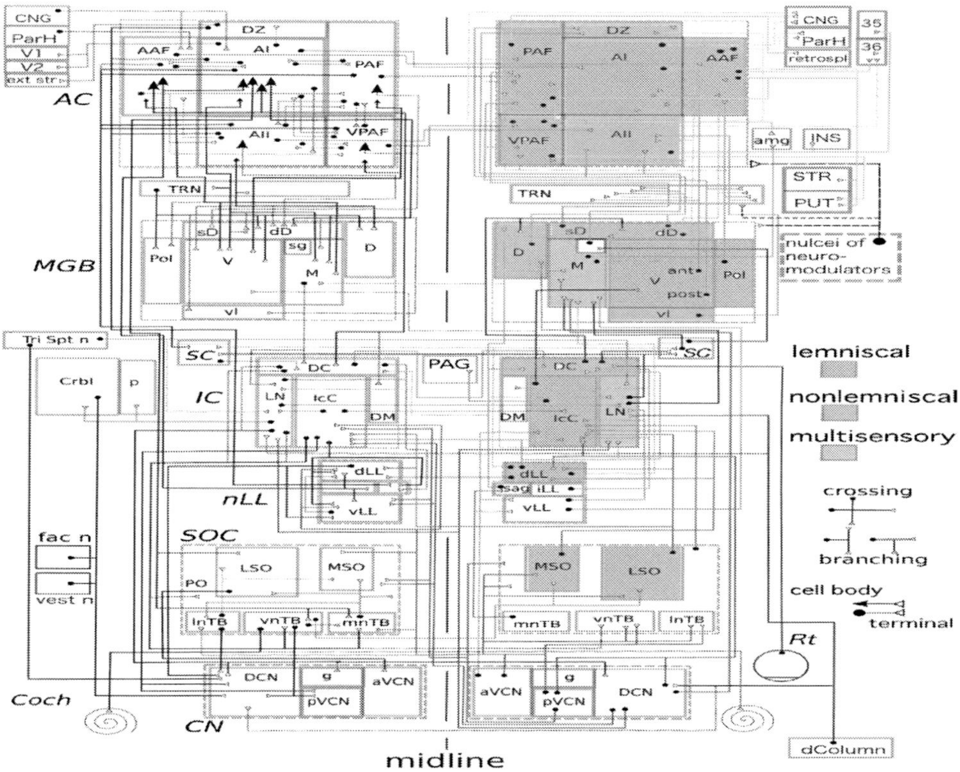


Figure 1. Wiring scheme of the auditory pathway. Left, intracortical (i.e., intrinsic and extrinsic corticocortical, and commissural) and descending projections. Right, ascending projections. Lines show connections, with filled circle(s) and open triangle(s) attached to them indicating the nuclei or field(s) of origin and projection target(s), respectively. Filled triangles, instead of the circles, are used if their laminar positions in the A1 is concerned. If connection is weak, inconsistent among authors or animal species, and/or simply inferred from the findings in other modalities, dotted line is used. AAF, anterior auditory field; AC, auditory cortex; aVCN, anteroventral cochlear nucleus; AI, primary auditory field; AII, secondary auditory field; CN, cochlear nucleus; DCN, dorsal cochlear nucleus; g, granule cell area; pVCN, posteroventral cochlear nucleus. amg, amygdala; CNG, cingulate cortex; Coch, cochlea; Crbl, cerebellum; D, dorsal and dorsocaudal nuclei of MGB; DC, dorsal cortex of IC (mostly overlapping with the external nucleus of Rockel and Jones, 1973a, b); dColumn, dorsal column nuclues; dD, deep dorsal nucleus of MGB; dLL, dorsal nucleus of lateral lemniscus; ext str, extrastriate areas; DM (of Rockel and Jones, 1973a, b), dorsomedial zone of IcC (corresponding to layers 3/4 of DC); DZ, dorsal zone; fac n, facial nucleus; IC, inferior colliculus; IcC, central nucleus of IC; iLL, intermediate nucleus of lateral lemniscus; INS, insular; Lem, lemniscal; LN, lateral nucleus of IC (external nucleus); lnTB, lateral nuclues of trapezoid body; LSO, lateral superior olive; M, medial nucleus of MGB; MGB, medial geniculate body; mnTB, medial nucleus of trapezoid body; MSO, medial superior olive; multi, multimodal; nLL, nuclei of lateral lemniscus; nonlem, nonlemniscal; p, pontine nucleus; PAF, posterior auditory field; PAG, periaquaductal gray; ParH, parahippocampal area; PO, periolivary nuclei; Pol, lateral part of the posterior thalamic nucleus; Prh, perirhinal cortex; PUT, putamen; retrospl, retrosplenial cortex; Rt, retina; sg, sagulum (belonging to tegmentum); SC, superior colliculus; sD, superficial dorsal nucleus of MGB; sg, suprageniculate nucleus; SOC, superior olivary complex; STR, striatum; Tri Spt n, spinal nucleus of trigeminal nerve; TRN, thalamic reticular nucleus; V, ventral nucleus of MGB (divided into anterior and posterior portions); vest n, vestibular nucleus; vnTB, ventral nucleus of trapezoid body; vl, ventrolateral nucleus of MGB; vLL, ventral nuclues of lateral lemniscus; ventral nucleus of trapezoid body; VPAF, ventroposterior field; V1 and V2, primary and secondary visual fields. Figure is a synthesis of papers [1, 83, 90, 91, 92], as well as following book chapters [93, 94] and books [95, 96].

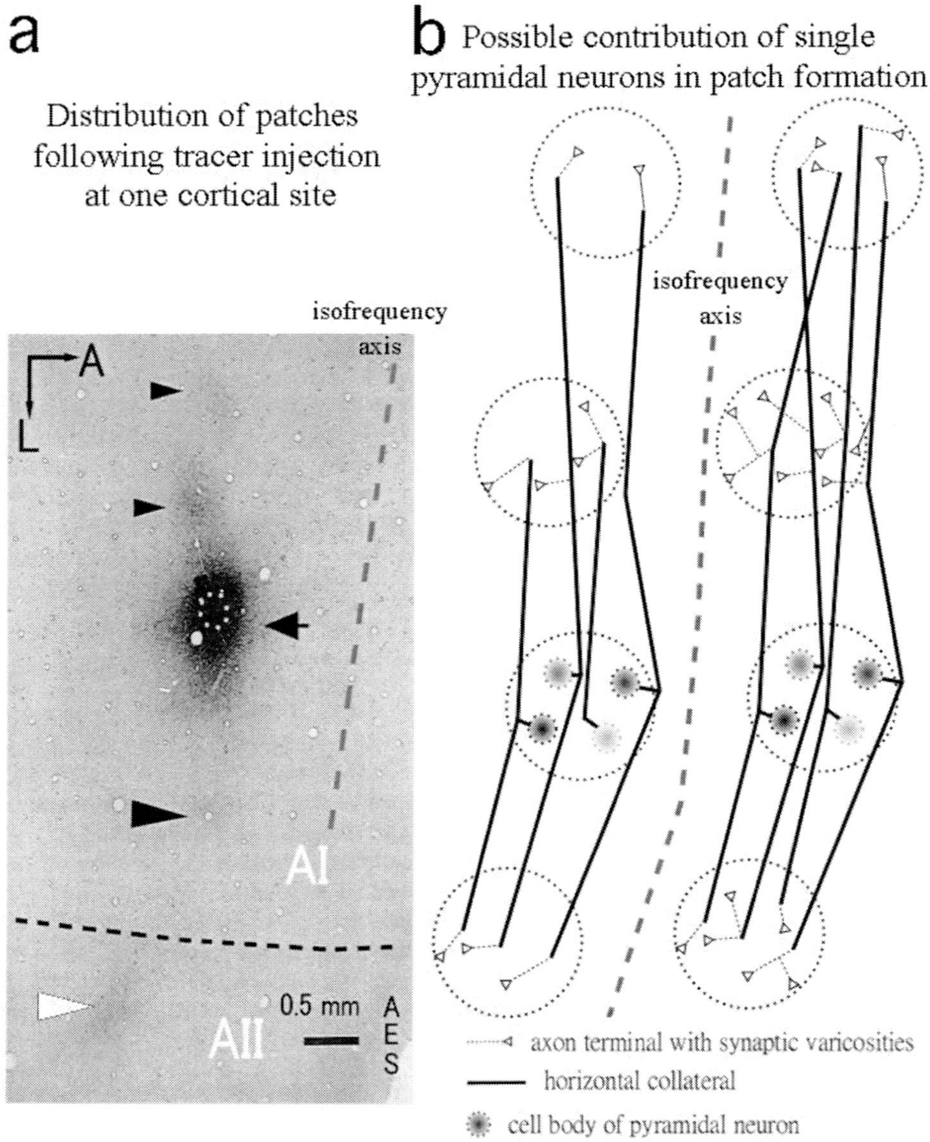


Figure 2. Local circuit revealed by extracellular injection of anterograde tracer at one cortical site (population labeling). Left; tangential layer 3 section of the cat middle ectosylvian gyrus on which a frequency (anteroposterior) and isofrequency (dorsoventral) axes can be mapped. Injection site is pointed by arrow with the injection center of labeled cells of origin (circle of white dots). The injection center is determined in layer 6 as a bundle of projecting axons that descend and leave the grey matter (circle of white dots). Dorsal and ventral to the injection site, 4 patches (remote patches, arrowheads) of labeled structures such as clustered axon terminals and a few cell bodies are formed. The most ventral patch (white arrowhead) resides in the secondary auditory cortex (AII). A well-circumscribed patch of highly dense axon terminals is formed at the injection site. AES, anterior ectosylvian sulcus. Right; two possible extremes of how individual constituent neurons within the patch at the injection site project to other remote patches. The left case shows that constituent neurons in the injection patch project to only some of the remote patches, while in the right case they project to all patches. Modified from Ojima and Takayanagi [29].

This is consistent with more recent studies showing the modulation by expectation [15] or brain state related to exploration [16]. Although the basic functional organization of A1 has been well established [17], the information carried by each of the segregated ascending systems as well as the role of each cortical layer, domain, and field in the processing of acoustic signals still remains to be elucidated [18, 19, 20, 21].

Modules can be demonstrated anatomically as well as functionally, though the latter may be ill defined. They have been characterized so far by several basic acoustic parameters such as frequency, intensity, binaurality and others in A1, therefore for the lemniscal projection system. However, they have not been defined for each of the triple ascending connection systems, i.e., nonlemniscal ascending system and multimodal connectivity. Besides, how elementary constituents contribute anatomically and functionally to the module formation in A1 has little been elucidated.

To clarify the mechanisms as to how basic acoustic parameters such as frequency and intensity represented by lower-order cortical neurons are integrated or cooperated to generate response preferences for naturalistic sounds such as vocalizations is a critical issue. There must be some anatomical substrates for transformation from responses to these basic parameters to those to more complex sounds. Fragmented knowledge on connections known so far for cortical areas as well as subcortical stations at the macro-to-micro level needs to be comprehensively synthesized for a global chart. That will be a purpose of the current review. The chart will give us a hint to notice what should be placed next as a new piece in this complicated system, so as a functional link.

## 1. Modules along the Frequency and Isofrequency Axes in the AI

As in the visual cortex, columns or modules (in a more anatomical sense, patches) have been demonstrated in AC, too (Figure 2). It is assumed that they are structural units of various acoustic parameters such as frequency, spectral bandwidth, intensity, and binaurality [22]. Across the surfaces of the cat AI and other tonotopic fields, neurons tuned to systematically changing frequencies are orderly arranged along one axis (frequency axis). This arrangement raises an obvious question about what is represented along the axis orthogonal to this frequency axis, since cochlea has only one-dimensional axis. Along the 2nd axis, especially prominent in the AI, parameters other than frequency must be represented, with the frequency selectivity of neurons kept almost similar (isofrequency axis). So far, along the isofrequency axis, different integration modes of spectrum and space are thought to take a pattern of alternating groups of neurons. These include the spectral bandwidth (spectral range of tuning of a neuron or neurons when driven at a sound intensity somewhat higher than threshold), the binaural interactions (how stimulation to both ears affects response magnitude induced by monaural stimulation to the dominant ear [23, 24, 25, 26]) and other [17]. Thus, it should be noted that single frequencies do not uniquely correspond to particular cortical modules in a one-to-one manner.

An injection of anterograde or retrograde tracers into a cortical site results in labeling of patches of clustered axons and/or cell bodies at remote sites, not forming continuous sheets of labeled structures. This anatomically demonstrated structure is believed to correspond to functional columnar architecture. The remote patches of labeled axons or cell bodies are separated from a source patch that is formed at the injection site. The outline of each patch is round or oval in shape, and their size is approximately 300 to 500 μm in diameter. The labeled axons and cell bodies in patches represent output from neurons at the injection site and source neurons providing output to the injection site, respectively. Distribution of such patches is anisotropic in the AC, being arranged mainly along the isofrequency axis. It is observed that remote patches are linked to the source patch by horizontal axon collaterals, coursing almost parallel to the cortical surface [27, 28]. In the cat AI, a small injection of tracers produces typically 3 to 4 remote patches across the field [left panel in Figure 2 of 29], while a large injection seems to generate more patches [27]. The center-to-center separation between nearby 2 patches is approximately 0.5 to 1-2 mm. Thus, in the cat AI, a population of neurons within a putative single module projects their output axons locally to other modules that are separated apart but so along an isofrequency axis on which the source module is also located.

Dispersed modules are interconnected along the isofrequency axis in the AI. It implies that there may be some acoustic parameters that are commonly shared among them. One possible parameter is the binaural interaction of neuronal responses, since, when stimulated binaurally, subsets of neurons showing facilitation (EE bands) and those showing suppression (EI bands) form separate multiple bands that alternate their location along the isofrequency axis. However, sharp segregation of different binaural interaction bands has been questioned. It was claimed on the basis of their own observations [30, 31, 32] that the organization along cortical depth was indeed columnar, but what was common among columnarly arranged neurons was not the binaural properties but simply a common ear-dominance. The fact that the ear-dominance is common among neurons within a single vertical module does not always guarantee the same type of binaural effect to obtain along the cortical depth.

A similar module/patch organization has been demonstrated in area 17 (V1) of the monkey [33, 34, 35] and cat [36, 37, 38, 39, 40]. It is also demonstrated in higher visual areas [monkey; 41, 42, 43, 44 and cat; 45]. Earlier studies combining the tracer-based anatomy with electrophysiological mapping and/or glucose utilization mapping for visual features show that patches of horizontal connections link cortical domains of the same eye as well as domains of the same or similar orientation preference [cat area 17, 46]. Interestingly, for the cat area 18, however, the opposite was resulted; anatomically connected patches preferentially link cortical domains of orthogonal orientation preference and are independent of the ocular dominance of the cortical cells [36, 37]. A single rule simply may not be applied to the local cortical organization.

Later studies employing combination of anatomical labeling with the optical imaging for functional organizations in the monkey V1 [47] suggested that horizontal connections linked both the common and different response properties; long-range horizontal connections only partially linked the ocular dominance columns of the same-eye or nearly one third of connections interconnect patches whose orientation preferences were not alike but were different by at least 45 degrees. They therefore noted that such connectivity had a limited precision. These results suggest that "multiplicity" rather than "specificity" might be the principal of the local cortical connectivity, implying that the response selectivity at a cortical domain, or probably also of a single neuron, could be determined by computation or competition of activities of presynaptic inputs carrying heterogeneous stimulus selectivity. Inhibitory circuitry would be involved in such computation. It is not fully addressed how specifically modules representing common response properties are interconnected in the auditory system. However, even if the multiplicity rule proposed for the visual system holds true for the auditory system, at least the specificity of frequency representation seems to be preserved within a tonotopic auditory field through the mutual linking of modules of like frequencies by horizontal collaterals (see below).

## 2. Correspondence between imaging of spectral preference and anatomical projections in the A1

In the auditory cortex, frequency organization can also be demonstrated by optical imaging employing both the intrinsic signals and voltage sensitive dyes (also see chapter IV). By these techniques, it was confirmed that areas activated with pure tones showed elongated contours along a line almost parallel to the isofrequency axis (prominently in the cat, see Figures 3, but also in ferrets and guinea pigs; [48, 49, 50, 51]), with their most peripheral portions extending beyond the borders between the AI and adjoining fields, such as the dorsal field dorsal to AI and the secondary auditory field ventral to it [50].

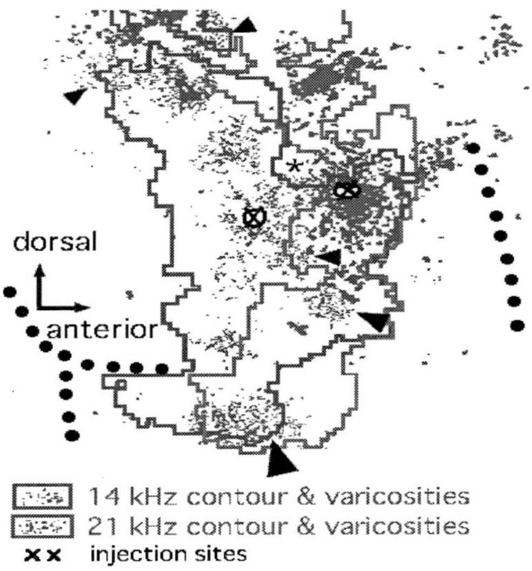


Figure 3. Optically detected areas of activation combined with anatomical visualized output axons originating from the center region of the activated areas (x). In the surface view of the cat AI, the isofrequency axis courses approximately in the dorsoventral direction. Binaural stimulations at 14 kHz and 21 kHz pure tones under isoflurane gas anesthesia showed dorsoventrally-elongated areas of activation, outlined by two different respective solid lines (one in blue and the other in red) with partial overlaps at various regions except for the center region (depicted by *). Separate injections of different tracers in the center of each area of activation of single hemispheres results in labeling of axon terminals that are originated from a population of neurons located at the injection sites (small dots, red from 21 kHz injection site and blue from 14 kHz injection site; also see Figure 2). At loci indicated by arrowheads, axon terminals of the two different origins are intermingled, suggestive of convergence of different spectral information. These are observed both in the border region between the two injection sites and at the periphery of the activation contours, probably outside of A1. Dotted lines indicate the posterior ectosylvian sulcus (left) and anterior ectosylvian sulcus (right). Modified from Ojima et al., [50].

If such isofrequency-like contours activated by two different pure tone pips with an approximately half octave separation were superimposed, they extensively overlapped on the cortical surface at several locations including those far peripheral portions (Figure 3). It contrasted the presence of non-overlap areas at more centrally located regions of the isofrequency contours of activation (* symbol in Figure 3).

Anatomical correspondence to these functionally defined areas of activation was also demonstrated after the optical imaging. Separate injection of different anterograde tracers into the center (two x in Figure 3) of each of the two different isofrequency contours of activation showed substantial separation in distribution of output axons (red and blue dots in Figure 3) of the different origins, but their occasional intermingling far dorsal and ventral (large arrowheads in Figure 3) to the injection sites, at or near the border zones between two injections and just outside of the A1 (small arrowheads). These regions of anatomical convergence were included in the overlap zones of activation demonstrated by optical imaging (Figure 3, also see [52]). From this convergent projection pattern, it is likely that certain integration of different spectral components obtains if information is transferred from the A1 to the next stage, but not within the A1.

# 3. Activation Spread from Single Cortical Modules

Differences in overall pattern of horizontal connectivity have been noted between the auditory and visual systems. Patches, one being at the injection site and others at remote locations, are altogether arranged along an imagery line, like a part of rosary, in the cat A1, while remote patches are arranged so as to surround one source patch at an injection site, like a set of satellites, in the cat and monkey V1. Although retinotopy tells us the spatial one-to-one relationship between the visual field and V1 in the subcortical projection, every cortical domain is mutually connected to several other cortical domains through the horizontal collateralization. This would let us image the occurrence of a progressively radiating wave of activation from a single cortical site when that site is adequately stimulated. In the visual system, the stimulus that activates single cortical sites is a small spot of flashing light fixed at the visual field or a small, high-contrast black-and-white drifting grating. On the basis of the one-to-one correspondence between the visual field and V1, stimulation with such a small flash or drifting light grating will activate a single cortical domain whose location is determined on the retinotopic relationship. According to the anatomical pattern of the spread of horizontal collaterals from one cortical site, activation at a single cortical domain might lead to spreading of activation to multiple remote patches connected horizontally to the original activation domain. Indeed, using voltage sensitive dye imaging, an activation spread was observed in monkey V1 following a drifting grating of a size 1° x 1°, but prominent activation peaks were observed at locations corresponding to remote patches around one major peak corresponding to the retinotopically-defined initial activation spot [53]. Instead, a few small peaks were formed, though the number of these peaks was much smaller than that of remote peaks generally observed for the V1 of the same animal species. So far, it has not been explored whether such minor activation peaks correspond to anatomically detected patches of horizontal collaterals.

How about in the AI? An adequate stimulus to arbitrarily activate one cortical site along the frequency axis could be determined according to the tonotopy if pure tone is used as stimulus at a relatively mild intensity. Imaging studies indeed showed the initial focal activation at a locus along the stimulus-matched isofrequency contour. However it was not stationary but rather propagated along the isofrequency axis, with some spread of the activation orthogonal to that axis [49, 50, 51, 54, 55]. The activity propagation along the isofrequency axis was in most cases unidirectional, with an initial activation spot emerging relatively dorsal and then propagating mostly in the ventral direction [51, 56]. As the activation propagated, a few peaks of later activation appeared to be formed [see 50], although their correspondence to anatomical patches was not explored yet. Strangely, spots in which the activation was initiated tended to vary from trial to trial. Thus, it is still not clear what is an adequate acoustic stimulus to activate a single domain along the isofrequency axis. This may be related to what properties or acoustic parameters are represented along the isofrequency axis.

Other than the binaurality, it is known that the stimulus bandwidth preference is represented along the isofrequency axis; that is, how broadly neuronal populations are tuned to stimulus frequencies [57]. In the cat, broadly and narrowly tuned regions alternate across the AI and divide it into 3 to 4 zones along the axis orthogonal to the frequency axis (i.e., along the isofrequency axis). Therefore, stimulation with broad range of frequency-step sounds (pure tone lasting for a short period shifts its frequency gradually within a broad range) is likely to activate the separate zones along the isofrequency axis. Indeed, regions of higher response magnitude to the frequency-step stimulation roughly overlapped with the tone-defined broadband zones [58]. This matching was probably due to the reduced effect of sideband inhibition by the use of the transient frequency step in which component frequencies were asynchronously presented, so minimizing the interaction of excitatory and inhibitory activities of neuron clusters. Thus, if standard narrowband or broadband noises had been used as stimulus, different results would have been yielded, since component frequencies are synchronously presented in these sounds.

Anatomical justification that cortical domains of similar spectral tuning properties were mutually connected by horizontal connections was made later [58]. Combination of electrophysiology and anatomical tracer injections, together with broadband frequency-step sounds as stimulus, provided evidence for the link between the patches of similar bandwidth; for example, a narrowly tuned patch located in the center AI was connected with the other narrowly tuned patch dorsal to the center one, with the lack of labeling in the in-between regions that corresponded to the broadly tuned patch. This series of experiments suggests that it might be possible to activate arbitrarily a specific cortical domain *along the isofrequency axis*. However, since resolution to segregate functional domains *along the frequency axis* is theoretically low because of the type of stimulus used (broad range!), it must be difficult or impossible to segregate the domains arranged *along the frequency axis*. Thus, we still have not any adequate stimuli to activate arbitrarily one cortical site across the AI. This was also the case when the AC fields of guinea pigs were explored for possible segregated binaural domains using stimuli including binaural cues. In trials of stimulation using tone pips with different stimulus intensities between left and right ears (interaural intensity difference), no specific activation was observed *along the isofrequency axis* [59, 60].

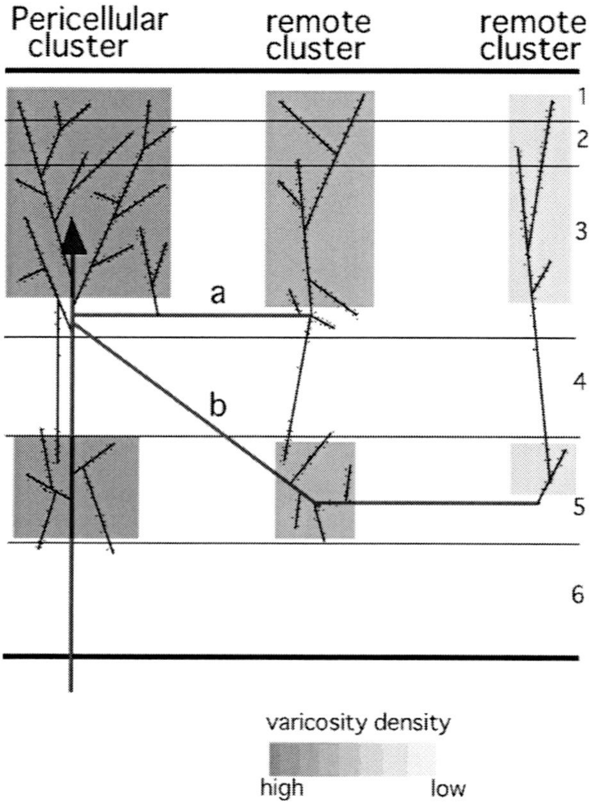


Figure 4. Schematic summary of axon collaterals with varicosities originating from layer 2/3 PNs labeled intracellularly with a diffusible tracer after confirmation of the responses to pure tones. Cell body (filled triangle) is located in layer 3. Horizontal axons (a and b) are emitted at layer 3 from its descending main axon that enters white matter and bifurcates thereafter. Secondary fine branches are derived from these horizontal axons and give rise to clustered axon terminals with varicosities (small dots) near the cell body and at distances from it. The Secondary branches are clustered to form a column and are higher in density in layers 2/3 and in layer 5 than in other layers. This laminar specificity seems to be common among the pericellular and remote clusters of single PNs. Though a substantial number of varicosities are found on remote clusters, the highest density of varicosities is always observed in the pericellular cluster. Modified from Ojima et al., [28].

## 4. Clustered Axon Terminals of Single Layer 2/3 PNs of AI

Intracellular labeling of single PNs with a diffusible dye of small molecular weight (biocytin or neurobiotin, MW ca. 350), followed by the reconstruction of axon with varicosities (morphological term suggesting synaptic boutons at the light microscopy level), can illustrate the full extent of intrinsic local collateralization of single PNs. It has pointed out three major characteristics as schematized in figure 4. In accordance with the population labeling following an extracellular tracer injection in the cat A1, clustering of axon terminals is formed at several loci; one prominent cluster around the cell body and 2 to 3 clusters at remote sites. The remote clusters are derived usually from horizontal collaterals, but sometimes from obliquely coursing collaterals. Second, the clustering occurs at relatively regular intervals (about 500-1500 μm). Laminar localization of axon terminals should also be noted as the 3rd characteristic. Supragranular PNs project exclusively to both layers 2/3 and layer 5 [61]. Interestingly, the similar laminar distribution pattern of axon terminals or varicosities was found both for the cluster near cell body as well as for clusters in remote loci. Thus, through horizontal collateralization, single PNs are able to activate the same layers at dispersed cortical loci.

Functional role of horizontal connection has not been fully evaluated. Although it is proposed for V1 [see 62 for the visual system], the role which horizontal collaterals parallel to an A1 isofrequency line play is still unknown, especially so from the view point of "hearing" mechanism. Nonetheless, it may be helpful to compare the weight of axon clusters that a single neuron forms in an attempt to evaluate local influences of the horizontal connectivity. Comparison of the varicosity number in the cluster near cell body and in remote clusters will give us an implication about how much impact single cells exert on different remote cortical domains. The number of remote clusters located within the cat AI (excluding one around the cell body) varied from 1 to 3 per single PN (average, 2.0 ± 0.7, S.D., n=5; see Table 1; [29]). The varicosity number of individual remote clusters varied considerably from cluster to cluster (41 to 956 varicosities per cluster), but had the average of 382 ± 350 (S.D., n=10; Table 1), while that of the pericellular clusters was 1338 ± 476 (n=5). Although the possibility might not be excluded that distal axons were insufficiently filled with tracer, this proximal-to-distal gradient of the synaptic number that single PNs had was consistent among all neurons examined. Besides, this local gradient could also be applied to a case of PN in which the furthest distal cluster, though not included in the quantification because of its location outside the AI, had as many varicosities as the pericellular cluster had. Thus, it is believed that our estimation was not biased toward counting more varicosities in the pericellular clusters because of the insufficient filling of distal axons. The comparison indicates that the varicosity number of the distant clusters is consistently smaller than that of the pericellular clusters, suggesting that synaptic driving force is weaker at locations far away from the first activated domain within a field.

**Table 1. Quantification of varicosities within remote and pericellular clusters (cluster at cell body) of axon terminals**

| | Number of varicosity per cluster | | |
|---|---|---|---|
| cell | cluster dorsal to cell body | cluster at cell body | cluster ventral to cell body |
| 1 | 106 | 881 | 126 |
| 2 | - | 1467 | 198 |
| 3 | 706 | 945 | 535, 41 |
| 4 | - | 1334 | 863, 86 |
| 5 | 206, 957 | 2063 | - |

Remote clusters are classified into those dorsal or ventral to the pericellular cluster formed around the cell body. Single PNs located in layers 2/3 of the cat AI are intracellularly labeled with biocytin. After the 2-dimensional reconstruction of the entire intrinsic collaterals together with the dendritic arbors and cell body of well-stained single PNs (n=5), varicosities are plotted and grouped to clusters by confirming microscopically their relative location in histological sections. Varicosities on the horizontal collaterals and clusters of varicosities located outside the AI field (e.g., one pointed by the ventral large arrowhead in Figure 2a) are excluded from quantification. Modified from Ojima and Takayanagi [29].

# 5. Contribution of Single PNs to Patch Formation

Individual patches labeled following a tracer deposition in a single cortical site are comprised of axons of multiple cells of origin (see Figure 2a). If this complexity is decomposed to axonal projection pattern of unitary neurons, it will be informative. Intracellular labeling studies have shown that distribution of clustered axon terminals derived from horizontal collaterals of single PNs matches topographically well with the patchy organization demonstrated by the population labeling; secondary branches with clustered axon varicosities are intermittently emitted along horizontal collaterals of PNs in the A1 [29] as well as V1 [63, 64]. Despite of this decomposition, it has not been answered yet to what extent individual PNs contribute to the formation of each patch (see Figure 2b). Does every neuron in the source patch contribute to the formation of all of remote patches or do single neurons in the source patch provide with terminal axons to only some of remote patches? Simply, by counting the number of axon clusters formed by individual PNs, we can compare that number with the number of patches formed by the population labeling and have found that the former number is slightly smaller than the latter (2.0 n=5 vs. 2.8 n=6; unpublished data). The comparison suggests that each PN in the source patch appears to project to most but not all remote patches surrounding it. Combined with the findings described in the preceding subsection, it can be said that PNs located even close project to different sets of target domains, with a tendency to exert a stronger impact on the home domain than on remote ones (i.e., lower number of varicosities). This appears to be also the case, based on the author's own evaluation, for the projection of PNs in the V1 of the same animal species [see 64]. Local connection rule might be the same between these two sensory systems.

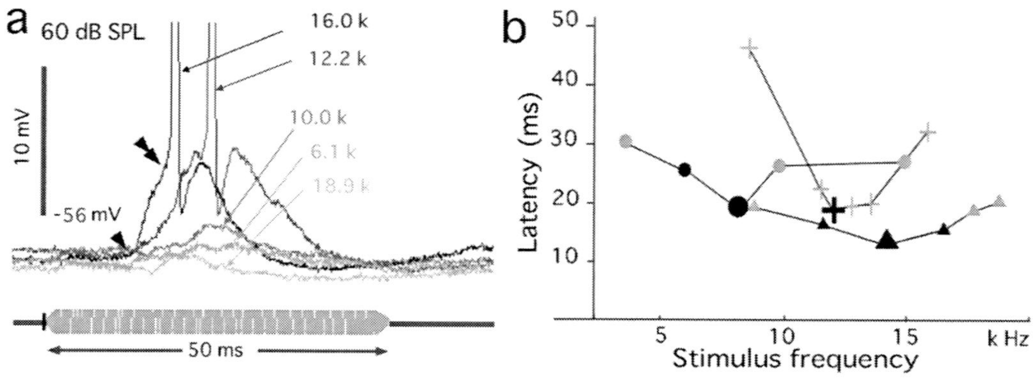


Figure 5. Subthreshold and suprathreshold behavior of membrane potentials recorded intracellularly from a single PN in the cat AI. Typical responses of layer 3 PNs to a set of pure tone pips applied at 60 dB SPL (*a*) at time 0 (left vertical bar). Note that the subthreshold synaptic responses evoked at stimulus frequencies of 6.1, 10.0 and 18.9 kHz cannot be detected by the conventional unit recording. Panel *b* shows the latency-frequency relationship of PNs stimulated at a set of pure tones. Three representative examples are recorded in middle layer 3. Individual neurons are designated by different symbols, with a larger symbol representing the response at the best frequency, and symbols in black and grey indicating suprathreshold and subthreshold responses, respectively. Onset time of the upward deflection of the membrane potential (single arrowhead in *a*) is regarded as latency of synaptic responses, while the time for membrane potential to cross the threshold level (double arrowhead) is regarded as latency of the unit discharge.

# 6. Synaptic Activation of AI Single PNs by Acoustic Stimulation

By inserting the tip of a fine glass micropipette into a cell (intracellular recording) or attaching it to the plasma membrane, thereafter peeling the attached part of membrane (patch clamping), potentials generated between the inside and outside of the plasma membrane of a cell can be measured. Potential changes from the resting state (resting membrane potential) consist of oppositely directed deflection of the membrane potential, positive deflection representing excitatory synaptic input (excitatory postsynaptic potential or current, EPSP or EPSC) and negative deflection representing inhibitory synaptic input (inhibitory postsynaptic potential or current, IPSP or IPSC) (Figure 5, [65]). Subthreshold EPSPs that do not grow to action potentials cannot be detected by extracellular recording in general.

As to the latency of the TC activity, it should be noted that since action potentials are generated on the rising phase of EPSP or at the peak of EPSP of a neuron, the onset of depolarizing deflection (EPSP onset), reflecting the arrival time of the earliest presynaptic activities, should precede the onset of the first evoked action potential (see single and double arrowhead in Figure 5a). The latter is generally evoked at the time for the neuron's membrane potential to cross the threshold level. Consequently, the latency measured conventionally, so defined for the first spike evoked by stimulation, should eventually be longer than the arrival time of the synaptic activity that initiates the first spike. Similarly, the onset time of the earliest activity measured by the voltage sensitive dye imaging, that is also believed to detect mainly subthreshold synaptic potentials, would be shorter than that of the first action potentials measured in the conventional way. It thus suggests that cortical activation following acoustic stimulation would be initiated earlier than traditionally thought on the basis of the time of the first spike occurrence.

In learning-associated plasticity, short-term plasticity following repetitive stimulation, and some suppression phenomena, measurement of synaptic activities can be a unique way to elucidate the contribution of input of different origins, i.e., computation through the integration of multiple subcortical and cortical sources. It is little known how subthreshold input of TC or CC afferents is involved in these types of response alterations. Indeed, in the conventional way, frequency receptive area (FRA) of a neuron has been defined on the basis of spikes count. However, subthreshold synaptic input also obtains in that recorded neuron at stimulus frequencies outside of its spike-based FRA (Fig. 5b). Such extra-FRA stimulus frequencies, by definition, do not evoke action potentials in the recorded neuron but might cooperate with other subthreshold input from different sources to generate action potentials. This would be possible if the neuron is stimulated by more than one frequency at an adequate synchrony, new input is recruited by learning, or the increased efficacy of the existing subthreshold input. Thus, subthreshold activities are potentially important in modulating the responseiveness of neuron.

# 7. Axonal Distribution of Single PNs in Different Layers

Detailed scheme of output of single cells in layers 2/3 of the cat AI has been demonstrated by intracellular labeling of axons of single PNs as described above. The same methodology can be applied to reveal proximal axons [61] and distal axons [28, 66] morphologies of neurons in other layers. On the basis of laminar distribution of pericellular axon branches, Mitani et al., [61] proposed a basic scheme of the local circuitry, showing that it appeared to be almost identical to that of V1. Their analysis was confined to the pericellular axon branches and did not resolve long distant trajectories of projection axons. At this resolution, neurons located in different layers but showing the same target or those located in the same layer but showing different targets could not be differentiated. Since PNs in layer 6 consists of multiform cells [67] and their projection targets are diverse [68], for example, it would be interesting to see if there are differences in arborization of cortical axon terminals among layer 6 PNs with different projection targets. Similarly, layer 5 is knwon to contain PNs projecting to several different subcortical targets including MGB, IC or striatum. Furthermore, unlike the visual [69, 70] and somatosensory [71, 72] primary cortices, eventually every part of the AI projects contralaterally across the corpus callosum; a major population being located in layer 3 and a minor one in layers 5 and 6 [73, 74, 75]. Here, author has presented a scheme in which the target variability of PNs in infragranular layer is incorporated (Figure 6). Furthermore, it is more informative to include the local axonal projection to the layer in which the cell of origin is located. This information was lacked in the original scheme proposed for the AI. Furthermore, to evaluate the putative targets of labeled single PNs, their main descending axon was simply followed, as far as possible, to the target or a structure that could be used as a milestone to identify the target [modified from 66]. This scheme suggests that there may be relationships between the local collateralization patterns of cortical PNs and the targets to which they project. This seems to be more prominent for infragranular PNs.

As summarized in Figure 7, TC afferents from the lemniscal thalamic nucleus, vMGC, terminate predominantly in layers 4 and 3 [61, 74, 77]. Unlike the V1 and somatosensory cortices, the major recipient zone of TC afferents is not only layer 4 but also lower layer 3. Furthermore, constituent neuronal elements are spiny neurons but are not stellate in shape (so, not spiny stellate neuron typical of V1), rather pyramid in shape in both layers [78, 79]. Evidence for the localization of the major TC recipient population in lower layer 3 and the minor one in layer 4 may suggest only a weak activation of layer 4 prior to the activation of supragranular layer 3 following the TC afferent stimulation. This could be seen in optical imaging when TC afferents in slices cut normal to the A1 surface were stimulated electrically at the border of layer 6 and white mater [51, 80]. Considering the stable extensive activation of supragranular layer, therefore, it is expected that excitatory synaptic input from layer 4 TC-recipient neurons to layer 2/3 PNs would be very powerful, probably substantiated by large amount of excitatory synaptic currents upon stimulation or the minimum divergence in projection pattern of layer 4-derived axon terminals. Indeed, the excitatory effects of layer 4 neurons on layer 2/3 PNs were powerful, as represented by larger synaptic currents at the synapses made by layer 4 neurons than by any other sources [79, 81]. Findings of the transient spot-like activation at layer 4 and the extensive horizontal spread of activation within layers 2/3 following TC afferent stimulation in *in vivo* optical imaging studies suggest that layer 4 neurons are responsible more for the vertical transfer of TC activation within a column, while layer 2/3 neurons more for horizontal transfer of cortical activation between columns in the AI. Recent studies showed differentiated influences of TC synaptic input onto layer 4 and layers 2/3 PNs in slices experiment of the rat AI [82]. It is said that synaptic input onto most layer 4 cells from the MGB is of "driver" type, carrying information critical for determining the receptive field of cortical neurons, including paired-pulse depression, all-or-none responses, and the absence of a metabotropic component. On the other hand, synaptic input onto most CC neurons in layers 2/3 is of 'modulator" type, characterized by its modulation effect on the receptive field properties of recipient neurons, including paired-pulse facilitation, graded responses, and a metabotropic component. Such differentiated influences onto the cortical neurons may suggest a certain type of filtering properties present already at the earliest stage of the synaptic transmission to the AI neurons (and probably also in other sensory cortices).

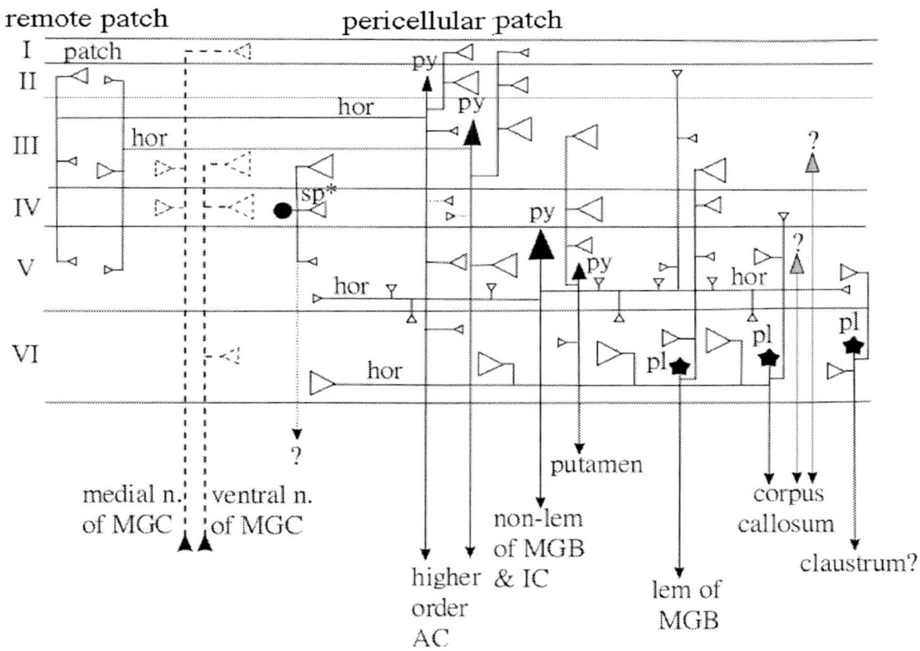


Figure 6. Laminar distribution of axon terminals derived from single pyramidal neurons (py) labeled intracellularly with biocytin (see *a* in Figure 6). Long horizontal projections indicate horizontal axons (hor) and vertical lines means the main descending axons (small arrowhead attached). Cell bodies are filled symbols, and terminals are represented by open triangles. Neurons in layer 6 do not take a pyramidal shape but multiple forms (pl). In the AI, it is known that spiny stellate neurons are very sparse and, instead, many star-like pyramids are present. These PNs in layer 4, as well as those in lower layer 3, are presumed to be the target of thalamocortical afferents. sp* represents the substitute for spiny stellate neuron as a tentative candidate of the TC recipient cell type. It is supposed that there are neuronal types in layers 3, 5 and 6 which project to the corpus callosum, but the last one has been characterized in this scheme. The others are putatively depicted by grey triangles with (?).

# 8. Interlaminar and Intercolumnar Interactions in the AI

Corticocortical patches are usually identified in tangential sections (cut parallel to the cortical surface). In sections cut perpendicular to the cortical surface, these patches are cylindrical in shape and contain labeled neurons/axons throughout the cortical depth except for TC-recipient layer 4. It is thought that neurons in such a columnar architecture are tightly interconnected. This was shown for neurons in mouse AI when interactions of supragranular and infragranular PNs in single columns were examined by focal laser activation of caged excitatory amino acid *in vitro* [81]. When columns arranged along the isofrequency axis were examined, PNs in both layers were in an input-output relationship within a common column. On the contrary, intercolumnar connections from infragranular to supragranular neurons were noted between adjoining columns when examined along the frequency axis. Thus, input to layer 3 PNs (but not in layer 2 PNs) in a column was derived preferentially from layer 6 PNs in different columns adjoining along the frequency axis. Since these columns neighboring along the frequency axis should show different frequency selectivity, it may represent connectional substrates for the preferred direction of frequency sweep (e.g., preference of either upward or downward frequency shifts).

# 9. AI as a Node of Interaction of Bottom-up and Top-down Streams

Recent anatomical findings showed that AC, even A1, was directly connected with lower order cortical areas of other modalities and multimodal subcortical stations [10, 11] (see Figure 1), suggesting that the AC may be essentially a site of multimodal processing or exert a priming effect on multimodal processing in later stages. Indeed, a small population of AI neurons could be driven by stimuli of other modalities or in a much larger population of AI neurons, their responses to acoustic parameters could be modulated when combined with non-auditory stimuli [9, 12, 13]. Anatomical findings in rodents also showed that A1 was directly connected even to association cortices [11] and limbic cortex [83]. Furthermore, according to the scheme proposed for the sequential connectivity throughout cerebral cortex [84], one cortical area theoretically could exert indirect influences onto every cortical area of any sensory modalities. Thus, this would be extended to a possibility that neurons in AC, even those in the AI, could be modulated by activation of higher order cortical fields such as those related to attention, expectation, emotion and exploration. Earlier work, for example, had already noticed that the AC, probably the AI, contained neurons that were driven only if animals attended to the sound source. Although data concerning the connectivity beyond the AC are extremely sparse [rat, 85; monkey, 86], anatomical evidence that projections of the second order or third order AC, namely, belt and parabelt cortex in monkeys, are reciprocally connected directly to higher order brain areas, such as prefrontal cortex and parietal cortex, may substantiate such top-down modulations to AI neurons. It is not impossible that even A1 may also be influenced by the activation of these higher order AC fields through top-down indirect routes.

Gradually increasing are experiments using freely moving animals in which they are engaged in goal-directed behaviors through training [87] or forced to shift their behavior in changing environment [16]. These experiments showed the modulations of receptive field properties or background firing activity probably by expectation, emotional states or attention. In an experiment using the guinea pig, for example, where their behavior was observed to change following the shift of environment illumination from the light to dark (or vice versa), it was found activities of single neurons in the AI-like field (field A) concomitantly changed. This light-to-dark shift of illumination almost always drove the animals to initiate an explorative behavior reflected by stepping forward from the stationary posture kept in the light. In concordance with the environment change, a mode of high background firing of neurons while animals were staying quietly in the light was changed to a mode of decreased firing (or sometimes increased) soon after the room light was turned off [16]. Simply, it appears to be possible that the change in background firing might be caused by the visual cue, somatosensory sensation associated with the initiated motion and/or motor activity itself. However, careful observation would be able to eliminate these possibilities. It is plausible to draw a conclusion that the shift of background firing is not simply linked to the environmental changes or the movement activity itself, but rather to changes in the internal brain state that is likely to be responsible for the explorative behavior. In further support for the unlikelihood of the somatosensory and/or motor cues as possible causes, this behavioral shift of the animal and the accompanying firing changes of neurons did occur even while the animal was actively engaged in eating in the light (i.e., body motion continuing virtually throughout the periods before and after the light off). Soon after the darkness, the animal stopped the continuing behavior of eating and initiated a new explorative behavior, as its attention was apparently shifted to something else (see video in supplemental data of [16]). Thus, irrespective of animal's posture or motion prior to the darkening, the shift in the background firing occurred at the illumination change. Considering that changes in animal's explicit behavior (e.g., from stationary to walking or vice versa) cannot be induced without shifts in the brain state, it is most plausible that the AI may be influenced by performance of cognitive functions. Indeed, if sounds to which such neurons were responsive were applied as acoustic stimuli, these sounds were more effective in the darkness than in the light, since the background firing of the neurons was in the decreased mode in the dark, leading to a higher S/N ratio. Interestingly, these neurons whose background firing was changed according to the animal's behavioral state, therefore, the internal brain state, were localized predominantly in upper layer 5, where descending, i.e., cortico-collicular and cortico-nonlemniscal thalamic PNs were located to serve as the mediator for transferring the cortically processed information to subcortical sensory stations (see [4]). In the similar context, another recent study has shown a different aspect of the cognitive function mediated by layer 5 PNs projecting down to the IC. When layer 5 corticocollicular neurons were pharmacologically eliminated in vivo using chromophore-targeted laser photolysis, the ability of intact animals to relearn the calibration of sound localization in the situation of one-ear clogging was lost without affecting the standard leaning of accurate sound localization [88]. Monitoring of cognitive, therefore behavioral, state seems to be utilized as a piece of information for subcortical neurons to modulate their responses via this corticocortical pathway.

## Conclusion

It is known that AC, including the AI, is activated without real acoustic signals or by viewing auditory scenes without sounds accompanying them, for example the lip reading [89]. The activity of the AC is also modified by other sensory stimuli belonging to the visual or somatosensory modality. It is also sensitive to a slight change in the acoustic parameter of a sound when the sound with the changed parameter (deviant) is sparsely distributed among a sequence of the frequently presented sound (standard). A question of how the AI utilizes such a deviant vs. standard relationship in tone detection for adaptive behaviors remains to be answered. Although such mismatch negativity is believed to be of subcortical or A1 origin, it does change animal's behavior, so via cognitive functions activated by such subtle changes detected in A1. If more experiments designed for cognitive aspects of the AI or higher order AC are to be made in future, it would reveal how much the AI is involved in the relationships between the acoustic detection and the induction of appropriate behavior. The current knowledge based on these recent anatomical and physiological experiments seems to extend the traditional view that the AI may be functioning already as an association cortex rather than an entrace to cortex for coding of spectral and temporal parameters of acoustic signals. Such a view would prompt us to step forward to opening the question of how the traditional auditory association cortex is different from the A1 and how information is modified in its transfer between the A1 and association auditory cortices.

## Acknowledgments

Author is grateful to Yamashita A. for critical reading of manuscript, Kishida T. for assistance in editing manuscript, and Tanifuji M. for discussion on activation of the visual cortex.

## References

[1] Winer, J.A. and Lee, C.C. (2007). The distributed auditory cortex. *Hear Res*. 229:3-13.

[2] Morel, A. and Imig, T.J. (1987). Thalamic projections to fields A, AI, P, and VP in the cat auditory cortex. *J. Comp. Neurol*. 265:119-144.

[3] Ojima, H. (1994). Terminal morphology and distribution of corticothalamic fibers originating from layers 5 and 6 of cat primary auditory cortex. *Cereb. Cortex*. 4:646-663.

[4] Ojima, H. and Rouiller, E.M. (2011) *Auditory cortical projections to the medial geniculate body*. In J.A. Winer, and C.E. Schreiner (Eds), *The Auditory Cortex* (pp.171-188). New York: Springer.

[5] Ojima, H. and Murakami, K. (2011). Triadic synaptic interactions of large corticothalamic terminals in non-lemniscal thalamic nuclei of the cat auditory system. *Hear Res*. 274:40-7.

[6] Malmierca, M.S. and Ryugo, D.K. (2011). *Descending connections of auditory cortex to the midbrain and brain stem.* In J.A. Winer, and C.E. Schreiner (Eds), *The Auditory Cortex* (p.p. 189-208). New York: Springer.

[7] Falchier, A., Clavagnier, S., Barone, P., and Kennedy, H. (2002). Anatomical evidence of multimodal integration in primate striate cortex. *J. Neurosci.* 22:5749-5759.

[8] Rockland, K.S. and Ojima, H. (2003). Multisensory convergence in calcarine visual areas in macaque monkey. *Int. J. Psychophysiol.* 50:19-26.

[9] Bizley, J.K., Nodal, F.R., Bajo, V.M., Nelken, I., and King A.J. (2007). Physiological and anatomical evidence for multisensory interactions in auditory cortex. *Cereb. Cortex.* 17:2172-189.

[10] Smiley, J.F.and Falchier, A. (2009). Multisensory connections of monkey auditory cerebral cortex. *Hear Res.* 258:37-46.

[11] Budinger, E. and Scheich, H. (2009). Anatomical connections suitable for the direct processing of neuronal information of different modalities via the rodent primary auditory cortex. *Hear Res.* 258:16-27.

[12] Brosch, M., Selezneva, E., and Scheich, H. (2005). Nonauditory events of a behavioral procedure activate auditory cortex of highly trained monkeys. *J. Neurosci.* 25:6797-6806.

[13] Lakatos, P., Chen, C.M., O'Connell, M.N., Mills, A., and Schroeder, C.E. (2007). Neuronal oscillations and multisensory interaction in primary auditory cortex. *Neuron.* 53:279-292.

[14] Hubel, D.H., Henson, C.O., Rupert, A., and Galambos, R. (1959). Attention units in the auditory cortex. *Science.* 129:1279-1280.

[15] Jaramillo, S. and Zador, A.M. (2011). The auditory cortex mediates the perceptual effects of acoustic temporal expectation. *Nat. Neurosci.* 14:246-251.

[16] Ojima, H., Taoka, M., and Iriki A. (2010). Adaptive changes in firing of primary auditory cortical neurons following illumination shift from light to dark in freely moving guinea pigs. *Cereb. Cortex.* 20:339-351.

[17] Linden, J.F. and Schreiner, C.E. (2003). Columnar transformations in auditory cortex? A comparison to visual and somatosensory cortices. *Cereb. Cortex.* 13:83-89.

[18] Malhotra, S., Hall, A.J., and Lomber, S.G. (2004). Cortical control of sound localization in the cat: unilateral cooling deactivation of 19 cerebral areas. *J. Neurophysiol.* 92:1625-1643.

[19] Malhotra, S. and Lomber, S.G. (2007). Sound localization during homotopic and heterotopic bilateral cooling deactivation of primary and nonprimary auditory cortical areas in the cat. *J. Neurophysiol.* 97:26-43.

[20] Lomber, S.G., Malhotra, S., and Hall, A.J. (2007). Functional specialization in non-primary auditory cortex of the cat: areal and laminar contributions to sound localization. *Hear Res.* 229:31-45.

[21] Lomber, S.G. and Malhotra, S. (2008). Double dissociation of 'what' and 'where' processing in auditory cortex. *Nat. Neurosci.* 11:609-616.

[22] Read, H.L., Winer, J.A., and Schreiner, C.E. (2002). Functional architecture of auditory cortex. *Curr. Opin. Neurobiol.* 12:433-40.

[23] Brugge, J.F. and Merzenich, M.M. (1973). Responses of neurons in auditory cortex of the macaque monkey to monaural and binaural stimulation. *J. Neurophysiol.* 36:1138-1158.

[24] Imig, T.J. and Adrián, H.O. (1977). Binaural columns in the primary field (A1) of cat auditory cortex. *Brain Res.* 138:241-257.
[25] Middlebrooks, J.C., Dykes, R.W., and Merzenich, M.M. (1980). Binaural response-specific bands in primary auditory cortex (AI) of the cat: topographical organization orthogonal to isofrequency contours. *Brain Res.* 181:31-48.
[26] Clarey, J.C., Barone, P., and Imig, T.J. (1994). Functional organization of sound direction and sound pressure level in primary auditory cortex of the cat. *J. Neurophysiol.* 72:2383-2405.
[27] Wallace, M.N., Kitzes, L.M., and Jones, E.G. (1991). Intrinsic inter- and intralaminar connections and their relationship to the tonotopic map in cat primary auditory cortex. *Exp. Brain Res.* 86:527-544.
[28] Ojima, H., Honda, C.N., and Jones, E.G. (1991). Patterns of axon collateralization of identified supragranular pyramidal neurons in the cat auditory cortex. *Cereb. Cortex.* 1:80-94.
[29] Ojima, H.and Takayanagi, M. (1999). Morphological characteristics of horizontal collaterals, with special reference to auditory cortex (*in Japanese*). *The Cell.* 31:304-308.
[30] Phillips, D.P.and Irvine, D.R. (1979). Methodological considerations in mapping auditory cortex: binaural columns in AI of cat. *Brain Res.* 161:342-346.
[31] Phillips, D.P.and Irvine, D.R. (1983). Some features of binaural input to single neurons in physiologically defined area AI of cat cerebral cortex. *J. Neurophysiol.* 49:383-395.
[32] Reser, D.H., Fishman, Y.I., Arezzo, J.C., and Steinschneider, M. (2000). Binaural interactions in primary auditory cortex of the awake macaque. *Cereb. Cortex.* 10:574-584.
[33] Rockland, K.S.and Lund, J.S. (1982). Widespread periodic intrinsic connections in the tree shrew visual cortex. *Science.* 215:1532-1534.
[34] Livingstone, M.S. and Hubel, D.H. (1984). Specificity of intrinsic connections in primate primary visual cortex. *J. Neurosci.* 4:2830-2835.
[35] Tanigawa, H., Wang, Q., and Fujita, I. (2005). Organization of horizontal axons in the inferior temporal cortex and primary visual cortex of the macaque monkey. *Cereb. Cortex.* 15:1887-99.
[36] Matsubara, J., Cynader, M., Swindale, N.V., and Stryker, M.P. (1985). Intrinsic projections within visual cortex: evidence for orientation-specific local connections. *Proc. Natl. Acad. Sci. USA* 82:935-939.
[37] Luhmann, H.J., Martínez Millán, L., and Singer, W. (1986). Development of horizontal intrinsic connections in cat striate cortex. *Exp. Brain Res.* 63:443-448.
[38] Matsubara, J.A., Nance, D.M., and Cynader, M.S. (1987). Laminar distribution of GABA-immunoreactive neurons and processes in area 18 of the cat. *Brain Res. Bull.* 18:121-126.
[39] Matsubara, J.A. (1988). Local, horizontal connections within area 18 of the cat. *Prog. Brain Res.* 75:163-172.
[40] Boyd, J. and Matsubara, J. (1991). Intrinsic connections in cat visual cortex: a combined anterograde and retrograde tracing study. *Brain Res.* 560:207-215.
[41] Maunsell, J.H. and van Essen, D.C. (1983). The connections of the middle temporal visual area (MT) and their relationship to a cortical hierarchy in the macaque monkey. *J. Neurosci.* 3:2563-2586.

[42] Yoshioka, T., Levitt, JB., and Lund, J.S. (1992). Intrinsic lattice connections of macaque monkey visual cortical area V4. *J. Neurosci.* 12:2785-2802.

[43] Lund, J.S., Yoshioka, T., and Levitt, J.B. (1993). Comparison of intrinsic connectivity in different areas of macaque monkey cerebral cortex. *Cereb. Cortex.* 3:148-162.

[44] Fujita, I.and Fujita, T. (1996). Intrinsic Connections in the macaque inferior temporal cortex. *J. Comp. Neurol.* 368:467-486.

[45] Villeneuve, M.Y., Vanni, M.P., and Casanova, C. (2009). Modular organization in area 21a of the cat revealed by optical imaging: comparison with the primary visual cortex. *Neuroscience.* 164:1320-1333.

[46] Gilbert, C.D. and Wiesel, T.N. (1989). Columnar specificity of intrinsic horizontal and corticocortical connections in cat visual cortex. *J. Neurosci.* 9:2432-42.

[47] Malach, R., Amir, Y., Harel, M., and Grinvald, A. (1993). Relationship between intrinsic connections and functional architecture revealed by optical imaging and in vivo targeted biocytin injections in primate striate cortex. *Proc. Natl. Acad. Sci. USA* 90:10469-10473.

[48] Horikawa, J., Hosokawa, Y., Kubota, M., Nasu, M., and Taniguchi, I. (1996). Optical imaging of spatiotemporal patterns of glutamatergic excitation and GABAergic inhibition in the guinea-pig auditory cortex in vivo. *J. Physiol.* 497:629-638.

[49] Versnel, H., Mossop, J.E., Mrsic-Flogel, T.D., Ahmed, B., and Moore, D.R. (2002). Optical imaging of intrinsic signals in ferret auditory cortex: responses to narrowband sound stimuli. *J. Neurophysiol.* 88:1545-1558.

[50] Ojima, H., Takayanagi, M., Potapov, D., and Homma, R. (2005). Isofrequency band-like zones of activation revealed by optical imaging of intrinsic signals in the cat primary auditory cortex. *Cereb. Cortex.* 15:1497-509.

[51] Song, W.J., Kawaguchi, H., Totoki, S., Inoue, Y., Katura, T., Maeda, S., Inagaki, S., Shirasawa, H., and Nishimura, M. (2006).Cortical intrinsic circuits can support activity propagation through an isofrequency strip of the guinea pig primary auditory cortex. *Cereb. Cortex.* 16:718-29.

[52] Takayanagi, M. and Ojima, H. (2006). Microtopography of the dual corticothalamic projections originating from domains along the frequency axis of the cat primary auditory cortex. *Neuroscience.* 142:769-80.

[53] Grinvald, A., Lieke, E.E., Frostig, R.D., and Hildesheim, R. (1994). Cortical point-spread function and long-range lateral interactions revealed by real-time optical imaging of macaque monkey primary visual cortex. *J. Neurosci.* 14:2545-2568.

[54] Taniguchi, I. and Nasu, M. (1993). Spatio-temporal representation of sound intensity in the guinea pig auditory cortex observed by optical recording. *Neurosci. Lett.* 151:178-181.

[55] Kubota, M., Sugimoto, S., and Horikawa, J. (2008). Dynamic spatiotemporal inhibition in the guinea pig auditory cortex. *Neuroreport.* 19:1691-1694.

[56] Nishimura, M., Shirasawa, H., Kaizo, H., and Song, W.J. (2007). New field with tonotopic organization in guinea pig auditory cortex. *J. Neurophysiol.* 97:927-932.

[57] Schreiner, C.E.and Mendelson, J.R. (1990). Functional topography of cat primary auditory cortex: distribution of integrated excitation. *J. Neurophysiol.* 64:1442-1459.

[58] Read, H.L., Winer, J.A., and Schreiner, C.E. (2001). Modular organization of intrinsic connections associated with spectral tuning in cat auditory cortex. *Proc. Natl. Acad. Sci. USA* 98:8042-8047.

[59] Hosokawa, Y., Horikawa, J., Nasu, M., and Taniguchi, I. (1999) Spatiotemporal representation of binaural difference in time and intensity of sound in the guinea pig auditory cortex. *Hear Res*. 134:123-132.

[60] Hosokawa, Y., Sugimoto, S., Kubota, M., Taniguchi, I., and Horikawa, J. (2004). Optical imaging of binaural interaction in multiple fields of the guinea pig auditory cortex. *Neuroreport*. 15:1093-1097.

[61] Mitani, A., Shimokouchi, M., Itoh, K., Nomura, S., Kudo, M., and Mizuno, N. (1985). Morphology and laminar organization of electrophysiologically identified neurons in the primary auditory cortex in the cat. *J. Comp. Neurol*. 235:430-447.

[62] Das, A.and Gilbert, C.D. (1999). Topography of contextual modulations mediated by short-range interactions in primary visual cortex. *Nature*. 399:655-661.

[63] Gilbert, C.D. and Wiesel, T.N. (1979). Morphology and intracortical projections of functionally characterised neurones in the cat visual cortex. *Nature*. 280:120-125.

[64] Gilbert, C.D. and Wiesel, T.N. (1983). Clustered intrinsic connections in cat visual cortex. *J. Neurosci*. 3:1116-1133.

[65] Ojima, H. and Murakami, K. (2002). Intracellular characterization of suppressive responses in supragranular pyramidal neurons of cat primary auditory cortex in vivo. *Cereb. Cortex*. 12:1079-1091.

[66] Ojima, H., Honda, C.N., and Jones, E.G. (1992). Characteristics of intracellularly injected infragranular pyramidal neurons in cat primary auditory cortex. *Cereb. Cortex*. 2:197-216.

[67] Tömböl, T. (1984). *Layer, VI cells*. In A. Peters, and E.G. Jones. (Eds.), *Cerebral Cortex, vol. 1*. (pp. 479-519). New York: Plenum Press.

[68] Katz, L.C. (1987). Local circuitry of identified projection neurons in cat visual cortex brain slices. *J. Neurosci*. 7:1223-12249.

[69] Shatz, C.J. (1977). Anatomy of interhemispheric connections in the visual system of Boston Siamese and ordinary cats. *J. Comp. Neurol*. 173:497-518.

[70] Harvey, A.R. (1980). A physiological analysis of subcortical and commissural projections of areas 17 and 18 of the cat. *J. Physiol*. 302:507-534.

[71] Jones, E.G., Coulter, J.D., and Wise, S.P. (1979). Commissural columns in the sensory-motor cortex of monkeys. *J. Comp. Neurol*. 188:113-135.

[72] Hayama, T. and Ogawa, H. (1997). Regional differences of callosal connections in the granular zones of the primary somatosensory cortex in rats. *Brain Res. Bull*. 43:341-347.

[73] Imig, T.J. and Brugge, J.F. (1978). Sources and terminations of callosal axons related to binaural and frequency maps in primary auditory cortex of the cat. *J. Comp. Neurol*. 182:637-660.

[74] Code, R.A. and Winer, J.A. (1986). Columnar organization and reciprocity of commissural connections in cat primary auditory cortex (AI). *Hear Res*. 23:205-222.

[75] Lee, C.C. and Winer, J.A. (2008). Connections of cat auditory cortex: II. Commissural system. *J. Comp. Neurol*. 507:1901-1919.

[76] McMullen, N.T. and de Venecia, R.K. (1993). Thalamocortical patches in auditory neocortex. *Brain Res*. 620:317-322.

[77] Huang, C.L. and Winer, J.A. (2000). Auditory thalamocortical projections in the cat: laminar and areal patterns of input. *J. Comp. Neurol*. 427:302-331.

[78] Smith, P.H. and Populin, L.C. (2001). Fundamental differences between the thalamocortical recipient layers of the cat auditory and visual cortices. *J. Comp. Neurol.* 436:508-519.

[79] Barbour, D.L. and Callaway, E.M. (2008). Excitatory local connections of superficial neurons in rat auditory cortex. *J. Neurosci.* 28:11174-11185.

[80] Kubota, M., Sugimoto, S., Horikawa, J., Nasu, M., and Taniguchi, I. (1997). Optical imaging of dynamic horizontal spread of excitation in rat auditory cortex slices. *Neurosci. Lett.* 237:77-80.

[81] Oviedo, H.V., Bureau, I., Svoboda, K., and Zador, A.M. (2010). The functional asymmetry of auditory cortex is reflected in the organization of local cortical circuits. *Nat. Neurosci.* 13:1413-1420.

[82] Viaene, A.N., Petrof, I., and Sherman, S.M. (2011). Synaptic properties of thalamic input to layers 2/3 and 4 of primary somatosensory and auditory cortices. *J. Neurophysiol.* 105:279-292.

[83] Namura, S., Takada, M., Kikuchi, H., and Mizuno, N. (1997). Collateral projections of single neurons in the posterior thalamic region to both the temporal cortex and the amygdala: a fluorescent retrograde double-labeling study in the rat. *J. Comp. Neurol.* 21;384:59-70.

[84] Scannell, J.W., Burns, G.A., Hilgetag, C.C., O'Neil, M.A., and Young, M.P. (1999).The connectional organization of the cortico-thalamic system of the cat. *Cereb. Cortex.* 9:277-299.

[85] Kimura, A., Donishi, T., Okamoto, K., Imbe, H., and Tamai, Y. (2007). Efferent connections of the ventral auditory area in the rat cortex: implications for auditory processing related to emotion. *Eur. J. Neurosci.* 25:2819-2834.

[86] Romanski, L.M., Tian, B., Fritz, J., Mishkin, M., Goldman-Rakic, P.S., and Rauschecker, J.P. (1999). Dual streams of auditory afferents target multiple domains in the primate prefrontal cortex. *Nat. Neurosci.* 2:1131-1136.

[87] Fritz, J., Shamma, S., Elhilali, M., Klein, D. (2003) Rapid task-related plasticity of spectrotemporal receptive fields in primary auditory cortex. *Nat. Neurosci.* 6:1216-1223.

[88] Bajo, V.M., Nodal, F.R., Moore, D.R., and King, A.J. (2010). The descending corticocollicular pathway mediates learning-induced auditory plasticity. *Nat. Neurosci.* 13:253-260.

[89] Calvert, G.A., Bullmore, E.T., Brammer, M.J., Campbell, R., Williams, S.C., McGuire, P.K., Woodruff, P.W., Iversen, S.D., David, A.S. (1997). Activation of auditory cortex during silent lipreading. *Science*. 1997 276:593-596.

[90] Rockel, A.J. and Jones, E.G. (1973a). The neuronal organization of the inferior colliculus of the adult cat. I. The central nucleus. *J. Comp. Neurol.* 147:11-60.

[91] Rockel, A.J. and Jones, E.G. (1973b). The neuronal organization of the inferior colliculus of the adult cat. II. The pericentral nucleus. *J. Comp. Neurol.* 149:301-334.

[92] Budinger, E. and Scheich, H. (2009). Anatomical connections suitable for the direct processing of neuronal information of different modalities via the rodent primary auditory cortex. *Hear Res.* 258:16-27.

[93] Malmierca, M.S. and Hackett, T.A. (2010). *Structural Organization of the Ascending Auditory Pathway.* In A. Rees and A.R. Palmer, (Eds.), *The Oxford Handbook of Auditory Science: The Auditory Brain* (pp. 9-41). New York: Oxford University Press.

[94] Schofield, B.R. (2010). *Structural organization of the descending auditory pathway*. In A. Rees and A.R. Palmer, (Eds.), *The Oxford Handbook of Auditory Science: The Auditory Brain* (pp. 43-64). New York, Oxford University Press.

[95] Ehret, G. and Romand, R. (2010). *The Central Auditory System*. New York, Oxford University Press

[96] Jones, E.G. (2007). *The Thalamus. Vol. 2*. ($2^{nd}$ edition). New York, Cambridge University Press.

In: Auditory Cortex: Anatomy, Functions and Disorders ISBN 978-1-62100-685-5
Editor: Mounya Elhilali 

Chapter III

# Infraslow Potentials of Primary Auditory Cortex: New Insights into Neocortical Mechanisms of Auditory Information Neuronal Processing in the Brain

***Igor V. Filippov,[1,*] Rudolf M. Khudoerkov,[2] Artem A. Krebs[1] and Konstantin S. Pugachev[1]***
[1]Department of Physiology and Biophysics,
Yaroslavl State Medical Academy (YSMA), Yaroslavl, Russia
[2]Head of Laboratory of Functional Morphochemistry, Brain Research Division,
Scientific Center for Neurology of Russian Academy of Sciences, Moscow, Russia

## Abstract

Several available reports demonstrate the presence of infraslow activity (< 0.5 Hz) in structures of the auditory system of the brain. It was demonstrated specific alteration of this activity in the domain of seconds (0.1 – 0.5 Hz) in the medial geniculate nucleus (MGN) in response to acoustic stimuli. The present work was performed to test three hypotheses: (1) that potentials in the domain of seconds in primary auditory cortex (A1) are related to specific mechanisms of acoustic information neural processing; (2) that potentials in the domain of seconds (0.1-0.5 Hz) reflect specific and direct interactions of the MGN and A1 during neural processing of sensory information; and (3) that low-frequency multisecond infraslow potentials in the A1 (0.0167-0.1 Hz) are related to the influences originating from the locus coeruleus (LC), dorsal raphe nucleus (DRN), and

* Main author's corresponding address and affiliation: I.V. Filippov (M.D., Ph.D. Associated Professor): Department of Physiology and Biophysics, Yaroslavl State Medical Academy (YSMA), Yaroslavl, Revolutsionnaya Street 5, Russia, 150000. Phone: +7(4852)305763; Fax: +7(4852)327915; E-mail: filippov@yma.ac.ru.

basal magnocellular nucleus (BMN). The experimental subjects were 25 adult rats with chronic stereotaxic electrodes implanted in the MGN, A1, LC, DRN and BMN. The animals were anesthetized and infraslow activity was recorded under several experimental conditions: (1) in the A1 under condition of silence and during rhythmical acoustic stimulation, (2) in the A1 before and after electrical stimulation of MGN, (3) in the A1 before and after sequential electrical stimulation of LC, DRN, and BMN. Different acoustic stimuli induced stimulus-related changes of activity in the range of seconds (0.1-0.3 Hz) in the A1; the effects of MGN stimulation were limited to overall increases in spectral powers in the frequency domain of 0.1-0.5 Hz. Specifically, power increased in the frequencies of 0.1-0.25, 0.35-0.4, and 0.45-0.5 Hz in the A1 after MGN stimulation. The electrical stimulation of LC, DRN, BMN affected only multisecond activity (0.0167-0.04 Hz) in the A1 in the similar way (alterations of powers of multisecond potentials), but there were no changes in the activity with the frequencies of 0.1-0.5 Hz in this structure. Obtained results support tentative conclusions that infraslow activity in the range of 0.1-0.5 Hz is implicated in specific mechanisms of acoustic information neural processing via interactions within the MGN-A1 thalamic–cortical system, whereas multisecond potentials (0.0167-0.04 Hz) in A1 are mainly attributed to the influences of brainstem nuclei (like LC and DRN) or basal forebrain structures (like BMN) on general neuronal excitability of primary auditory cortical area.

## 1. Introduction

In accordance with current data there are several frequency or spectral domains in spontaneous brain bioelectrical activity, these are: ultra-fast and fast bioelectrical brain potentials (with the frequencies from 40 Hz up to several hundreds of Hz), classical EEG oscillations (0.5-40 Hz), and slow or infraslow brain potentials with frequencies of below of 0.5 Hz [1-3, 27, 38, 45, 47, 60]. Although ultra-fast and EEG potentials of the brain have been studied in a numerous works, slow and infraslow brain oscillations remain poorly documented and their functional significance is obscure yet [7]. However, available experimental evidence demonstrates universal properties and importance of infraslow brain potentials in the functions of the brain [18-25]. Additionally, it was shown that infraslow brain potentials consist of several types (domains): potentials in the domain of seconds (frequencies of 0.1-0.5 Hz, periods of singular waveform from 10 to 2 seconds); multisecond activity (frequencies of 0.0167-0.1 Hz, periods from 60 to 10 seconds); potentials in the domain of minutes (frequencies of below of 0.0167 Hz, periods from 1 minute and more); and relatively stable potential of millivolt scale [2, 3, 18-25, 32,33]. Moreover, it was documented previously that different domains of infraslow brain potentials recorded from the same area of the brain carry different neurophysiological information and are associated with different types of neuronal information processing in the pertinent CNS structures [2, 3, 18-25, 32,33].

In the previous studies of our laboratory on visual thalamic-cortical sensory system of the brain (lateral geniculate nucleus – primary visual cortex), we found specific changes of infraslow brain potentials in these sites in response to different visual stimuli [18-21]. These changes were manifested as statistically significant stimulus-specific spectral pattern alterations of infraslow oscillations in the domain of seconds (0.1-0.25 Hz) in response to darkness, continuous illumination and rhythmic photostimulation in lateral geniculate nucleus and primary visual cortex. Additionally we found statistically significant changes of multisecond activity (0.02-0.05 Hz) in both the lateral geniculate nucleus and primary visual cortex but only in response to rhythmic photostimulation (there were no changes of this activity in darkness vs. constant illumination conditions). It was demonstrated that activity in the domain of seconds and multisecond oscillations in lateral geniculate nucleus – primary visual cortex system are involved in the mechanisms of bidirectional (thalamic-cortical and cortical-thalamic) interactions of thalamic and cortical sites of the visual system of the brain [18-21]. Later we studied infraslow activity of main thalamic auditory center – medial geniculate nucleus – under condition of silence and during rhythmical acoustic stimulation, and it was detected that presentation of different acoustic stimuli induced stimulus-dependent changes of activity in the domain of seconds (0.1-0.3 Hz).

As a result of these experiments, we proposed that in the primary auditory cortex (A1) there are existing infraslow potentials and that this activity is probably involved in some mechanisms of acoustic information processing [18-25]. Several available literature reports (although very limited) favor this idea. In example, in non-lemniscal division of the medial geniculate nucleus there were found slow neuronal oscillations with the frequencies of 0.03-0.25 Hz, and their dynamics were sensitive to acoustic and electrical stimulation of A1 [28]. It was also shown the cyclical top-down neuronal fluctuations in the domain of dozens of seconds in the medial geniculate nucleus and A1 during the processing of the acoustic stimuli [53]. It was found that some central sites of auditory system of the brain are periodically changing the type of neuronal activity from burst to tonic type and vice versa, with the time periods from several seconds to the dozens of seconds [64]. Finally, the studies of auditory evoked potentials associated with acoustic stimulus exposure revealed slow potentials shifts in time scale of seconds after presentation of auditory stimuli [63].

Based on aforementioned findings of our laboratory, their interpretation, available literature data, and pertinent hypothesis, we decided to perform those studies that are described in this chapter. Specifically, our aim was to test three hypotheses: (1) that potentials in the domain of seconds in primary auditory cortex (A1) are related to specific mechanisms of acoustic information neural processing; (2) that potentials in the domain of seconds (0.1-0.5 Hz) reflect specific and direct interactions of the MGN and A1 during neural processing of sensory information; and (3) that low-frequency multisecond infraslow potentials in the A1 (0.0167-0.1 Hz) are related to influences originating from the locus coeruleus (LC), dorsal raphe nucleus (DRN), and basal magnocellular nucleus (BMN).

## 2. General Methodological Notes (Materials and Methods)

In this part only general methodological design will be described; it was identical for all experiments. Other important experimental modifications will be mentioned particularly in the beginning of each subsection of the part 'Results' of this chapter under the rubric 'Methodological Aspects'; as well as technical details of our experiments were described in our previous publications [18-25].

The subjects were adult male albino rats. All procedures were conducted in strict accordance with humane principles of laboratory animal care [14].

## 2.1. Animal Preparations and Surgery

The first step was to prepare animals for chronic intracerebral recordings. Under general anesthesia (sodium pentobarbital, 40 mg/kg i.p.), and in accordance with rat brain stereotaxic atlas [58], long-term gold electrodes were implanted in the pertinent sites of the brain. Our previous studies and literature review [18-25] indicated that both bipolar and monopolar electrode commutations are appropriate for recordings of infraslow brain potentials (ISBP). We used monopolar scheme of electrode commutation. Recordings were obtained with high impedance (200 MΩ) differential multi-channel low-noise (internal noise in 0-0.5 Hz band-pass, less than 3 μV), low bias current (less than $10^{-12}$A), universal AC/DC-amplifier with precisely graduated DC-offset compensation (model UU-93, IEM, St.-Petersburg, Russia). It is necessary to specially note herein that metal (and gold) electrodes are adequate for ISBP recordings when they are connected to high input impedance amplifier [18-25, 31-33, 59]. Gold electrodes are non-toxic [56]; whereas non-polarized electrodes (like silver/silver chloride) are impossible to use as chronic brain implants due to their extremely toxic impact on the tissues [8, 26, 34, 65]. We took several counter-measures aimed to diminish the chance of possible artifacts in ISBP recordings, among these measures were: (1) All electrodes were absolutely identical by material, construction, and size. (2) Careful individual selection of electrode pairs was used for implantation: all electrodes were tested in physiological saline, and only those pairs were used as implants that had the stable standing inter-electrode potential without any spontaneous transient shifts, fluctuations, noise, etc. (3) Infraslow potentials were recorded in animals after lethal injection of sodium pentobarbital. It was found that dramatically altered ISBP existed in the recordings of comatose paralyzed animals. But this activity disappeared irreversibly in all recordings (isoelectric line) after confirmed cerebral death. These facts allow the conclusion that observed infraslow activity is from the brain and is not due to artifacts.

## 2.2. Electrophysiological Recording Technique

The second step was to perform experimental tests in chronic experiments. Experimental sessions and extracellular recordings were started not earlier than 14 days after implantation procedure. This time period was necessary to avoid temporary post-traumatic post-operational responses of the brain after the injury that was associated with electrode implantation procedure [18-25, 39]. The rat was placed in double-shielded Faraday's chamber and isolated in the special separate sound-proof cage with non-transparent walls.

After the end of experimental series, the rats were killed using an injection of sodium pentobarbital (100 mg/kg i.p.). Electrode positions were determined, post mortem, using Nissl's staining method for serial brain slices and light microscopy according to commonly accepted technique [62].

During recordings summary bioelectrical signal was artificially separated into 3 frequency domains using corresponding high- and low-pass amplifier filter settings: 0.1-0.5 Hz (activity in the range of seconds), 0.0167-0.1Hz (multisecond activity), and 0.001-0.0167 Hz (fluctuation in the range of minutes). It should be reiterated here that this artificial frequency separation was done guiding by three facts. The first one concerns the phenomenon that different ISBP domains contain different kind of neurophysiological information [18-25]. The second one [18-25] is about relative independence and simultaneous presence of aforementioned activities in the recordings (when one type of fluctuations is superimposed on the others). The third one [18-25] is explaining by significant amplitude difference between most slow ISBP (i.e. fluctuations in the domain of minutes) and faster ISBP activities (e.g. in the domain of seconds). Therefore, the attempt to plot general fast Fourier transformation (FFT) curve with the same proportional frequency resolution (identical number of point per octave) for the whole spectrum usually leads to the graph where significant differences in faster but low-amplitude activities will be masked by constant but high-amplitude activities of the slowest ISBP domains. In order to avoid these pitfalls we plotted different FFT graphs (although with different frequency resolution) for the different known domains of ISBP [18-25].

Amplified signals were continuously digitized on-line (at a sampling frequency of 1 Hz) by analog-to-digital converter (model KPCI-3101, Keithley Instruments, Inc., Cleveland, Ohio, USA) and stored on computer disk for pre-processing and further off-line analysis.

There were selected the following data sets (epochs) for subsequent analyses: (a) ISBP in the domain of seconds, 256 data points=256 seconds, (b) multisecond ISBP band, 512 data points=512 seconds, and (c) ISBP in the domain of minutes, 1024 data points=1024 seconds, respectively. Each segment was subjected to the ordinary FFT and power spectral analysis [62], and after that we compared pre-stimulus spectra with stimulus-on spectra or pre-stimulus spectra were compared with post-stimulus spectra.

### 2.3. Statistical Procedures

The statistical procedures of this study included averaging of the results of the sessions per animal. After that mean values per animal were obtained, and the statistical procedures were performed over the animals. Obtained differences were analyzed by one-way, repeated-measures ANOVA. An alpha level of $P<0.05$ was adopted for all significance tests. When statistical significance was indicated, post-hoc analysis was performed using multiple-range Duncan's test.

## 3. Results

In general, the primary auditory cortex exhibited different types of ongoing infraslow potentials in anesthetized animals under all experimental conditions that were used: e.g., under condition of silence and during rhythmic acoustic stimulation (Figure 1), before and after electrical stimulation of the MGN (Figure 3), LC, DRN and BMN (Figure 5, 7, 9). Specifically, there were infraslow potentials in the domain of seconds (frequencies of 0.1–0.3 Hz), multisecond potentials (approximately 0.02–0.035 Hz), and irregular fluctuations in the domain of minutes (< 0.0035 Hz). It is necessary to note here that such infraslow brain potentials were complexly organized in terms of their permanent ongoing dynamics, when oscillations in the domain of seconds were superimposed on multisecond waves and these multisecond phenomena were superimposed on the slowest occasional fluctuations in the range of minutes and dozens of minutes. These infraslow waves were observed on constant background level of millivolt scale potential. As a result, the A1 expressed different by their frequencies and time scales infraslow brain potentials, although with different periods and amplitudes.

## 3.1. Infraslow Brain Potentials in the Primary Auditory Cortex during Silence and Acoustic Stimulation

*Methodological Aspects:* This part of the work was performed on 15 anaesthetized rats (n=45 experimental repetitions). Chronic recordings from A1 region were used for analyses. The rats were randomly exposed to silence and to acoustic stimulation with the following parameters: ‘clicks’ with sound intensity level of 80 dB (by standard pressure level scale); sound tone frequency, 2000 Hz; single ‘click’ duration time, 60 msec; stimulus presentation frequency, 8 Hz.

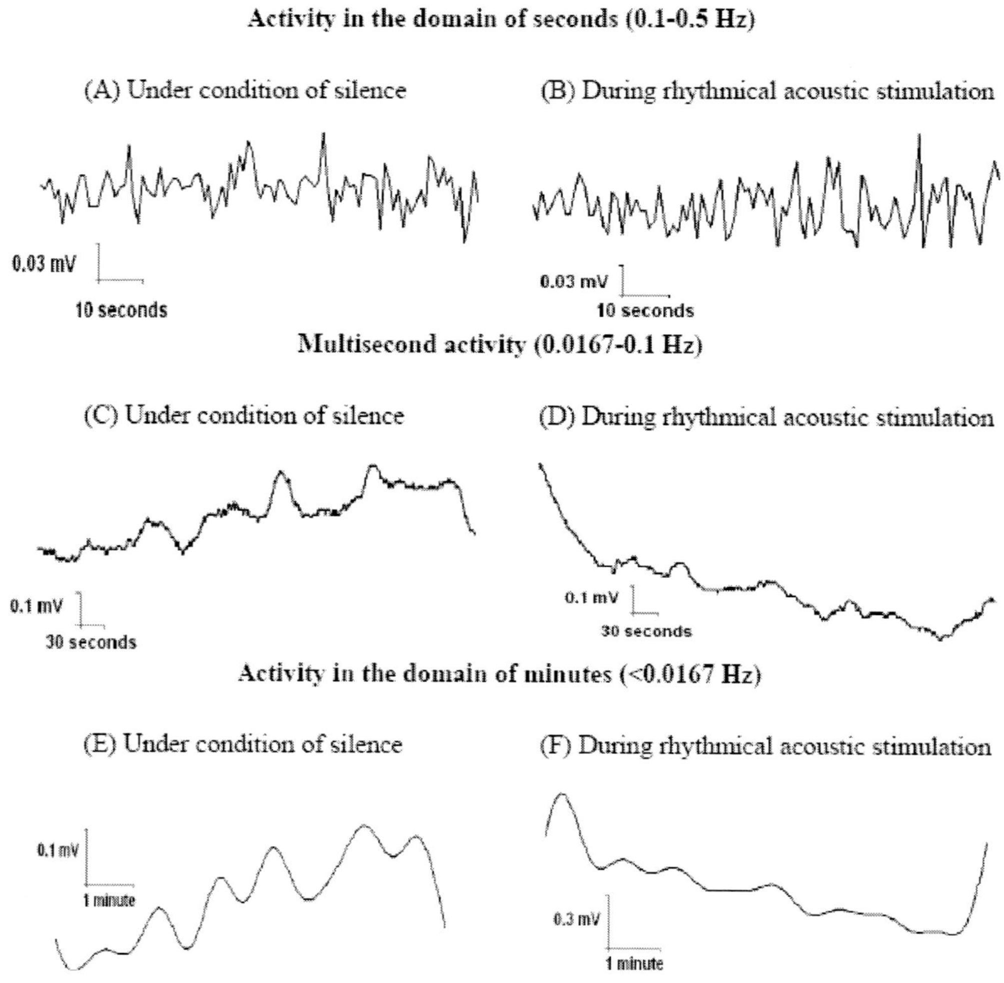


Figure 1. Representative examples of different frequency domains of typical infraslow brain potentials in the primary auditory cortex of the rat under different conditions of acoustic environment.

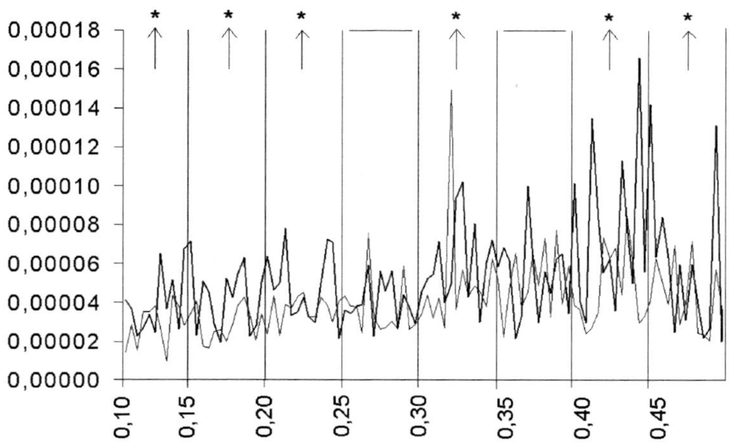


(A) Activity in the domain of seconds (0.1-0.5 Hz)

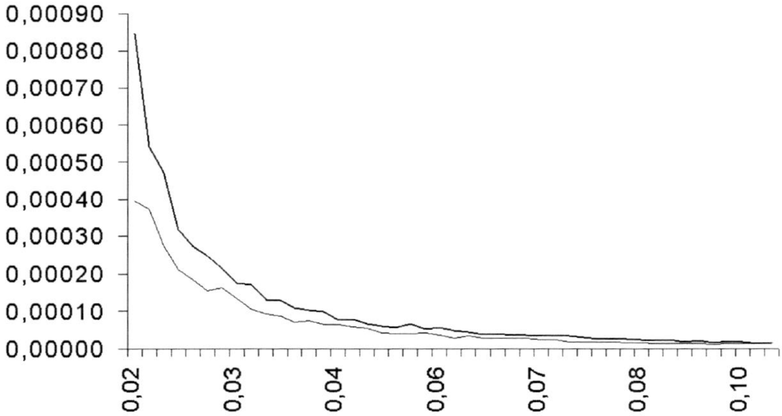


(B) Multisecond activity (0.0167-0.1 Hz)

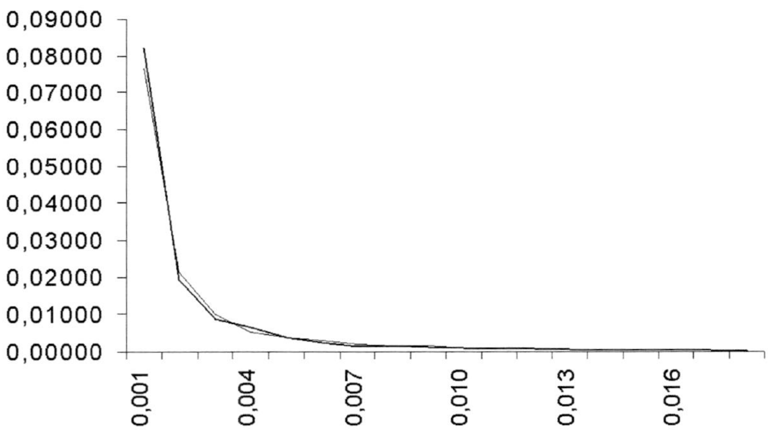


(C) Activity in the domain of minutes (<0.0167 Hz)

Figure 2. Graphical results of power spectral analysis. Mean (algebraically summarized overall 45 repeated experiments) power spectra patterns of different frequency domains of infraslow brain potentials in the primary auditory cortex of rats under different conditions of acoustic environment: thin line – under condition of silence, thick line – under rhythmic acoustic stimulation.

Silence and phonostimulation were maintained without changes for 1024 seconds. A1 ISBP power spectra within the same frequency domain were compared with each other under different acoustic conditions (i.e., silence vs. rhythmic acoustic stimulation). In these experiments the rats were exposed only to acoustic stimuli and were maximally isolated from other types of accident sensory stimulation by means of special methodological approach [25].

*Results:* Spectral power analysis of ISBP in A1 indicated that rhythmical acoustic stimulation induced statistically significant ($p < 0.00001$) shifts of infraslow activity in the domain of seconds in A1 (Figure 1). Specifically, power in the range of seconds tended to increase (Figure 2 A), though several frequencies in the range of seconds diminished or remained the same. Frequencies in the domain of seconds were subdivided into 8 equal sub-domains, creating frequency windows of: 0.1 - 0.15 Hz, 0.15 - 0.2 Hz, 0.2 - 0.25 Hz, 0.25 - 0.3 Hz, 0.3 - 0.35 Hz, 0.35 - 0.4 Hz, 0.4 - 0.45 Hz, and 0.45 - 0.5 Hz. This was done in order to obtain more precise information about the direction of power change in these windows (Figure 2 A) and also to determine whether the changes were statistically significant. Powers as sums of squares were calculated for each window during silence and during rhythmical acoustic stimulation. This approach permitted the detection of significant increases of powers in the sub-domains of 0.1 - 0.35 Hz and 0.4 - 0.45 Hz in A1 (Figure 2 A).

There were no significant changes in responses to acoustic stimuli in the domains of multisecond fluctuations (Figure 2 B) and activity in the range of minutes in A1 (Figure 2 C), and these spectra (Figure 2 B and C) were not subjected to the more detailed statistical analyses. Additionally there were no significant changes in response to acoustic stimuli in relatively stable potential of millivolt scale of A1.

On all graphs on X-line are frequencies (Hz), whereas on Y-line are absolute power densities (mV per Hz). Vertical lines mark borders of sub-domains, arrow up – increase of powers, horizontal line – no significant changes, asterisk indicate that the changes are statistically significant ($p<0.05$).

## 3.2. Infraslow Brain Potentials in the Primary Auditory Cortex before and after Electrical Stimulation of the Medial Geniculate Nucleus

*Methodological Aspects:* This part of the work was performed on 15 anesthetized rats (n=45 experimental repetitions). Chronic monopolar recordings from A1 region were used for analysis. Recordings from A1 were randomly obtained before electrical stimulation of the MGN and after electrical stimulation of this thalamic nucleus (not during stimulation!). Before, during, and after intracerebral stimulation the animal was under constant condition of darkness (illumination intensity, 0 lx) and silence. Electrical stimulation parameters were as following: rectangular bipolar pulses, amplitude 80 μA; frequency, 100 Hz; impulse duration 0.4 ms; electrical stimulation duration, 10 seconds). Pre-stimulation ISBP recordings from the A1 were compared with post-stimulus ISBP recordings from this CNS site. Each recording length (both pre- and post-stimulus) was 1024 seconds. In these experiments the rats were exposed only to electrical stimulation and were maximally isolated from any types of accident sensory stimulation by means of special methodological approach [25].

*Results:* There were prominent differences in infraslow potentials between pre-stimulus and post-stimulus recordings obtained from A1 (Figure 3). There were easily discernable increases in spectral power in the domain of seconds in A1 after stimulation of MGN. These changes can be seen in Figure 4 (A). Specifically, there was an increase in powers in the dominant frequencies of 0.1–0.25 Hz in A1 after MGN stimulation (Figure 4 A). These spectral changes were statistically significant. Nevertheless, some particular frequencies in the range of seconds decreased or remain unchanged after the stimulation of MGN (Fig 4 A). For more accurate description, previously mentioned frequency bandwidth of 0.1–0.5 Hz was subdivided into 8 equal frequency sub-domains (frequency windows of 0.1–0.15 Hz, 0.15–0.2 Hz, 0.2–0.25 Hz, 0.25–0.3 Hz, 0.3–0.35 Hz, 0.35–0.4 Hz, 0.4–0.45 Hz, and 0.45–0.5 Hz), see Figure 4 (A). Mean powers (as sums of power squares of proportionally normalized averaged spectra) were calculated for each of these sub-domains for pre-stimulation and post-stimulation spectra. We also evaluated the direction of change. The analysis performed with sub-domains recorded from A1 after stimulation of MGN revealed significant increases in five out of eight sub-domains; specifically, 0.1 – 1.25 Hz, 0.35 – 0.4 Hz, and 0.45 – 0.5 Hz. Apparent increases in the remaining three sub-domains were not significant (Figure 4 A).

There were no statistically significant shifts in the frequency range of 0.001-0.1 Hz (multisecond activity and fluctuations in the range of minutes) in the A1, see Figure 4 B and C. Therefore, these spectra were not subjected to further detailed analysis mentioned above. Additionally there were no significant changes in the responses of A1 to MGN contact electrical stimulation in the range of relatively stable potential of millivolt scale.

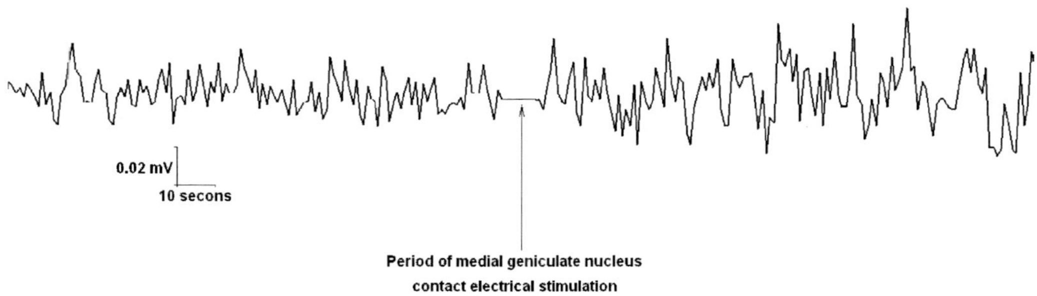


(A) Activity in the domain of seconds (0.1-0.5 Hz)

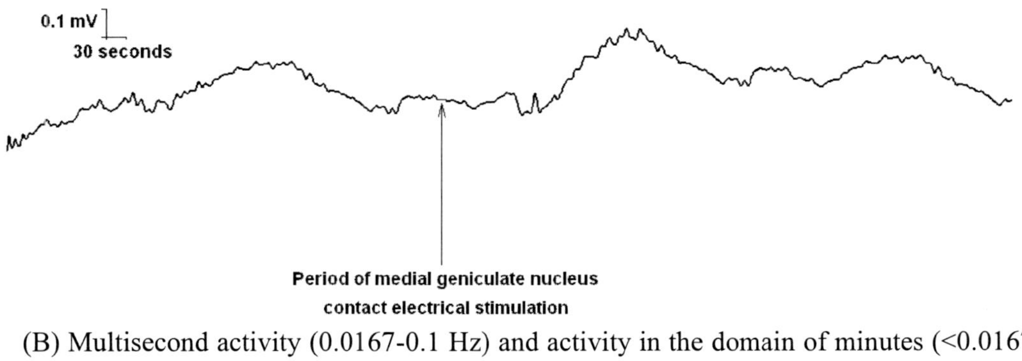


(B) Multisecond activity (0.0167-0.1 Hz) and activity in the domain of minutes (<0.0167 Hz)

Figure 3. Representative examples of different frequency domains of typical infraslow brain potentials in the primary auditory cortex of the rat before and after contact electrical stimulation of the medial geniculate nucleus.

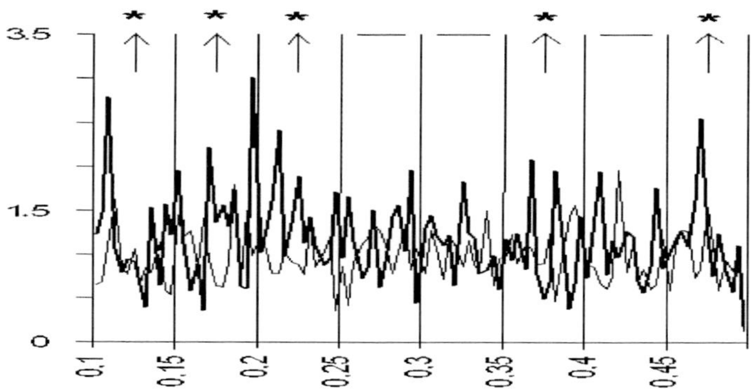


(A) Activity in the domain of seconds (0.1-0.5 Hz)

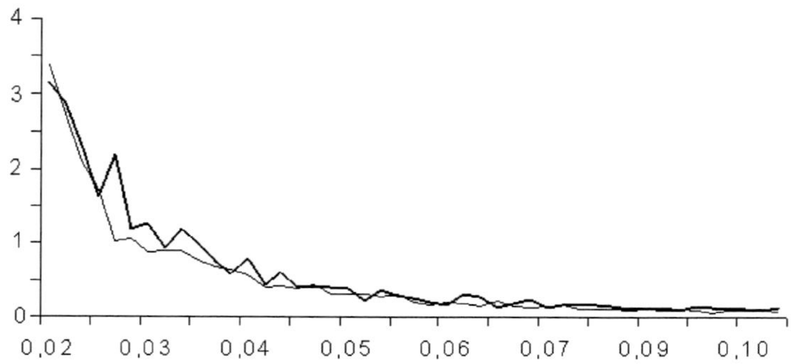


(B) Multisecond activity (0.0167-0.1 Hz)

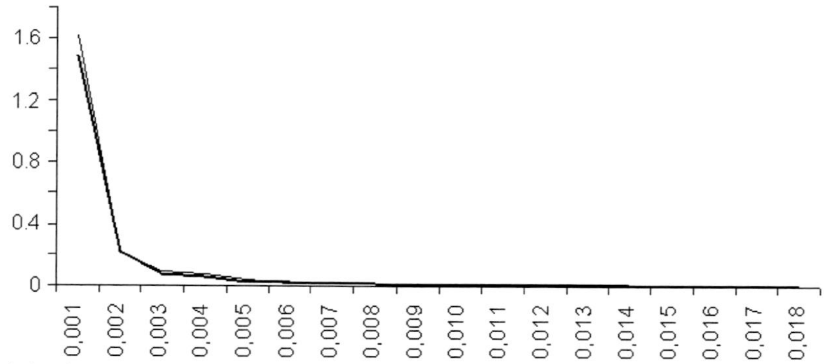


(C) Activity in the domain of minutes (<0.0167 Hz)

Figure 4. Graphical results of power spectral analysis. Mean (algebraically summarized overall 45 repeated experiments) power spectra patterns of different frequency domains of infraslow brain potentials in the primary auditory cortex of rats before (thin line) and after (thick line) contact electrical stimulation of medial geniculate nucleus.

On all graphs on X-line are frequencies (Hz), whereas on Y-line are absolute power densities (mV per Hz). Vertical lines mark borders of sub-domains, arrow up – increase of powers, horizontal line – no significant changes, asterisk indicate that the changes are statistically significant ($p<0.05$).

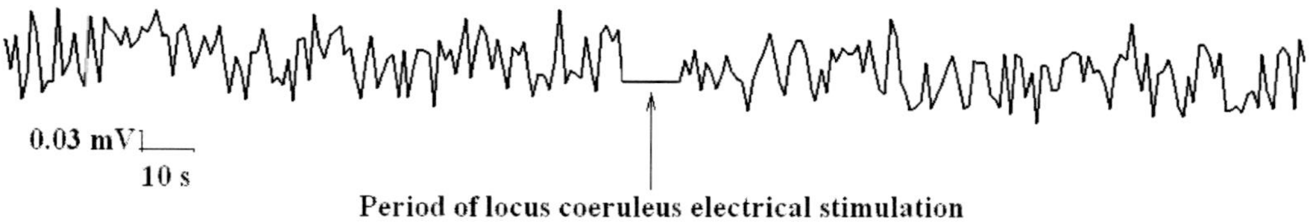


(A) Activity in the domain of seconds (0.1-0.5 Hz)

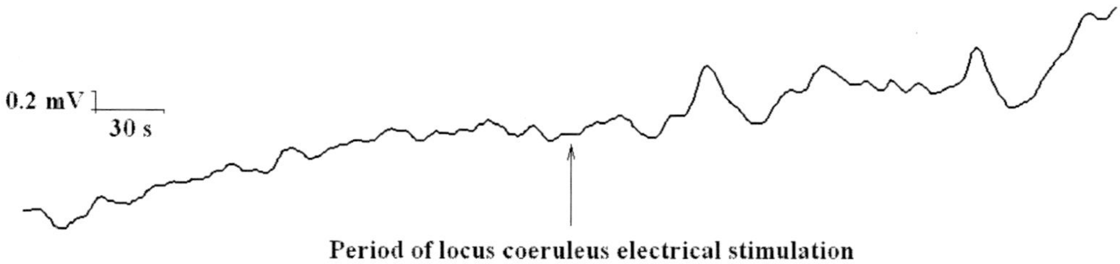


(B) Multisecond activity (0.0167-0.1 Hz) and activity in the domain of minutes (<0.0167 Hz)

Figure 5. Representative examples of different frequency domains of typical infraslow brain potentials in the primary auditory cortex of the rat before and after locus coeruleus contact electrical stimulation.

### 3.3. Infraslow Brain Potentials in the Primary Auditory Cortex before and after Electrical Stimulation of the Locus Coeruleus, Dorsal Raphe Nucleus, and Basal Magnocellular Nucleus

*Methodological Aspects:* This part of the work was performed on anesthetized rats: 15 rats were used for studies of LC influences on A1 infraslow activity (n=45 experimental repetitions); 15 rats were used for studies of DRN influences on A1 infraslow activity (n=45 experimental repetitions); and 15 rats were used for studies of BMN influences on A1 infraslow activity (n=45 experimental repetitions). Chronic monopolar recordings from A1 region were used. Recordings from the A1 were randomly obtained before electrical stimulation of the LC and after electrical stimulation of this brainstem site (not during stimulation!). Recordings from the A1 were randomly obtained before electrical stimulation of DRN and after electrical stimulation of this nucleus (not during stimulation!). Recordings from the A1 were randomly obtained before electrical stimulation of BMN and after electrical stimulation of this basal forebrain nucleus (not during stimulation!). Before, during and after intracerebral stimulations the animal was under constant condition of darkness (illumination intensity, 0 lx) and silence. Electrical stimulation parameters were as following: rectangular bipolar pulses, amplitude 80 μA; frequency, 100 Hz; impulse duration 0.4 ms; electrical stimulation duration, 10 seconds). Pre-stimulation ISBP recordings from the A1 were compared with post-stimulus ISBP recordings of this area (before and after LC activation, before and after DRN stimulation, before and after BMN stimulation, respectively). Each recording length (pre- and post-stimulus) was 1024 seconds. In these experiments the rats were exposed only to electrical stimulation and were maximally isolated from any types of accident sensory stimulation by means of special methodological approach [18, 20, 25].

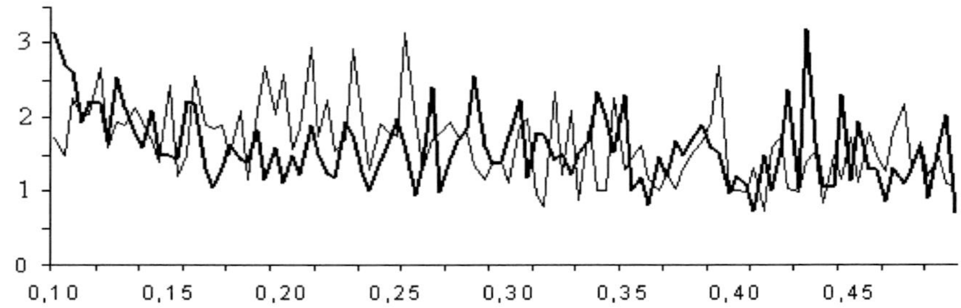


(A) Activity in the domain of seconds (0.1-0.5 Hz)

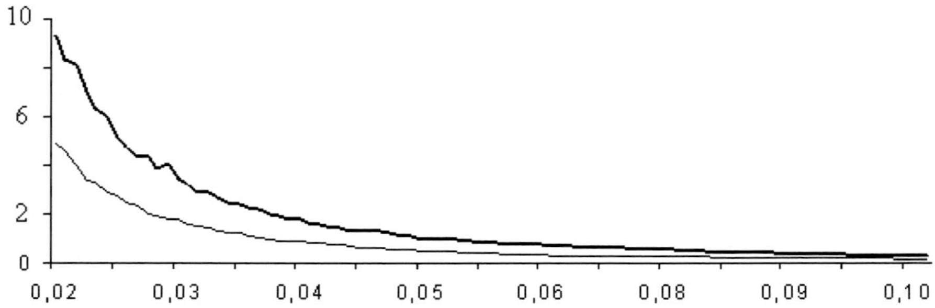


(B) Multisecond activity (0.0167-0.1 Hz)

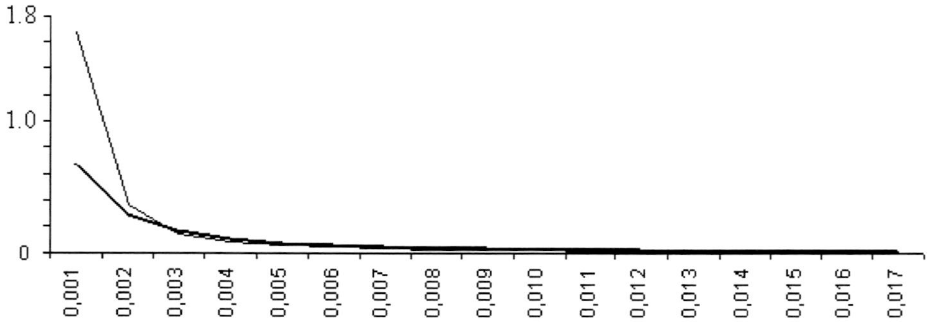


(C) Activity in the domain of minutes (<0.0167 Hz)

Figure 6. Graphical results of power spectral analysis. Mean (algebraically summarized overall 45 repeated experiments) power spectra patterns of different frequency domains of infraslow brain potentials in the primary auditory cortex of rats before (thin line) and after (thick line) contact electrical stimulation of locus coeruleus.

*Results:* We found no statistically significant differences in A1 infraslow potentials in the range of seconds between pre-stimulus and post-stimulus recordings obtained both before and after LC and/or DRN and/or BMN stimulation, respectively (Figure 6 A, 8 A, and 9 A). In addition, there were no statistically significant shifts in the frequency range of 0.001-0.0167 Hz in the A1 before and after LC stimulation, before and after DRN electrical activation, before and after BMN electric activation, see (Figure 6 C, 8 C, and 9 C). These results were confirmed by sufficient statistical tests. Therefore, these A1 spectra in the domain of seconds and in the range of minutes were not subjected to further detailed analyses. In addition, there were no significant changes of A1 relatively stable potential of millivolt scale in response to LC, DRN, and BMN contact electrical stimulation.

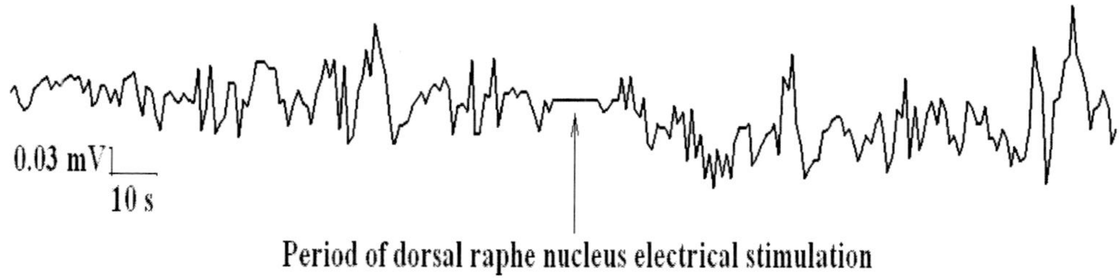


(A) Activity in the domain of seconds (0.1-0.5 Hz)

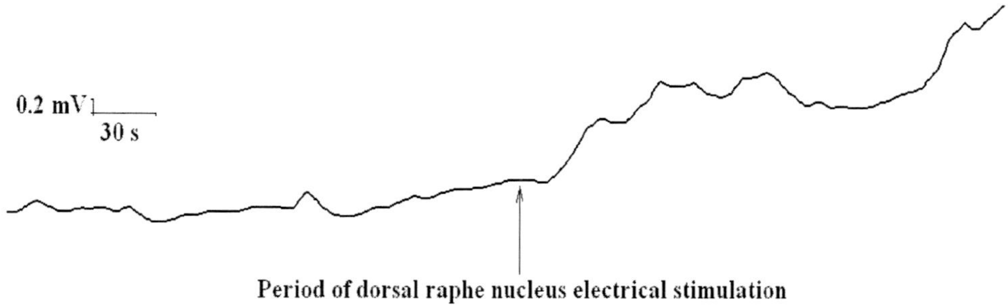


(B) Multisecond activity (0.0167-0.1 Hz) and activity in the domain of minutes (<0.0167 Hz)

Figure 7. Representative examples of different frequency domains of typical infraslow brain potentials in the primary auditory cortex of the rat before and after dorsal raphe nucleus contact electrical stimulation.

However, there were differences in multisecond recordings that were manifested as the prominent significant increases in spectral power in the multisecond activity in A1 after stimulation of LC and DRN (Figure 6 B and 8 B). Moreover, these increases were identical by their directions. We detected prominent increases in powers of multisecond activity observed in the A1 both after LC and DRN electrical stimulation (compared to pre-stimulus conditions, respectively). These spectral changes were statistically significant. The directions of these changes are clearly visible on the spectral graphs, because there were no frequency sub-domains in the A1 that were decreased or remained unchanged after these manipulations (Figure 6 B and 8 B).

On all graphs on X-line are frequencies (Hz), whereas on Y-line are amplitudes (power spectral densities), these amplitudes are proportionally normalized by percentage method.

Although electrical stimulation of BMN also affected the multisecond activity in A1, these changes were opposite to those that we observed in primary auditory cortex after LC and DRN electrical activations (Figure 9 B and 10 B). These alterations were manifested as statistically significant decrease of powers of multisecond potentials after electrical activation of BMN (Figure 9 B and 10 B).

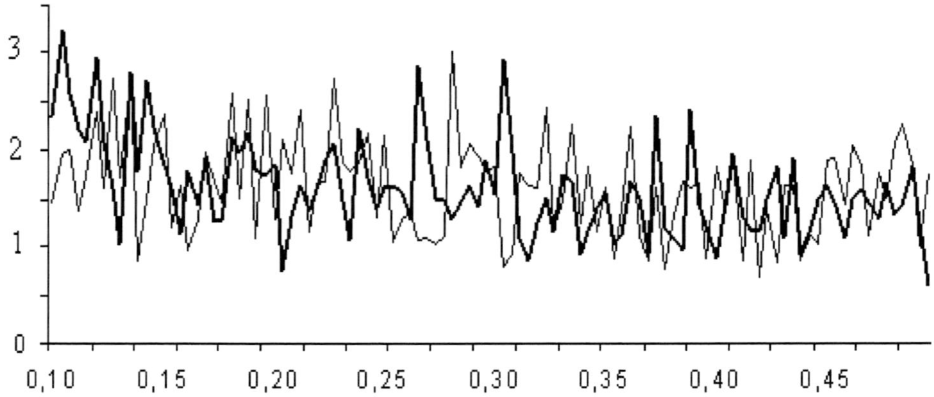


(A) Activity in the domain of seconds (0.1-0.5 Hz)

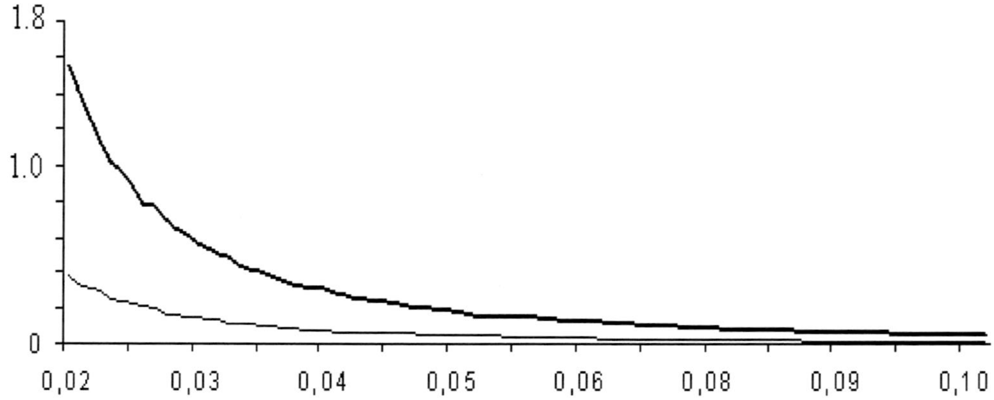


(B) Multisecond activity (0.0167-0.1 Hz)

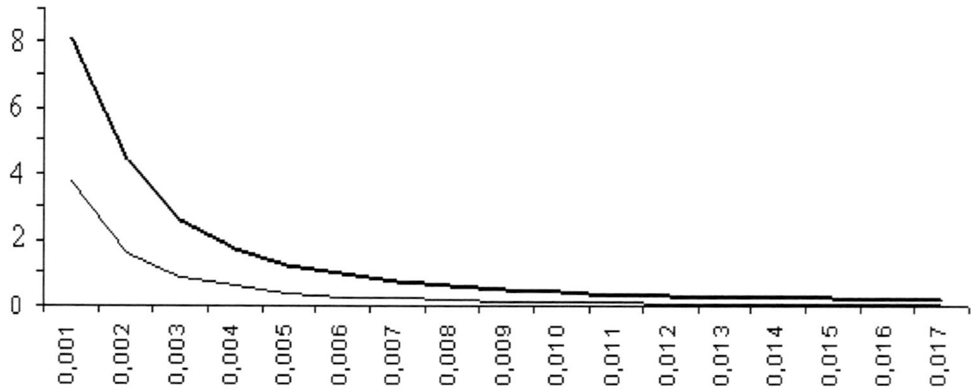


(C) Activity in the domain of minutes (<0.0167 Hz)

On all graphs on X-line are frequencies (Hz), whereas on Y-line are amplitudes (power spectral densities), these amplitudes are proportionally normalized by percentage method.

Figure 8. Graphical results of power spectral analysis. Mean (algebraically summarized overall 45 repeated experiments) power spectra patterns of different frequency domains of infraslow brain potentials in the primary auditory cortex of rats before (thin line) and after (thick line) contact electrical stimulation of dorsal raphe nucleus.

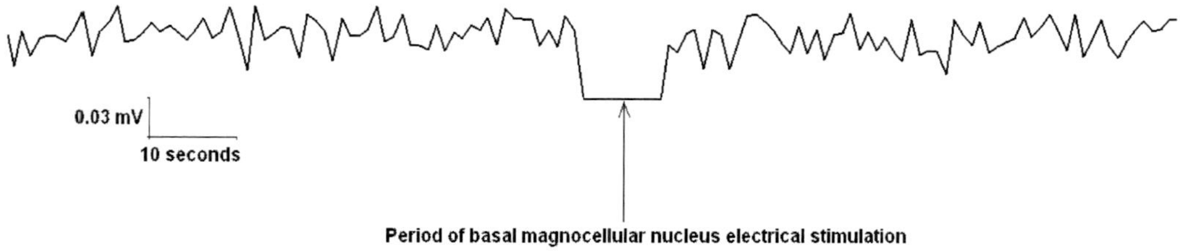


(A) Activity in the domain of seconds (0.1-0.5 Hz)

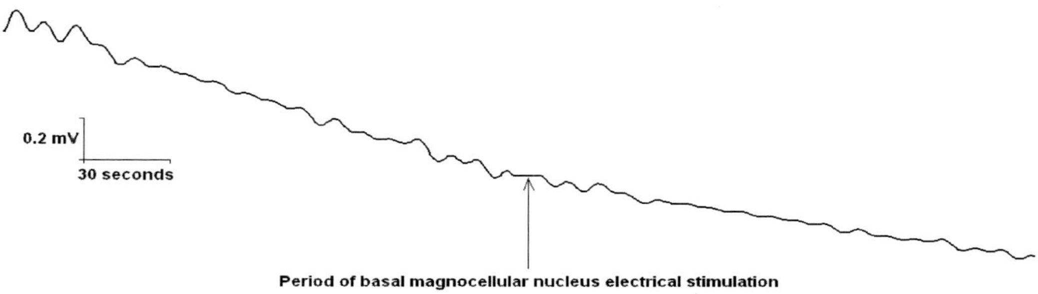


(B) Multisecond activity (0.0167-0.1 Hz) and activity in the domain of minutes (<0.0167 Hz)

Figure 9. Representative examples of different frequency domains of typical infraslow brain potentials in the primary auditory cortex of the rat before and after basal magnocellular nucleus contact electrical stimulation.

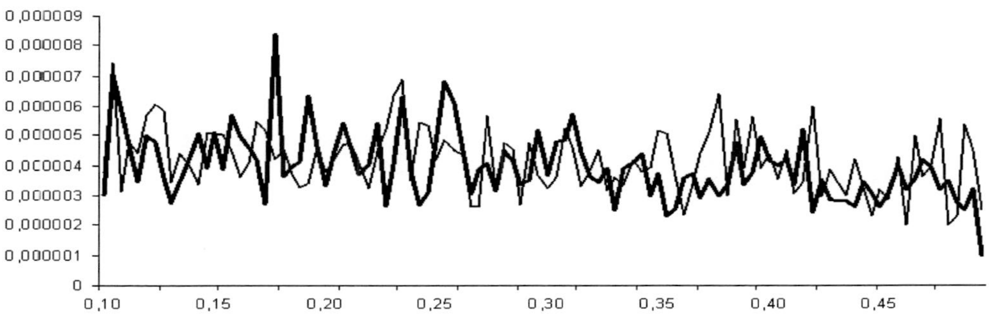


(A) Activity in the domain of seconds (0.1-0.5 Hz)

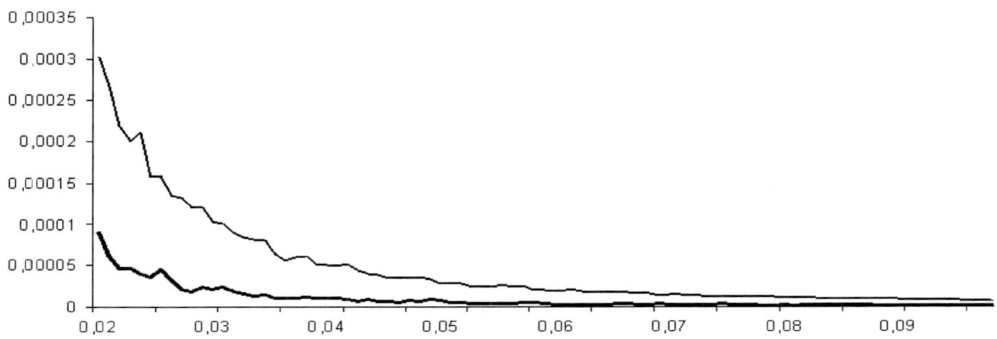


(B) Multisecond activity (0.0167-0.1 Hz)

Figure 10. (Continued on next page).

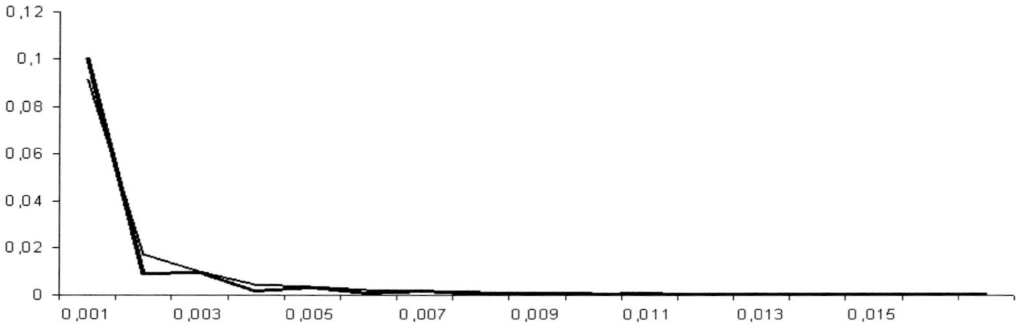


(C) Activity in the domain of minutes (<0.0167 Hz)

On all graphs on X-line are frequencies (Hz), whereas on Y-line are absolute power densities (mV per Hz).

Figure 10. Graphical results of power spectral analysis. Mean (algebraically summarized overall 45 repeated experiments) power spectra patterns of different frequency domains of infraslow brain potentials of primary auditory cortex of rats before (thin line) and after (thick line) contact electrical stimulation of basal magnocellular nucleus.

# Conclusion

Based on the results of our experiments described in this chapter and on the analysis of the literature, it is possible to make several final general conclusions.

1. Oscillations in the domain of seconds (frequencies of 0.1-0.3 Hz) are related to the mechanisms of specific auditory sensory information processing in the A1, as well as this activity is tightly connected with neurophysiological mechanisms of functional bidirectional interactions within thalamic-cortical-thalamic axis (MGN-A1-MGN system) during the process of central hearing. These results are in line with available literature data about 'up and down' neuronal processing in the cortex that is modulated by intra-cortical and thalamic-cortical-thalamic mechanisms [4, 9, 10, 28, 29, 48, 50, 57, 67]. We also suppose that oscillations in the domain of seconds could reflect low frequency periodic cyclical receptive field alterations (frequency tuning changes) of neurons of A1.
2. Multisecond activity in the A1 is mainly attributed to the mechanisms of global neuronal excitability fluctuations in auditory neocortical neurons. Such fluctuations are not directly related to specific process of auditory stimulus processing. However, they might affect this neuroprocessing indirectly. These global processes in the A1 are, obviously, governed both by inputs from the MGN and by ascending projections from noradrenergic and serotoninergic brainstem nuclei (like the LC and DRN, respectively) and from cholinergic basal forebrain nucleus (like BMN). These findings, on one hand, coincide with the concept that aforementioned sites have auditory stimulus sensitive neurons [11, 30, 40, 41, 54]. On another, these data correspond to available notions that structures of the brainstem are responsible for slow EEG modulations [44] and that LC, DRN, and BMN (in other words noradrenergic, serotoninergic, and cholinergic mechanisms) are involved in the

process of neuronal excitability modulation in the auditory cortex [5, 6, 11, 13, 15-17, 35-37, 40-43, 46, 49, 51, 52 61, 66]. Additionally, it is possible to suggest that multisecond waves may be involved in the mechanisms of periodic short-term neuronal plasticity modulation in the A1.

3. Fluctuations in the range of minutes and relatively stable potential of millivolt scale in the A1 are not sensitive to auditory stimulation that is incoming into the auditory cortex; these fluctuations are also not correlated with the physiological states that are induced by MGN, LC, DRN or BMN electrical activation, since there were no changes from this type of activity in response to all of these manipulations. Therefore, it is possible to assume that activity in the domain of minutes and millivolt scale potential in the A1 attributes either to some basic neural metabolic processes or to those that are taking place on the liquor-brain and blood-brain barriers boundaries in the primary auditory cortex. This idea is in agree with available in the literature interpretation of functional significance of this slowest types of brain activity [18-25, 55, 60].
4. Finally, our experiments on visual sensory thalamic-cortical-thalamic system of the brain (lateral geniculate nucleus-primary visual cortex-lateral geniculate nucleus) and our findings on auditory sensory thalamic-cortical-thalamic system of the brain (medial geniculate nucleus-primary auditory cortex-medial geniculate nucleus) allow the pertinent conclusion about common principles and mutual mechanisms of involvement and participation of dynamics of infraslow brain potentials in some general physiological processes of afferent sensory information neural processing in the brain [18-21, 24, 25].

## Acknowledgments

This exploration scientific-research study was performed in the context of realization of Federal Special-Purpose Program “Scientific and scientific-pedagogical personnel of innovative Russia” for 2009-2013 years.

## References

[1] Adey, WR. Slow electrical phenomena in the central nervous system. *Neuroscience Research Program Bulletin,* 1969, 7, 75-180.

[2] Aladjalova, NA. Infra-slow rhythmic oscillations of the steady potential of the cerebral cortex. *Nature.* 1957, 179, 957-959.

[3] Aladjalova, NA. *Psychophysiological aspects of brain infra-slow rhythmical activity.* Moscow: Nauka; 1979.

[4] Belitski, A; Panzeri, S; Magri, C; Logothetis, NK; Kayser, C. Sensory information in local field potentials and spikes from visual and auditory cortices: time scales and frequency bands. *Journal of Computational Neuroscience,* 2010, 29, 533-545.

[5] Bottjer, SW; Brady, JD; Cribbs, B. Connections of a motor cortical region in zebra finches: relation to pathways for vocal learning. *Journal of Comparative Neurology,* 2000, 420, 244-260.

[6] Budinger, E; Laszcz, A; Lison, H; Scheich, H; Ohl, FW. Non-sensory cortical and subcortical connections of the primary auditory cortex in Mongolian gerbils: bottom-up and top-down processing of neuronal information via field AI. *Brain Research,* 2008, 1220, 2-32.

[7] Bullock, TH. Slow potentials in the brain: still little understood but gradually getting analytical attention. *Brain Research Bulletin,* 1999, 50, 315-316.

[8] Cooper, R; Crow, HJ. Toxic effects of intra-cerebral electrodes. *Journal of Medical and Biological Engineering and Computing,* 1966, 4, 575-581.

[9] Cordes, D; Haughton, VM; Arfanakis, K; Wendt, GJ; Turski, PA; Moritz, CH; Quigley, MA; Meyerand, ME. Mapping functionally related regions of brain with functional connectivity MR imaging. *AJNR American Journal of Neuroradiology,* 2000, 21,1636-1644.

[10] Cossart, R; Aronov, D; Yuste, R. Attractor dynamics of network UP states in the neocortex. *Nature,* 2003, 423, 283-288.

[11] Cransac, H; Cottet-Emard, JM; Hellstrom, S; Peyrin, L. Specific sound-induced noradrenergic and serotoninergic activation in central auditory structures. *Hearing Research,* 1998, 118, 151-156.

[12] Crochet, S; Fuentealba, P; Cisse, Y; Timofeev, I; Steriade, M. Synaptic plasticity in local cortical network in vivo and its modulation by the level of neuronal activity. *Cerebral Cortex,* 2006, 16, 618-631.

[13] Dimova, RN; Usunoff, KG. Cortical projection of giant neostriatal neurons in the cat. Light and electron microscopic horseradish peroxidase study. *Brain Research Bulletin,* 1989, 22, 489-499.

[14] Directive 2010/63/EU of the European Parliament and of the Council on the protection of animals used for scientific purposes, dated by September 22, 2010. *Official Journal of European Union*, 20.10.2010, L 276, 33-79.

[15] Dringenberg, HC; Sparling, JS; Frazer, J; Murdoch, J. Generalized cortex activation by the auditory midbrain: Mediation by acetylcholine and subcortical relays. *Experimental Brain Research,* 2006, 174, 114-123.

[16] Edeline, JM; Manunta, Y; Hennevin, E. Induction of selective plasticity in the frequency tuning of auditory cortex and auditory thalamus neurons by locus coeruleus stimulation. *Hearing Research,* 2011, 274, 75-84.

[17] Everitt, BJ; Robbins, TW; Gaskin, M; Fray, PJ. The effects of lesions to ascending noradrenergic neurons on discrimination learning and performance in the rat. *Neuroscience,* 1983, 10, 397-410.

[18] Filippov, IV. Infraslow potentials in the primary visual cortex: The new approach to neurophysiology of neocortical visual sensory information processing. In: Portocello TA, Velloti RB, editors. *Visual Cortex: New Research*. New-York: Nova Science Publishers; 2008, 355 pp.

[19] Filippov, IV. Power spectral analysis of very slow brain potential oscillations in primary visual cortex of freely moving rats during darkness and light. *Neurocomputing,* 2003, 52-54, 505-510.

[20] Filippov, IV. Very slow brain potential fluctuations (<0.5 Hz) in visual thalamus and striate cortex after their successive electrical stimulation in lightly anesthetized rats. *Brain Research,* 2005, 1066, 179-186.

[21] Filippov, IV; Frolov, VA. Very slow potentials in the lateral geniculate complex and primary visual cortex during different illumination changes in freely moving rats. *Neuroscience Letters,* 2005, 373, 51-56.

[22] Filippov, IV; Williams, WC; Frolov, VA. Very slow potential oscillations in locus coeruleus and dorsal raphe nucleus under different illumination in freely moving rats. *Neuroscience Letters,* 2004, 363, 89-93.

[23] Filippov, IV; Williams, WC; Gladyshev, AV. Role of infraslow (0-0.5 Hz) potential oscillations in the regulation of brain stress response by the locus coeruleus system. *Neurocomputing,* 2002, 44-46, 795-798.

[24] Filippov, IV; Williams, WC; Krebs, AA; Pugachev, KS. Sound-induced changes of infraslow brain potential fluctuations in the medial geniculate nucleus and primary auditory cortex in anesthetized rats. *Brain Research,* 2007, 1133, 78-86.

[25] Filippov, IV; Williams, WC; Krebs, AA; Pugachev, KS. Dynamics of infraslow potentials in the primary auditory cortex: Component analysis and contribution of specific thalamic-cortical and non-specific brainstem-cortical influences. *Brain Research,* 2008, 1219, 66-78.

[26] Fisher, G; Sayre, GP; Bickford, RG. Histologic changes in cat's brain after introduction of metallic and coated wire used in electroencephalography. *Proceedings of Mayo Clinic,* 1957, 32, 14-21.

[27] Gumnit, RJ. DC potential changes from auditory cortex of cat. *Journal of Neurophysiology,* 1960, 23, 667-675.

[28] He, J. Slow oscillation in non-lemniscal auditory thalamus. *Journal of Neuroscience,* 2003, 23, 8281-8290.

[29] He, Y; Wang, J; Wang, L; Chen, ZJ; Yan, C; Yang, H; Tang, H; Zhu, C; Gong, Q; Zang, Y; Evans, AC. Uncovering intrinsic modular organization of spontaneous brain activity in humans. *PLoS One,* 2009, 4, e5226.

[30] Heym, J; Trulson, ME; Jacobs, BL. Raphe unit activity in freely moving cats: effects of phasic auditory and visual stimuli. *Brain Research,* 1982, 232, 29-39.

[31] Ikeda, A; Nagamine, T; Yarita, M; Terada, K; Kimura, J; Shibasaki, H. Reappraisal of the effect of electrode property on recording slow potentials. *Electroencephalography and Clinical Neurophysiology,* 1998, 107, 59-63.

[32] Iliukhina, VA. *Human brain in the mechanisms of information and regulation interactions of the organism and environment.* St. Petersburg: Russian Academy of Sciences, Institute of the human brain, 2004.

[33] Iliukhina, VA. *Neurophysiology of human functional states.* Leningrad: Nauka, 1986.

[34] Jackson, WF; Duling, BR. Toxic effects of silver-silver chloride electrodes on vascular smooth muscle. *Circulation Research,* 1983, 53, 105-108.

[35] Juckel, G; Hegerl, U; Molnar, M; Csepe, V; Karmos, G. Auditory evoked potentials reflect serotoninergic neuronal activity – a study in behaving cats administered drugs acting on 5-HT1A autoreceptors in the dorsal raphe nucleus. *Neuropsychopharmacology,* 1999, 21, 710-716.

[36] Klepper, A; Herbert, H. Distribution and origin of noradrenergic and serotonergic fibers in the cochlear nucleus and inferior colliculus of the rat. *Brain Research,* 1991, 557, 190-201.

[37] Levitt, P; Moore, RY. Noradrenaline neuron innervation of the neocortex in the rat. *Brain Research,* 1978; 139, 219-231.

[38] Lickey, ME. Localization and habituation of sensory evoked DC responses in cat cortex. *Experimental Neurology,* 1966, 15, 437-454.

[39] Maxwell, WL; Follows, R; Ashhurst, DE; Berry, M. The response of cerebral hemisphere of the rat to injury. I. The mature rat. *Philosophical Transactions of the Royal Society. London B,* 1990, 328, 479-500.

[40] Metherate, R; Ashe, JH. Ionic flux contributions to neocortical slow waves and nucleus basalis-mediated activation: whole-cell recordings in vivo. *Journal of Neuroscience,* 1993, 13, 5312-5323.

[41] Metherate, R; Cox, CL; Ashe, JH. Cellular bases of neocortical activation: modulation of neural oscillations by the nucleus basalis and endogenous acetylcholine. *Journal of Neuroscience*, 1992, 12, 4701-4711.

[42] Miyazato, H; Skinner, RD; Garcia-Rill, E. Locus coeruleus involvement in the effects of immobilization stress on the p13 midlatency auditory evoked potential in the rat. *Progress in Neuropsychopharmacology and Biological Psychiatry,* 2000, 24, 1177-11201.

[43] Muck-Seler, D; Diksic, M. DL-fenfluramine increases the 5-HT synthesis rate in the terminals while decreasing it in the cell bodies of the rat brain. *Brain Research,* 1996, 737, 45-50.

[44] Novak, P; Lepikovska, V. Slow modulations of EEG. *Neuroreport,* 1992, 3, 189-192.

[45] O'Leary, JL; Goldring, S. DC-potentials of the brain. *Physiological Review,* 1964, 44, 91-125.

[46] Oleshko, NN; Maisky, VA. Topographical organization of the sources of discrete cortical projections within the striatum as determined by a retrograde fluorescence tracing technique in the cat. *Neuroscience,* 1993, 57, 683-695.

[47] Ozaki, I; Hashimoto, I. Neural mechanisms of the ultrafast activities. *Clinical EEG and Neuroscience, 2005*, 36, 271-277.

[48] Riecke, L; Esposito; F; Bonte, M; Formisano, E. Hearing illusory sounds in noise: the timing of sensory-perceptual transformations in auditory cortex. *Neuron,* 2009, 64, 550-561.

[49] Rouiller, EM; Hornung, JP; De Ribaupierre, F. Extrathalamic ascending projections to physiologically identified fields of the cat auditory cortex. *Hearing Research,* 1989, 40, 233-246.

[50] Saleem, AB; Chadderton, P; Apergis-Schoute, J; Harris, KD; Schultz, SR. Methods for predicting cortical UP and DOWN states from the phase of deep layer local field potentials. *Journal of Computational Neuroscience,* 2010, 29, 49-62.

[51] Salgado, H; Garcia-Oscos, F; Patel, A; Martinolich, L; Nichols, JA; Dinh, L; Roychowdhury, S; Tseng, KY; Atzori, M. Layer-Specific Noradrenergic Modulation of Inhibition in Cortical Layer II/III. *Cerebral Cortex,* 2011, 21, 212-221.

[52] Savaki, HE; Kadekaro, M; McCulloch, J; Sokoloff, L. The central noradrenergic system in the rat: metabolic mapping with alpha-adrenergic blocking agents. *Brain Research,* 1982, 234, 65-79.

[53] Schonwiesner, M; Krumbholz, K; Rubsamen, R; Fink, GR; von Cramon, DY. Hemispheric asymmetry for auditory processing in the human auditory brain stem, thalamus, and cortex. *Cerebral Cortex,* 2007, 17, 492-499.

[54] Shinba, T; Briois, L; Sara, SJ. Spontaneous and auditory-evoked activity of medial agranular cortex as a function of arousal state in the freely moving rat: interaction with locus coeruleus activity. *Brain Research,* 2000, 887, 293-300.

[55] Shvets-Teneta-Gurii, TB. Electrochemical activity at implanted metal electrodes as a response of the brain to injury. *Zhurnal Vysshei Nervnoi Deiatelnosti Imeni I P Pavlova,* 1981, 31, 148-157.

[56] Stensaas, SS; Stensaas, LJ. Gold implants and the brain. *Acta Neuropathologica (Berl),* 1978, 41, 145-155.

[57] Steriade, M; Nunez, A; Amzica, F. A novel slow (<1 Hz) oscillation of neocortical neurons in vivo: depolarizing and hyperpolarizing components. *Journal of Neuroscience,* 1993, 13, 3252-3265.

[58] Swanson, LW. *Brain Maps: Structure of the rat brain.* Amsterdam-Tokyo: Elsevier; 1998.

[59] Tallgren, P; Vanhatalo, S; Kaila, K; Voipio, J. Evaluation of commercially available electrodes and gels for recording of slow EEG potentials. *Clinical Neurophysiology,* 2005, 116, 799-806.

[60] Vanhatalo, S; Voipio, J; Kaila, K. Full-band EEG (FbEEG): an emerging standard in electroencephalography. *Clinical Neurophysiology,* 2005, 116, 1-8.

[61] Wenk, H; Bigl, V; Meyer, U. Cholinergic projections from magnocellular nuclei of the basal forebrain to cortical areas in rats. *Brain Res.* 1980; 2(3):295-316.

[62] Windhorst, U., Johansson, H. (Eds). *Modern Techniques in Neuroscience Research.* Berlin, Heidelberg, New-York: Springer-Verlag; 1999.

[63] Wong, PS; Bernat, E; Snodgrass, M; Shevrin, H. Event-related brain correlates of associative learning without awareness. *International Journal of Psychophysiology,* 2004, 53, 217-31.

[64] Xu, M; Liu, CH; Xiong, Y; He, J. Corticofugal modulation of the auditory thalamic reticular nucleus of the guinea pig. *J Physiol.* 2007; 585(Pt 1):15-28.

[65] Yuen, TG; Agnew, WF; Bullara, LA. Tissue response to potential neuroprosthetic materials implanted subdurally. *Biomaterials,* 1987, 8,138-141.

[66] Zhang, JS; Kaltenbach, JA; Wang, J; Kim, SA. Fos-like immunoreactivity in auditory and nonauditory brain structures of hamsters previously exposed to intense sound. *Experimental Brain Research,* 2003, 153, 655-60.

[67] Zhou, Y; Wang, X. Cortical processing of dynamic sound envelope transitions. *Journal of Neuroscience,* 2010, 30, 16741-16754.

In: Auditory Cortex: Anatomy, Functions and Disorders
Editor: Mounya Elhilali
ISBN 978-1-62100-685-5


*Chapter IV*

# Auditory Cortex in Guinea Pigs: Subfield Organization and Functional Domains

***Wen-Jie Song, Masataka Nishimura and Kazuya Saitoh***
Department of Sensory and Cognitive Physiology, Graduate School of Medical Sciences, Kumamoto University, Kumamoto, Japan

## Abstract

The guinea pig produces a variety of vocalizations, providing a suitable mammalian model for auditory research. The organization of the auditory cortex in guinea pigs, however, remains to be elucidated. We have examined this issue over the past several years using *in vivo* optical imaging techniques. Our results indicate that guinea pig auditory cortex is comprised by a core area, consisting of the primary area (AI) and a field dorsocaudal to the AI. A number of belt regions have been found around the core, which exhibit different functional characteristics. By examining the spatiotemporal response patterns in the AI to tone stimulation and electrical stimulation, we show that an isofrequency strip in the AI appears to operate as a functional domain. Evidence from spontaneous activity in the AI also supports this notion. The functional domain of an isofrequency strip has implications for the development of auditory prostheses involving cortical stimulation.

## Introduction

The precise role of the auditory cortex in hearing remains contentious. However, an increasing body of evidence indicates that the auditory cortex is essential in the analysis of complex sounds and the processing of spatial cues (Schnupp et al. 2001; Lomber and Malhotra, 2008), as well as in the perception of elementary sound (Talwar et al., 2001). Regarding the organization of the auditory cortex, Kaas and colleagues have proposed that in monkeys the auditory cortex has a core area and surrounding belt regions, with the belt regions being further surrounded by parabelt regions (Kaas and Hackett 2000; Hackett et al., 2001). Such core-belt organization also appears to apply to cats (Reale and Imig 1980) and rodents (Horikawa et al., 2001; Nishimura et al., 2007; Polley et al., 2007). Although the function of auditory cortical areas has not been fully elucidated, it is possible that each area plays a specialized role in the processing of acoustic information. It is thus important to identify all cortical fields related to acoustic information processing.

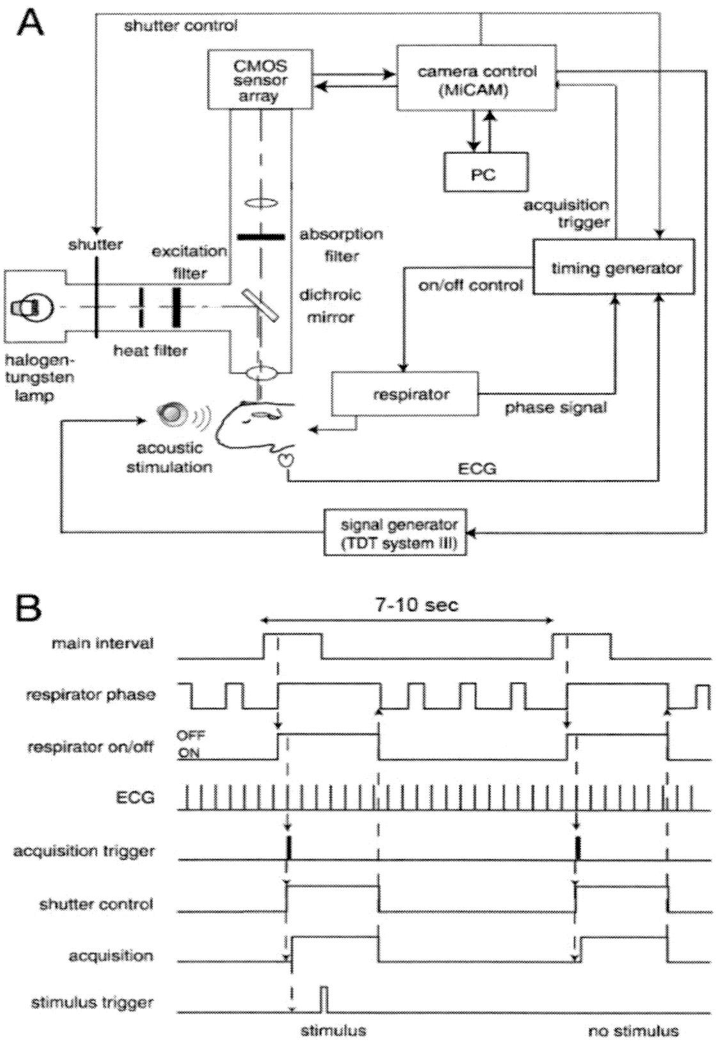


Figure 1. Schematic diagrams of our system for *in vivo* optical recording and a timing chart for the control of recording. (A) The recording system. For suppression of heartbeat and respiration interferences, ECG and the phase signal of the respirator were monitored and used for the control of recording and stimulation. (B) Timing chart for control of recording and stimulation. An oscillation signal (main interval) was used to gate the phase signal of the respirator to control the on/off of the respirator. The on/off signal was used to gate the ECG signal to produce a trigger signal for shutter control, recording, and stimulation with increasing delays. The trigger signal is synchronized to the first R wave gated by the respirator on/off signal. Tone stimulus was triggered in one of two successive recordings to allow separation of evoked responses by subtraction.

The guinea pig, a commonly used laboratory animal, produces a variety of vocalizations (Berryman, 1976), and is therefore an appropriate model for auditory research. Microelectrode mapping in guinea pigs has revealed two fields in the core area, the primary area (AI) and a dorsocaudal field (DC, dorsocaudal to the AI), as well as several belt areas around the core area (Hellweg et al. 1977; Redies et al. 1989; Wallace et al. 1999).

Optical imaging *in vivo* using voltage-sensitive dyes has confirmed the existence of AI and DC (Fukunishi et al. 1992; Taniguchi et al. 1992; Song et al. 2006), and has further revealed propagating activity in the AI (Song et al. 2006). Recently, Horikawa et al. (2001) imaged tone-evoked activities at multiple sites of the auditory cortex and identified seven or eight spot-like areas in the belt regions. There are, however, discrepancies in the size and location of auditory subfields in the literature.

We examined the auditory cortex of guinea pigs with a high-resolution *in vivo* imaging system using the voltage-sensitive dye RH-795 (Grinvald et al. 1994), revealing the entire organization of the auditory cortex. Within the AI, we obtained evidence suggesting that an isofrequency strip appears to operate as a functional domain.

## Materials and Methods

All experiments were carried out according to the Guidelines for Use of Animals in Experiments of Kumamoto University. Hartley guinea pigs were prepared for imaging under anesthesia with a mixture of ketamine (46 mg/kg) and xylazine (24 mg/kg). Our experimental procedures have been described in detail previously (Song et al. 2006; Nishimura et al. 2006; Nishimura et al. 2007; Saitoh et al., 2010). The skull over the left auditory cortex, ~12 mm in rostrocaudal direction and ~10 mm in the dorsoventral direction, was removed, and the dura mater was resected. The cortex was then stained for one hour with the voltage-sensitive dye RH-795 (0.7 mg/ml in saline; Invitrogen, Carlsbad, CA).

The principles of optical imaging using voltage-sensitive dyes have been described elsewhere (Cohen et al. 1978). We used a high-resolution complementary metal oxide semiconductor (CMOS) imaging system (100 × 100 pixels; MiCAM Ultima, BrainVision, Tokyo, Japan) to detect optical signals at a sampling interval of 1.0 msec. The recording system and optics are schematically illustrated in Figure 1A. In our optical imaging system, the sensor array covered a cortical area of $6.25 \times 6.25\ mm^2$. It is possible to cover a larger area of the cortex if a low magnification optical system is used. However, for optical imaging, it is always necessary to consider the trade-off among imaging area size, spatial resolution, and signal-to-noise ratio.

The optical signal recorded *in vivo* is severely interfered by heartbeat and respiration. To suppress these types of noise, we stopped respiration during recording and synchronized recording with heartbeat. A subtraction procedure then allowed the separation of evoked responses (Song et al., 2006). The timing chart for control of recording is shown in Figure 1B, and was implemented with a microcomputer. Pure tones (50 msec; 10 msec onset and offset cosine ramps, 30 msec plateau; 250 Hz to 16 kHz) at sound pressure level (SPL) between 50 to 70 dB (re. 20 μPa) were generated and presented to the right ear of the animal in a double-walled soundproof room. Data acquired with the CMOS imaging system were analyzed with custom-made software programmed in C++ or Matlab. The mean fractional fluorescence (ΔF/F) signal in 16 consecutive recordings was calculated and filtered with a Gaussian-windowed sinc temporal filter (cutoff frequency: 500 Hz). The latency of tone-evoked responses was defined as the time interval from stimulus onset to when the signal exceeds triple the standard deviation (SD) of the baseline (50 msec recording before stimulus application).

To study spontaneous activity in the cortex, we obtained recordings that were each several tens of seconds long, and used independent component analysis to isolate neural activity from heartbeat and respiration interferences (Inagaki et al., 2003; Maeda et al., 2001).

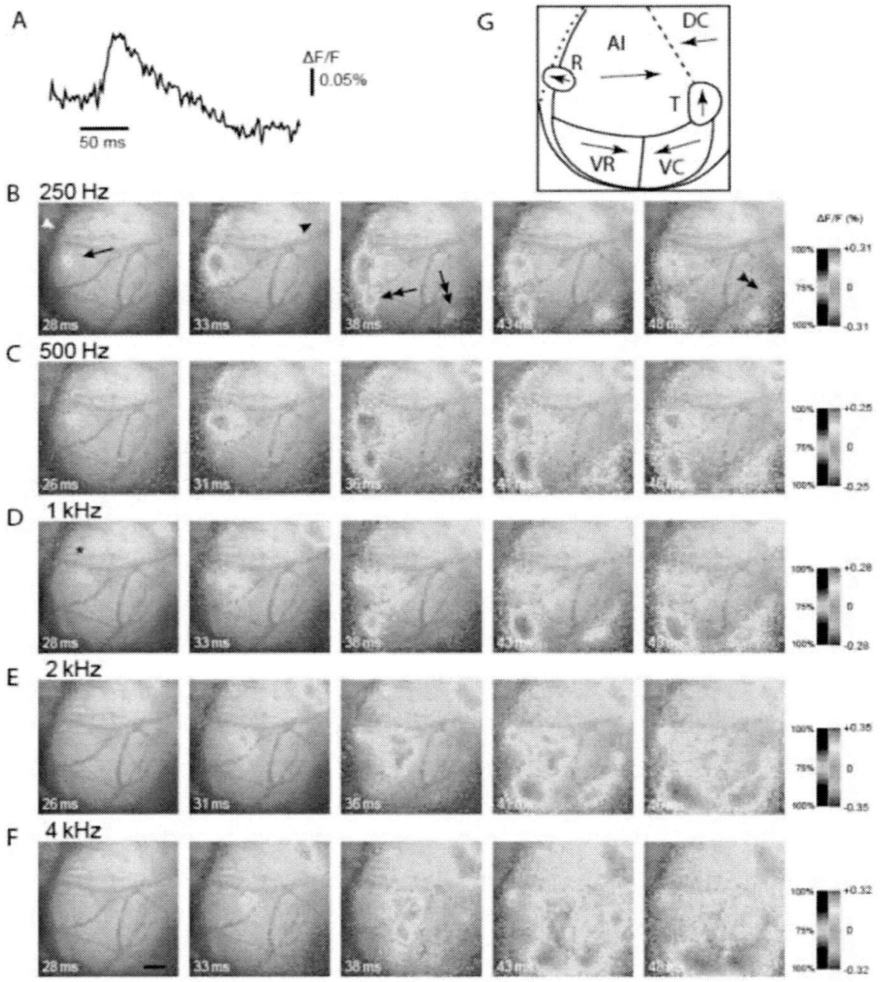


From Nishimura et al., 2007.

Figure 2. Parcellation of the rostroventral portion of the auditory cortex. (A) a representative response from a single channel, to stimulation of a pure tone. The time scale bar also shows the timing of tone stimulation. (B–F) Spatio-temporal responses of the cortex to pure tones of 250 Hz, 500 Hz, 1 kHz, 2 kHz, and 4 kHz, respectively. The responses were encoded by color using the color bar shown to the right of each figure, and were superimposed on the cortical surface with transparency defined by the transparency bar accompanying the color bar. The white arrowhead in B points to the pseudosylvian sulcus. (G) A summary of subfields in rostroventral portion of the auditory cortex. Arrows show the direction of shift of activation with increase of tone frequency.

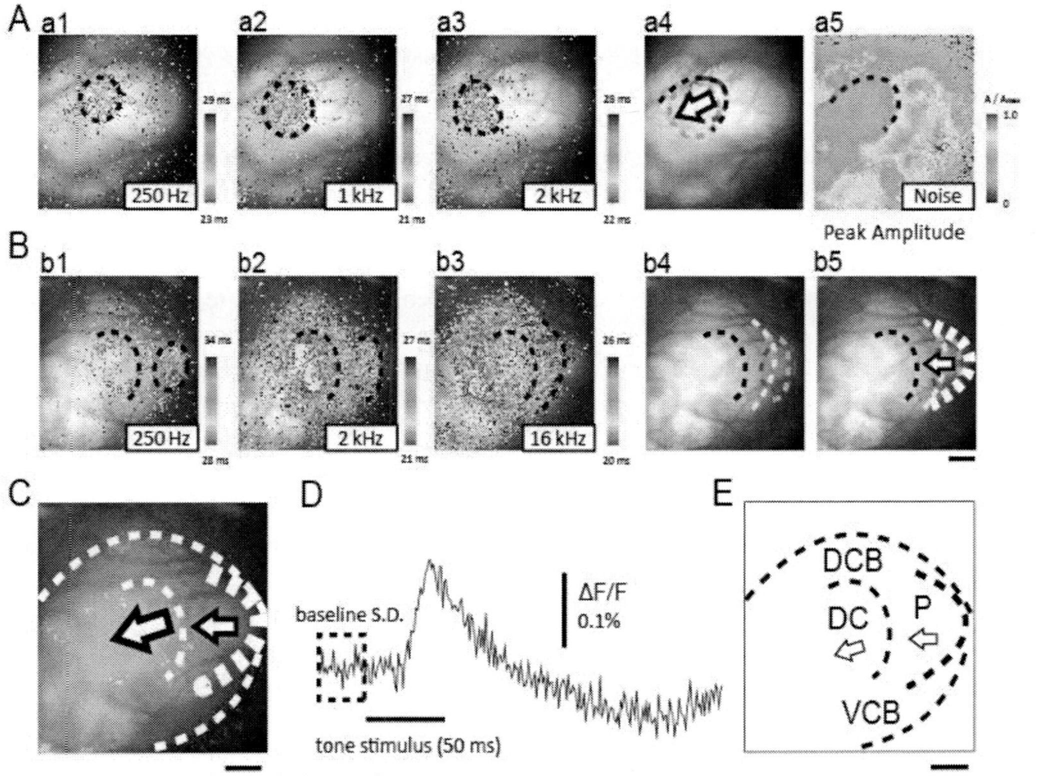


Nishimura et al., unpublished observations.

Figure 3. Parcellation of the dorsocaudal portion of the auditory cortex. (A) Defining the dorsal, caudal, and ventral border of DC. (a1–a3) Latency maps constructed using responses to pure tones of frequencies of 250 Hz, 1 kHz, and 2 kHz, respectively. (a4) Superposition of the contour of the latency maps in a1-a3 revealed tonotopy (arrow) and the border of DC field. Also superimposed is the border of DC (dotted black line) defined in a5. (a5) Peak amplitude map of responses to a wide-band noise stimulus. Such a map delineated the dorsal, caudal, and ventral border of DC (dotted line). (B) Field P. (b1-b3) Latency maps constructed using responses to pure tones of frequencies of 250 Hz, 2 kHz, and 16 kHz, respectively. An area caudal to DC is evident. This area was termed P following Horikawa et al. (2001). The dotted lines were drawn by eye to show the approximate border of DC and P. Superposition of the borders in b4 and b5 shows tonotopy in P (arrow in b5) and the caudal border of P. (C) The responses to a wide-band noise were binarized to reveal the size of the dorsocaudal portion of the auditory cortex. The borders of DC and P are superimposed (thicker dotted line). The arrows show tonotopy. (D) An illustration of the time interval used for calculation of baseline SD. Such SD values were used for the measurement of latency and as a part for the definition of a significant response. (E) Summary of the dorsocaudal portion of the auditory cortex. Arrows show tonotopy in each field. Bar = 1 mm.

# Results

Our sensor array covered a cortical area of $6.25 \times 6.25$ mm$^2$, an area smaller than the size of the guinea pig auditory cortex. It was thus necessary to study the cortex in separate recordings. We first studied the rostro-ventral half of the cortex.

We recorded from an area including the pseudosylvian sulcus and the ventral edge of the cortex, with the sulcus at the rostral end of the imaged area, and the ventral edge of the cortex at the ventral end of the imaged area (see the background image in Figure 2B–F). In response to tone stimulation, the optical signal exhibited an initial transient decrease and a later increase with a slower time course, as exemplified in Figure 2A. The initial fast transient decrease was found to be suppressed by glutamatergic antagonists, while the subsequent slower transient change could be suppressed or reversed by GABAergic antagonists in a concentration dependent manner (data not shown). The polarity here is reversed to show that the initial fast transient change reflects cortical excitation and the following, slower, transient change represents inhibition. In all following figures, the response amplitude of each pixel was represented with a pseudocolor, as shown by the color bars shown to the right in Figure 2B–F.

Shown in Figure 2B is an example of cortical response to stimulation with a 250 Hz tone. At 28 msec after the onset of the stimulus, a small area near the pseudosylvian sulcus was activated (Figure 2B, left most panel, arrow). Five msec later, an area at the upper right corner was activated (Figure 2B, 2nd panel from left, arrowhead). Two isolated areas were activated at the bottom of the imaged area at 38 msec after the stimulus onset (Figure 2B, 3rd panel from left, double arrows). A small area close to the caudal one of the two isolated areas was discernable 10 msec later (Figure 2B, right most panel, double arrowhead).

Stimulations with tones of higher frequencies elicited similar patterns of activation, as shown in Figure 2C–F. The activated areas, however, exhibited clear spatial shifts with the change of tone frequency. While the activation with the shortest latency shifted towards caudal direction, the activation at the upper right corner shifted towards the center of the imaged area. Such spatial shifts of activation according to stimulus tone frequency reflect tonotopy in each activated area. A detailed analysis revealed the existence of six cortical fields in the imaged area, as illustrated in Figure 2G (Nishimura et al., 2007). From the location, size, and tonotopy of each field, the primary area (AI) and the dorsocaudal field (DC) could be easily identified. Ventral to AI, only one belt area was reported in previous studies (Wallace et al., 2000), but the evidence shown here clearly demonstrates the existence of two separate fields. We named them VR and VC respectively.

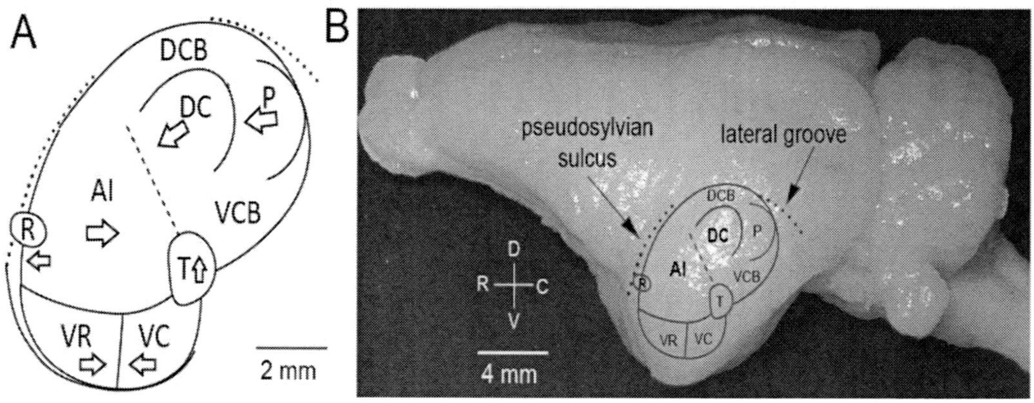


Figure 4. Parcellation and location of the auditory cortex in guinea pigs. (A) A combination of Figure 2G and Figure 3E, showing the parcellation of the auditory cortex. Arrows show tonotopy in each field. (B) Superposition of the A on the cortical surface. The auditory cortex is encompassed by the pseudosylvian sulcus and the lateral groove.

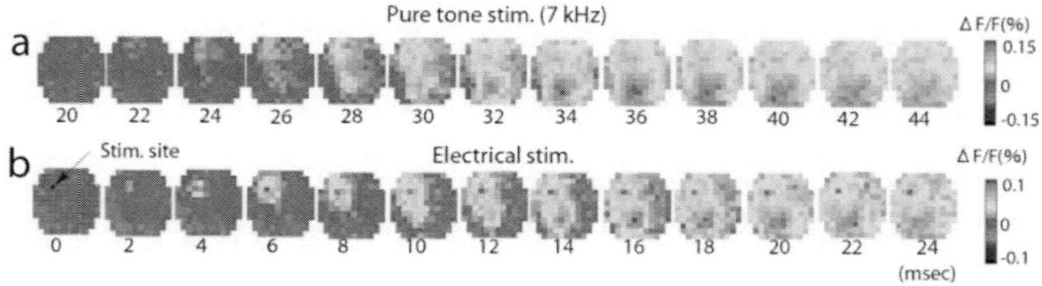


From Song et al., 2006.

Figure 5. In the AI, a pure tone stimulation evoked activity propagation along an isofrequency strip (a). Focal electrical stimulation evoked similar pattern of activity (b).

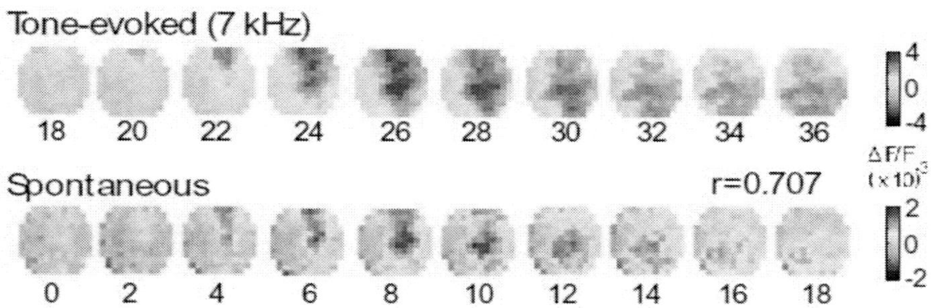


From Saitoh et al., 2010.

Figure 6. Spontaneous activity showing spatio-temporal pattern highly similar to tone-evoked activity was found in the AI.

Rostral to AI, a small area, which appeared to exhibit tonotopic organization, was also identified, and we termed the area R. An area at the junction of AI, DC, and VC, reported in a previous study (Wallace et al., 2000), was also identified here (area T). This finding provided a novel demonstration of the existence of tonotopy in this area.

Next, we shifted our camera to the dorsocaudal portion of the auditory cortex. Response-amplitude-based analyses, such as those applied to the rostroventral portion of the auditory cortex, did not readily reveal the border between sub-fields in the dorsocaudal portion. We thus analyzed both the latency and amplitude of responses to both tones and wide-band noises. Figure 3 illustrates an example of such analyses. Shown in Figure 3Aa1–a3 are latency maps of responses to tones of different frequencies. The response latency was defined as the time interval between the onset of stimulus to the time when the response amplitude exceeds three times of the base line SD (Figure 3D). In each case of Figure 3Aa1–a3, an isolated area of short latency could be defined. Superposition of these areas, as shown in Figure 3Aa4, revealed a shift towards the rostroventral direction with increasing tone frequency. This is characteristic to the field DC. The superposition also roughly defines the border of DC (Figure 3Aa4). In response to stimulation of wide-band noise, DC appeared to show less a response compared to areas dorsal, caudal, and ventral to it, revealing a border between DC and these neighboring areas (Figure 3Aa5). This border coincided well with that obtained from the superposition of latency maps (Figure 3Aa4).

Examining responses with longer latencies revealed an area caudal to DC that also showed tonotopy (Figure 3B). This area corresponds to the P area reported in Horikawa et al. (2001). Occasionally, an area ventral to P was observed, but this was not consistent among animals. To determine the total size of the dorsocaudal portion of the auditory cortex, responses to a wide-band noise stimulus were binarized based on two criteria: 1) the response amplitude exceeded three times of the baseline SD, and 2) the response peak exceeded 10% of the maximum response. An example of this type of analysis is shown in Figure 3C, with the caudal border of DC and P superimposed. The dorsocaudal portion of the auditory cortex thus consisted of DC, P, a belt area dorsal to DC and P (DCB), and a belt area ventral to DC and P (VCB) (Figure 3E). DCB and VCB did not appear to exhibit tonotopy.

Combining results of the rostroventral portion (Figure 2G) and the dorsocaudal portion (Figure 3E) provided a complete illustration of the parcellation of guinea pig auditory cortex (Figure 4A). Superposition of the parcellated areas onto the surface of the cortex using blood vessels as landmarks, revealed that guinea pig auditory cortex is encompassed by the pseudosylvian sulcus, the lateral groove, and the ventral border of the temporal cortex (Figure 4B), and consists of multiple areas with or without tonotopy.

With a total of nine identified fields in the auditory cortex, it is natural to ask why guinea pigs have so many fields and what the function of each field might be. The answers to these questions are currently unclear. To investigate the functional connections among the fields, we stimulated the AI with a single electrical pulse. These experiments, however, revealed that an isofrequency strip within the AI appears to operate as a functional domain. As shown in Figure 5b, focal electrical stimulation of the AI induced autonomous activity propagation, resulting in activity patterns that were highly similar to those evoked by a pure tone in the same animal (Figure 5a). Stimulation at sites along the isofrequency strip evoked the same pattern of activity (Song et al., 2006). These observations suggest that the whole isofrequency strip is activated when a small portion of it is activated. That is, neurons in the isofrequency strip tend to fire together as a functional domain. Consistent with this notion, we also found spontaneous activity in the AI that showed a similar pattern to tone-evoked activity in the same animal (Figure 6; Saitoh et al., 2010). Such spontaneous activity cannot be explained by random processes, and is likely related to anisotropic functional connections within the AI.

# Discussion

We examined the parcellation of guinea pig auditory cortex using an *in vivo* optical imaging technique. The guinea pig auditory cortex is comprised of a core area consisting of the AI and DC field, and belt areas consisting of at least seven fields. Our results largely agree with those obtained with the single electrode mapping method reported by Wallace et al. (2000), but also provide a novel demonstration of the existence of VR and VC.

One unique feature of the guinea pig auditory cortex is that the belt areas surrounding AI exhibit clear tonotopy, while those surrounding DC exhibit less prominent tonotopy. This finding indicates that the rostroventral and dorso-caudal belt areas may be functionally segregated. It is also possible that each subfield defined in this study plays a specialized role in the processing of acoustic information. Further investigating these questions is the most important challenge for future studies.

Our finding that an isofrequency strip appears to operate as a functional domain will have important implications for the development of auditory prostheses. For patients who have lost bilateral auditory nerves, it is necessary to stimulate structures along the central auditory pathway for functional auditory prosthesis. The AI appears to provide a suitable candidate area. Because of the two dimensional structure of the cortex, a two-dimensional electrode array may be useful for stimulation of the cortex. However, our current findings suggest that a single line of electrodes set along the frequency axis of the AI should be sufficient to activate the whole area of the AI.

## Conclusion

The guinea pig auditory cortex is comprised of a core area consisting of the AI and the DC field, and a belt area consisting of at least seven fields. All fields surrounding the AI exhibit clear tonotopy, while the fields surrounding the DC exhibit no clear tonotopy, except field P. Cells within an isofrequency strip in the AI appear to be functionally interconnected, working together as a functional domain. Such a functional structure may make it possible to control the activity of the AI with a single row of electrodes along the frequency axis.

## Acknowledgments

This work was supported by Japan MEXT grants.

## References

Berrymann, J.C. (1976). Guinea pig vocalization: Their structure, causation and function. *Z. Tierpsychol.*, 41, 80-106.

Cohen, L.B., Salzberg, B.M. and Grinvald, A. (1978). Optical methods for monitoring neuron activity. *Annu. Rev. Neurosci.*, 21, 171-182.

Fukunishi, K., Murai, N. and Uno, H. (1992). Dynamic characteristics of the auditory cortex of guinea pigs observed with multichannel optical recording. *Biol. Cybern.*, 67, 501-509.

Grinvald, A., Lieke, E.E., Frostig, R.D. and Hildesheim, R. (1994). Cortical point-spread function and long-range lateral interactions revealed by real-time optical imaging of macaque monkey primary visual cortex. *J. Neurosci.*, 14, 2545-2568.

Hackett, T.A., Preuss, T.M. and Kaas, J.H. (2001). Architectonic identification of the core region in auditory cortex of macaques, chimpanzees, and humans. *J. Comp. Neurol.*, 441, 197-222.

Hellweg, F.C., Koch, R. and Vollrath, M. (1977). Representation of the cochlea in the neocortex of guinea pigs. *Exp. Brain Res.*, 29, 467-474.

Horikawa, J., Hess, A., Nasu, M., Hosokawa, Y., Scheich, H. and Taniguchi, I. (2001). Optical imaging of neural activity in multiple auditory cortical fields of guinea pigs. *Neuroreport*, 12, 3335-3339.

Inagaki, S., Katura, T., Kawaguchi, H. and Song, W.J. (2003). Isolation of neural activity from respiratory and heartbeat noises for in vivo optical recordings using independent component analysis. *Neurosci. Lett.*, 352, 9-12.

Kaas, J.H. and Hackett, T.A. (2000). Subdivisions of auditory cortex and processing streams in primates. *Proc. Natl. Acad. Sci. USA*, 97, 11793-11799.

Lomber, S.G. and Malhotra, S. (2008). Double dissociation of 'what' and 'where' processing in auditory cortex. *Nat. Neurosci.*, 11, 609-616.

Maeda, S., Inagaki, S., Kawaguchi, H. and Song, W.J. (2001). Separation of signal and noise from in vivo optical recordings using independent component analysis. *Neurosci. Lett.*, 302, 137-140.

Nishimura, M., Shirasawa, H. and Song, W.J. (2006). A light-emitting diode light source for imaging of neural activities with voltage-sensitive dyes. *Neurosci. Res.*, 54, 230-234.

Nishimura, N., Shirasawa, H., Kaizo, H. and Song, W.J. (2007). New Field With Tonotopic Organization in Guinea Pig Auditory Cortex. *J. Neurophysiol.*, 97, 927-932.

Polley,• D.B., Read, H.L., Storace, D.A. and Merzenich, M.M. (2007). Multiparametric auditory receptive field organization across five cortical fields in the albino rat. *J. Neurophysiol.*, 97, 3621-3638.

Reale, R.A. and Imig, T.J. (1980). Tonotopic organization in auditory cortex of the cat. *J. Comp. Neurol.*, 192, 265-291.

Redies, H., Sieben, U. and Creutzfeldt, O.D. (1989) Functional subdivisions in the auditory cortex of the guinea pig. *J. Comp. Neurol.*, 282, 473-488.

Saitoh, K., Inagaki, S., Nishimura, M., Kawaguchi, H. and Song, W.J. (2010). Spontaneous activity resembling tone-evoked activity in the primary auditory cortex of guinea pigs. *Neurosci. Res.*, 68, 107-113.

Schnupp, J.W., Mrsic-Flogel, T.D. and King, A.J. (2001) Linear processing of spatial cues in primary auditory cortex. *Nature*, 414, 200-204.

Song, W.J., Kawaguchi, H., Totoki, S., Inoue, Y., Katura, T., Maeda, S., Inagaki, S., Shirasawa, H. and Nishimura, M. (2006). Cortical intrinsic circuits can support activity propagation through an isofrequency strip of the guinea pig primary auditory cortex. *Cereb. Cortex*, 16, 718-729.

Talwar, S.K., Musial, P.G. and Gerstein, G.L. (2001). Role of mammalian auditory cortex in the perception of elementary sound properties. *J. Neurophysiol.*, 85, 2350-2358.

Taniguchi, I., Horikawa, J., Moriyama, T. and Nasu, M. (1992). Spatio-temporal pattern of frequency representation in the auditory cortex of guinea pigs. *Neurosci. Lett.*, 146, 37-40.

Wallace, M.N., Rutkowski, R.G. and Palmer, A.R. (2000). Identification and localisation of auditory areas in guinea pig cortex. *Exp. Brain Res.*, 132, 445-456.

In: Auditory Cortex: Anatomy, Functions and Disorders
Editor: Mounya Elhilali
ISBN 978-1-62100-685-5


*Chapter V*

# Feature Extraction at Multiple Time-Scales in Primary Auditory Cortex

***Didier A. Depireux*[1,*] *and Barak Shechter*[2]**
[1]Institute for Systems Research, University of Maryland, College Park, US
[2]Department of Biology, University of Maryland, College Park, US

## Abstract

Perception of natural sounds such as speech is a complex task: the spectro-temporal content of speech (and in general, most natural sounds) changes over multiple time-scales, from a few tens of milliseconds to tens of seconds, and must often be attended to in the presence of competing background noise which must be ignored.

Primary auditory cortex (AI) is the first cortical recipient of auditory information, and plays a key role in detection, feature extraction, and further segmentation of the auditory scene. The computations performed by AI neurons are in large part determined by their integration of a diverse population of subcortical and intracortical inputs; the functional anatomy giving rise to these computations is not yet fully understood at present.

The standard systems-oriented approach to studying auditory processing primarily utilizes linear methods, such as the now standard spectro-temporal receptive field theory, which provides a-good first approximation. However, cortical processing is complex in nature; this can be uncovered through novel analyses of neural data taken in response to presentations of tailored complex sounds.

AI extracts and enhances biologically relevant information in the auditory environment; for example, enhancing features relevant to processing communication sounds including speech. The neural representation at this stage is ideal for further abstraction.

---

* Contact Information: Didier A Depireux, Institute for Systems Research, University of Maryland, College Park, College Park, MD 20742. E-mail: depireux@umd.com.

In this chapter we review recent experimental results demonstrating that AI provides the basic constructs necessary to process 1. rapid spectral transitions (e.g., consonant-vowel transitions), 2. contrast/signal enhancement (e.g., extracting speech in noise, as in the cocktail party effect and adapting to ongoing background sounds), 3. feature generalization (e.g., speaker invariance).

Altogether, our research points to higher order encoding schemes that generalize the linear models--with most cells showing evidence for multiple coding schemes.

For instance, phase-dependent and phase-independent tuning can occur simultaneously, potentially conveying separate information, or alternatively, conveying the same information cooperatively. These encoding schemes allow AI to generate specialized higher order representations of the spectro-temporal modulations of sounds at very short and long timescales and in noisy environments.

These studies shed light on the organizational principles at work in AI and constrain the space of plausible models of early cortical processing.

# 1. Introduction

The auditory system has been a subject of research for over a century, from investigating the mechano-transduction of sounds into a traveling wave in the cochlea, all the way to the neural responses in multiple auditory cortical areas [1]. The different stages along the auditory pathway from the cochlea through to auditory cortex were found to be organized along multiples axes, the most prominent of which is *tonotopy,* a spatial arrangement of frequency representation, whereby tones close in frequency elicit a maximal response in neurons close in physical distance in each of the stations of this auditory pathway. To a very good approximation, the axis of tonotopy follows the organization of the basilar membrane of the cochlea, i.e. a logarithmic frequency axis wherein a doubling of the frequency of the input is translated into a constant distance along the tonotopic axis. This is much like the arrangement of the keys of a piano, where a given spacing between keys (say, an octave) corresponds to a fixed multiplicative factor of frequency (an octave corresponding to a multiplication by a factor of 2 in frequency).

Neurons in the auditory pathway have been characterized by their responses to a variety of stimuli. Early on, the simplest controlled stimuli consisted in pure tones of different frequency and intensity. While pure tones do not resemble natural sounds, they are easy to produce and provide information about parameters that determine neural *tuning*; that is, characteristics of sounds that elicit strong neural responses such as the tones' frequency and intensity. Pure tones are obviously very narrowband; true natural sounds, on the other hand, are generally characterized by a large bandwidth and contain fast dynamics in both their spectral and temporal aspects, which carries important information.

The spectro-temporal modulations found in speech [2], music [3] and natural sounds [4] are in the same range as the modulations to which AI neurons respond most effectively. Neurons of the primary auditory cortex (AI) fundamentally seem to encode information regarding the modulation of the spectro-temporal envelope of sounds [5-10]. To better understand the cortical encoding of natural sounds (including speech and music), methods of characterization more encompassing than those based on pure tones and click trains were recently developed to describe neural responses to complex sounds. A framework for system characterization, based on the Volterra and the Wiener kernel analysis, was developed by

Marmarelis and Marmarelis [11]. Briefly, a linear descriptor of a system can be obtained by averaging stimulus (input) history weighted by system output. In the case of neurons, this was reduced to a spike triggered average (or reverse correlation), for which an average of the variable(s) under study, measured over the relevant time window of recent stimulus history, is averaged for every neural spike (action potential) generated. In this manner, particular features in the stimulus which consistently preceded a neural spike (presumably eliciting it) summed constructively whereas features which were uncorrelated with spiking averaged out. The neural coding or representation of spectro-temporally rich sounds has been the subject of intense research using these reverse-correlation techniques with the use of complex but well-parameterized broad-band sounds, which measure simultaneously both the spectral and temporal response properties of auditory neurons [12]. The details of how the sounds that are used as probing stimuli are constructed vary greatly, but their general properties remain the same, though this deserves further consideration [7, 13-17]. The results described in this chapter are based on the responses to stimuli called auditory gratings (also called ripples). These gratings comprise a set of well structured, spectro-temporally rich broadband sounds: each has a spectro-temporal profile which is modulated sinusoidally in time and in log spectrum (the log spectrum being the natural dimension of the tonotopic axis, as mentioned above). We characterize the spectro-temporal modulations of gratings, in spectrum by their *spectral density* $\Omega$ (cycles/octave), in time by their *temporal periodicity* $w$ (Hz), and in amplitude by the excursions away from the mean level of the stimulus (modulation depth $\Delta A$ , % of mean). The spectro-temporal modulation envelope of a grating stimulus $S(x,t)$, where $x$ corresponds to frequency $f$ as $x = \log_2(f / f_0)$ with $f_0$ the lower edge of the spectrum and time $t$ is then

$$S(x,t) = L\left[1 + \sum_i \Delta A \cdot \cos\left(2\pi\left(\Omega_i \cdot x + w_i \cdot t\right) + \phi_i\right)\right], \tag{1}$$

for a linear modulation. $L$ is the average level of the envelope (measured as the root-mean-square (RMS) of the stimulus with reference to a 1kHz sine tone) and $\phi$ is the starting phase of the grating (see Figure 1A).

This neural characterization obtained through reverse correlation is termed the spectro-temporal receptive field (STRF). It reveals the *features* in the modulation envelope of sounds to which a neuron is tuned (i.e., responds), where features are defined as a function of both frequency and time. Unlike the responses to pure tones for which one usually studies only the response in the first few milliseconds of the response (*onset response*), the STRF typically characterizes modulations in the neural firing in response to the modulations of an *on-going* sound of constant level or intensity, and in which only the spectro-temporal content (i.e. envelope) changes in time. The inherent assumption of the STRF is that the firing rate of the neuron it characterizes is linearly related to the details of the modulation of the spectro-temporal envelope away from a mean, flat level. This method provides a representation of the neural response as a function of spectrum, but also includes temporal aspects, thus making it a joint spectro-temporal quantification. Furthermore, the (linear) STRF can be used to predict the response of the neuron to fairly arbitrary on-going sounds (Figure 1B).

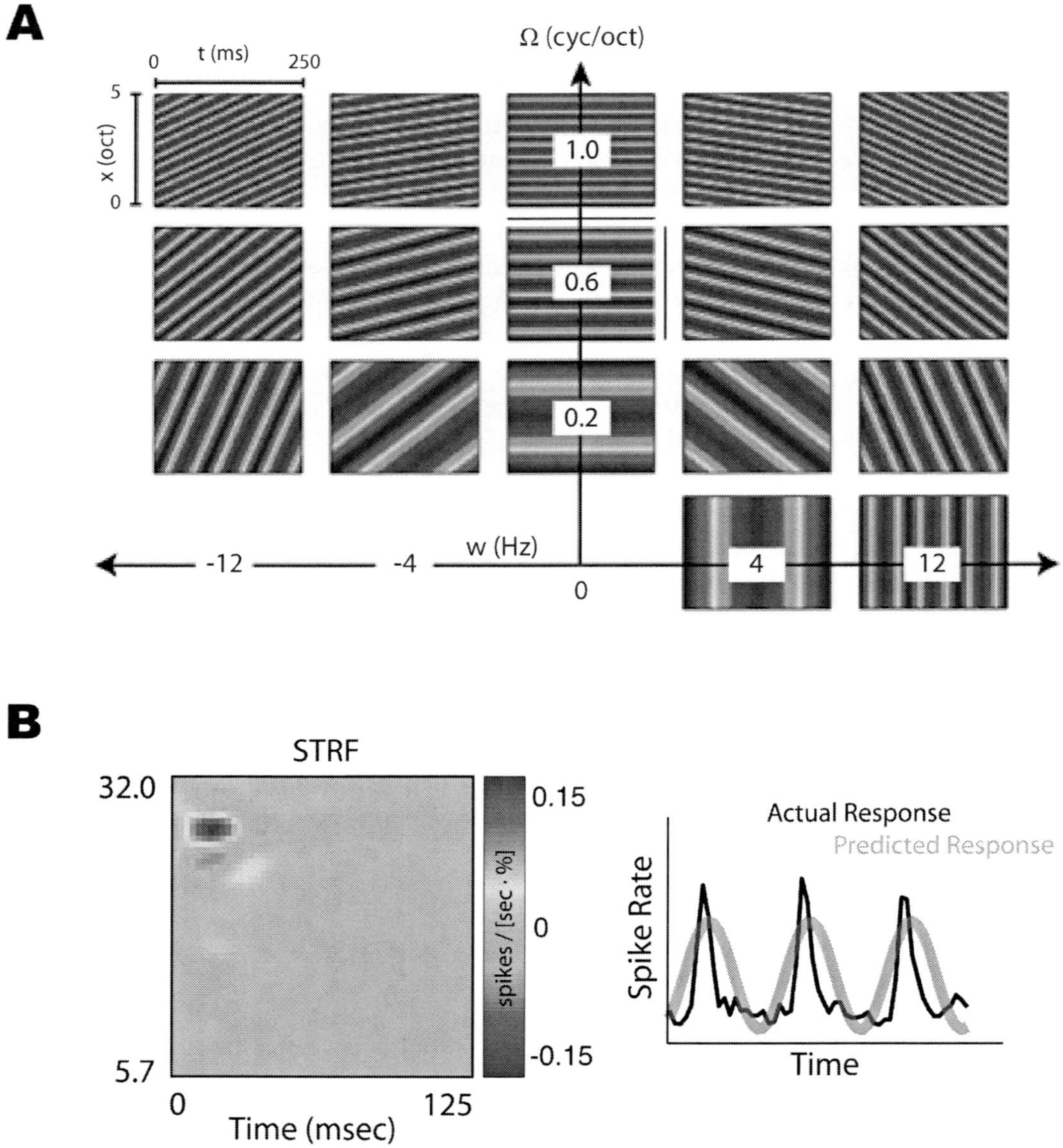


Figure 1. A. The auditory gratings are a set of well structured, spectro-temporally rich broadband stimuli that are modulated sinusoidally in log spectrum and in time. Their modulation is characterized by a spectral density Ω (cycles/octave) and temporal periodicity *w* (Hz). This plot shows spectro-temporal envelopes of auditory gratings obtained by varying Ω and *w* . The units of the ordinates of each grating are of log frequency (octaves) and the units of the abscissas are of time (ms). The auditory gratings form a complete and efficient Fourier basis onto which arbitrary spectro-temporal content can be decomposed. B. Spectro-temporal receptive field (STRF) characterization of an auditory neuron (Left). The STRF characterizes the response of a neuron in both spectrum and time to modulations in the spectro-temporal envelope of sound. Each point corresponds to a particular frequency and delay: Modulations at that frequency will evoke a change in the firing rate of the neuron after the corresponding delay. The change in firing rate is specified by the value of the STRF at that point. Using the STRF, one can predict the steady-state response of the neuron to fairly arbitrary on-going sounds (Right). The plot on the right shows an example response to an auditory grating (Black) and the predicted response obtained via the STRF (Blue).

As mentioned, STRFs are typically measured in a steady-state regime of the neural response --i.e., they characterize the neural preference for *ongoing* spectro-temporal features in a long duration sound. Given that natural sounds and speech typically have rapidly changing spectro-temporal content and silent epochs, it is unclear how sufficient such a characterization with respect to the processing of natural sounds. Longer duration cortical responses obtained in awake preparations exhibit a large variety of response characteristics. As early as 1964, Evans and Whitfield [18] demonstrated not only instantaneous tuning in the *onset response* but also tuning in the sustained responses to pure tones. More recently, Wang et al [19] showed that single neurons in AI exhibit an onset and sustained response to preferred stimuli, and onset-only response to non-preferred stimuli. This dichotomy of responses suggests complementary encoding schemes at multiple timescales during the response.

In this chapter, we review recent experimental results characterizing the processing of AI along multiple timescales. We first explore how AI processes rapid spectro-temporal transitions, such as those that continuously occur in running speech. From there, we summarize results showing the stability of responses in the steady state regime over long periods of time. Finally, we demonstrate complex responses with no absolute timescale, and discuss how these might be important for signal contrast enhancement and perhaps even a higher level of encoding, such as coding invariance with respect to translation on the frequency axis, which for instance would allow for coding of speech characteristics independently of the speaker (man vs boy).

## 2. Short Timescale Dynamics of Tuning

While tuning to sound *features* is often characterized on timescales of hundreds of milliseconds to several seconds, input coming from the outside world is usually very dynamic. Neural responses are remarkably plastic, whereby neural processing can be rapidly modified by its input history. The short-term dynamics of tuning have been studied in a number of sensory systems, including auditory and visual pathways. Bredfeldt and Ringach [20] studied dynamics of neural tuning in visual cortex; they measured the dynamics of spatial frequency tuning using reverse correlation with respect to rapidly changing spatial luminance gratings. They found that tuning in most cells becomes more selective over the course of the response, and the preferred spatial frequency shifts from low to higher spatial frequencies within the first tens of milliseconds of the neural response. In the auditory system, we expect the cortical STRF to evolve in time (see [21, 22]). We found that neurons in AI of the awake ferret respond in a phase dependent manner to feature transient gratings, and their spectral density-temporal periodicity tuning changes as a function of lag post feature onset. This supports an extension of the STRF model to include lag dependence, in which for sufficiently large lags (steady-state), the model reduces to the standard STRF model.

Since natural sounds such as speech are inherently non-stationary, it is especially important to characterize temporal tuning dynamics in addition to spectral tuning dynamics. Sound *level* and spectro-temporal *content* are two independent aspects of sound that are concurrently represented in cortical responses. We use the terms *level transient* to describe a change in level that occurs on a short time scale (typically resulting in a change in perceived loudness), and *feature transient* to describe a change in spectro-temporal content on a short time scale. The introduction of almost any broadband sound from silence induces a cortical response because of the level transient. As mentioned earlier, the STRF is useful both in characterizing the steady-state response of a neuron, and for predicting its response to arbitrary on-going stimuli. However, the onset response to an auditory grating is often not well predicted from the STRF, which is derived using steady-state responses to a sound of constant level [23]. As such, STRFs describe and predict responses best in the context of stimulus deviations away from a constant mean level and, by design, are not expected to aptly characterize the response to sudden changes in level or spectro-temporal content.

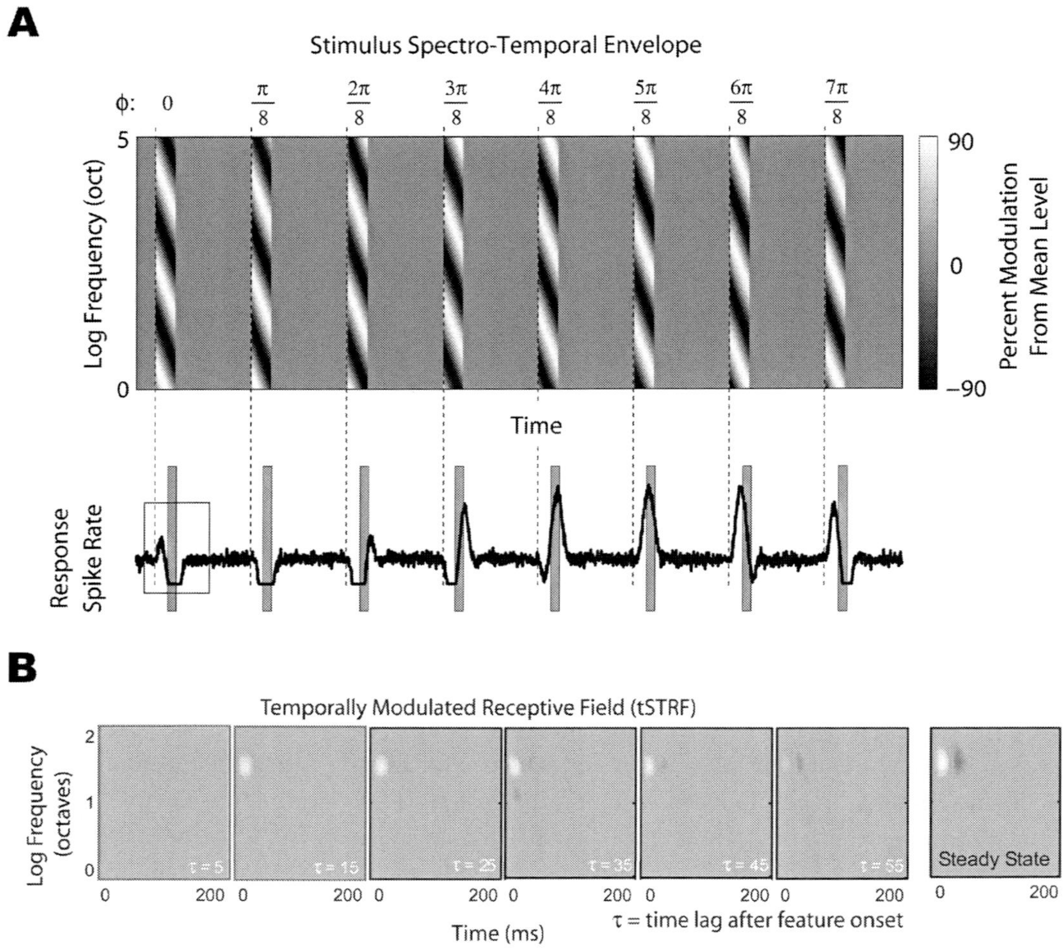


Figure 2. A. Spectro-temporal envelope of an example transient grating stimulus. The stimulus has a flat envelope with eight 50 ms transient segments of grating modulation interspersed. Each transient has the same density (Ω) and temporal periodicity (*w*), but starts at a different phase (ϕ). The stimuli used in practice have random inter-transient intervals. The response of a neuron to the transient grating stimulus is shown below with analysis windows shown in gray. These analysis windows are combined to measure the response to this grating at for a single delay after feature onset. B Temporally Modulated Receptive Fields (tSTRFs) for a representative cell in auditory cortex. Each frame depicts the tuning as it develops at 10 ms interval lags. Sideband inhibitory regions are present at intermediate lags (from 25 ms to 45 ms), but these regions are not seen in the steady-state receptive field, shown at right.

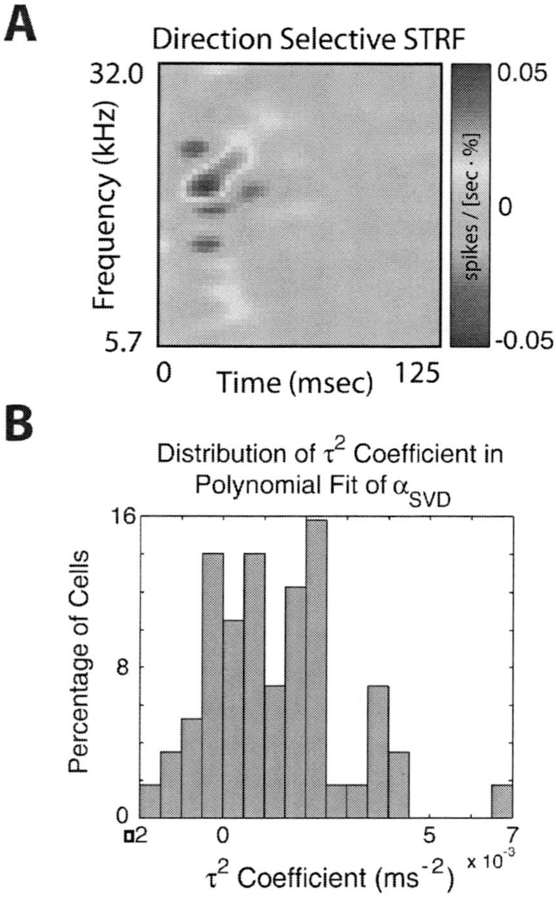


Figure 3. A. Direction selectivity arises when a neuron responds preferentially to spectro-temporal content that moves either up or down with time. This STRF corresponds to a neuron which responds preferentially to a frequency content that moves down in time. Note that STRFs represent the neural response to sound content at a given delay. In this sense, the neuron is first excited by high frequency modulation at longer delay and then by low frequency modulation at short delays—thus down-going modulations. B. The time course of $\alpha_{SVD}$ for the temporally modulated receptive field was fit to a polynomial, and the distribution of the second order coefficients are shown in the histogram. The majority of cells (73%) had a positive second order coefficient, corresponding to a concave behavior, in which $\alpha_{SVD}$ first decreases and then rises back to either a steady-state or continues to increase.

The difficulty in characterizing the encoding of feature transients separately from that of level transients lies in dissociating the two components of the response. The traditional stimuli used in probing the neural response have feature and level transients intertwined, and therefore, STRFs are measured during the steady-state response (after the responses to transients have subsided). However, a conceptually simple modification to the stimulus set can bypass this limitation: level and feature transients can be dissociated by constructing stimuli with a constant average sound level of flat spectral noise and well-defined spectro-temporal modulations at random times away from that reference (flat) level. In this respect, feature transients are presented independently of level transients, and the dynamics of tuning to spectro-temporal features can be studied from their onset response. Here, the feature transient is simply a well-defined spectro-temporal modulation that is turned on over a few milliseconds. In terms of Eq.(1), the $\Delta A\%$ modulation depth is changed from zero (flat noise) to a large value (say, 90%) over 3 ms, kept at 90% for 50 ms and brought back to zero over another 3 ms.

Figure 2A depicts an example of such a stimulus with multiple features. Using a modification of the reverse correlation technique for steady state STRFs using short stimulus history windows (for details see [24]), we can characterize the instantaneous tuning of a neuron at different times after the onset of a feature transient. These characterizations of instantaneous tuning are termed transient STRFs (tSTRFs). An example temporal progression of tuning is depicted in Figure 2B alongside its steady state STRF.

## Emergence of Direction Selectivity

As mentioned above, natural sounds are dynamic; their spectral content changes as a function of time (spectral motion). Since neural responses are not static either (i.e., they change as a function of time, even in their steady state), they can respond best to certain frequency transitions. This preference for a spectral change is called direction selectivity (Figure 3A). More specifically, direction selectivity arises when a neuron responds preferentially to spectro-temporal content which moves either up or down with time. A simple example of a sound with spectral motion is that of the changing spectro-temporal content is during phonemic transitions, such as the transition from /o/ to /i/ in the pronunciation of the word “boy”.

Despite statements of the ‘linear system’ properties of the STRF, it is not a first order Volterra or Wiener kernel. Rather, it can be viewed as a collection of linear systems, one per frequency band, the outputs of which are summed together to produce a probably density of firing. In this view, the STRF can be considered as a series of temporal profiles arranged along the tonotopic axis (their output then being summed). Direction selectivity requires a precise organization of these profiles along that spectral axis, such that their arrangement determines the preferred direction for stimulus spectral content (Figure3A). Hence spectral and temporal processing are interdependent in direction selective cells. Spectral and temporal independence can be measured by the separability of the STRF (which is a function of both frequency and time) into a product of spectral and a temporal functions:

$$STRF(x,t) = RF(x) \cdot IR(t) \tag{2}$$

An STRF which satisfies Eq.2 (i.e., which is separable) cannot be direction selective because of the spectral and temporal independence. i.e. all temporal profiles are identical except for an overall multiplication factor. However, separability need not be an all-or-none property, but rather we can talk of partial separability; we assess the property of separability in a graded fashion by using a singular value decomposition (SVD). This method decomposes the STRF into a sum of fully separable functions; a detailed explanation is available in [25]. Briefly, SVD decomposes the STRF into the product of a *diagonal* matrix $\Lambda$ and two unitary matrices $U$ and $V$ so that $U \times \Lambda \times V^T$. $\Lambda$ has the same dimensions as the STRF with nonnegative *decreasing* diagonal elements $\lambda_i$, so that the STRF gets decomposed into a sum of the outer products of the rows of *U* and *V*, each term of the sum being in the fully separable representation of Eq.2. In other words, SVD decomposes the STRF into a weighted sum of fully separable components, where each component is the product of a spectral and a temporal transfer function weighted by a diagonal element $\lambda_i$ of $\Lambda$.

We define

$$\alpha_{SVD} = \left(1 - \lambda_1^2 \Big/ \left(\sum_i \lambda_i^2\right)\right) \tag{3}$$

as a measure of the separability of the STRF. $\alpha_{SVD}$ measures the fraction of power contained in the first (and since the elements $\lambda_i$ are in decreasing order, the greatest contributing) SVD component. If the majority of power is accounted for by the first component, $\alpha_{SVD} \approx 0$ and the STRF is separable (to within measurement noise). Such an STRF is not direction selective. As we define $\alpha_{SVD}$ to be 0 for separable STRFs and to approach 1 for inseparable STRFs, we call it the *degree of inseparability*.

Direction selectivity in a cell's steady-state response does not imply direction selectivity in the response close to a feature onset. Depending on the spectral density and temporal periodicity of the grating, one expects that the direction of the grating, although well defined from its spectro-temporal envelope, cannot be *initially* determined with confidence given only the sound waveform. Note that there is an inherent time/frequency compromise resulting in uncertainty when determining the spectro-temporal content from a sound pressure waveform; this contributes to the uncertainty in the spectro-temporal analysis when given only a short segment of the sound: the concept of spectro-temporal envelope is not well defined over very short timescales.

We therefore studied the response of cortical cells to auditory gratings for which the modulation depth was non-zero for short periods of time. The modulation was "turned on" (from 0% to 90%) so that each spectral density and each temporal frequency was presented at 8 different phases for 50ms. The sound starts out with a flat spectro-temporal modulation ( $\Delta A = 0$ ), so that initially, the cell is responding only to the white noise segment of the stimulus. The analysis window for the neural response is of short but non-zero duration, which makes the neural response measure an average value over that window as opposed to a true instantaneous value. Therefore, the measure of the neural response transitions from response to noise to response to signal as the cell begins to respond. As our analysis starts at the onset of the change from flat noise to a specific spectro-temporal content—i.e., before the neural conduction time—the initial tSTRF is composed of random noise, with uniform power. Noise, by definition, is inseparable, and therefore, the value of $\alpha_{SVD}$ for this initial period will be random with a high mean. At the beginning of the neural response to the feature transients, it is not possible for a cell to distinguish between upward and downward moving gratings, because of the ambiguity in measuring spectral and temporal content at the time, and therefore in measuring the direction of the grating's envelope from a short sample of the stimulus. Therefore, the tSTRF should be highly separable at small lags with correspondingly small values of $\alpha_{SVD}$.

In [24], we showed that the majority of cells (73%) had $\alpha_{SVD}$ which started from an initial [high] random value, which then decreased shortly after the onset of the feature transient. This corresponds well with the prediction and suggests an inability to determine the direction spectral motion of a feature transient during the first few milliseconds of the response. Following this initial decrease, $\alpha_{SVD}$ then increased over a short period and leveled off over a period of 20 to 40 ms.

This trend is characterized by a concavity in $\alpha_{SVD}$ (see Figure 3B). When fit to a second order polynomial as a function of delay $\tau$ after the onset of a feature transient, this concavity translates into a positive coefficient for the second order term in $\tau^2$ of the polynomial. We show the distribution of second-order coefficients, with a heavy bias towards positive values. The temporal progression of inseparability implied by this distribution show that the majority of cells (73%) acquired some direction selectivity with increasing lag (Figure3B). The absence of highly negative values confirms that no cells had a progression from separability before feature onset, to inseparability during the first few milliseconds after feature onset, and then a return to separability at long lags; the absence of such behavior confirms the physical intuition that direction selectivity (as measured by inseparability) does not appear at short lags.

In addition to examining the emergence of direction selectivity, we considered the dynamics of tuning in terms of the features that elicited the strongest responses. In other words, did the spectral densities and temporal periodicities to which neurons were tuned change as a function of time from the onset of a feature transient? The preferred stimulus was defined as the center of mass of tuning in the conjugate space of the STRF (see below), in which the dimensions are spectral density and temporal periodicity. The dynamics of the center of mass were tracked in terms of the best spectral density and temporal periodicity. Spectral density and temporal periodicity center of mass ($\Omega_{CM}$, $w_{CM}$), were computed as the response power weighted average of all spectral densities and temporal periodicities presented, respectively.

To examine the change in center of mass, we extracted the slope of the best linear fit (as a function of delay after stimulus feature onset) to the center of mass (both in spectral density and temporal periodicity). Center of mass was increasing with lag in 70% of cells for spectral density ($\Omega$) and in 68% of cells for temporal periodicity ($w$). To understand what this increase in center of mass translates to in tuned feature space, it must be related to the breadth of tuning around that center of mass. More concretely, an overall increase in the center of mass of tuning corresponds to a sharpening of the tuned features if the breadth of tuning (about the center of mass) does not change.

To analyze breadth of tuning with respect to spectral density and temporal periodicity, we computed $\alpha_b$, which quantifies the spread of power around the center of mass. $\alpha_b$ is effectively a weighted measure of variance and is defined as

$$\alpha_b = \sum_i \sum_j P(\Omega_i, w_j) \sqrt{\left(\frac{\Omega_i - \Omega_{CM}}{\Omega_{max}}\right)^2 + \left(\frac{w_j - w_{CM}}{w_{max}}\right)^2} \tag{4}$$

where $P(\Omega_i, w_j)$ is the power of modulation in response to a grating of spectral density $\Omega_i$ and temporal periodicity $w_j$; $\Omega_{CM}$, $w_{CM}$ are the response center of mass for spectral density and temporal periodicity, respectively; and $\Omega_{\max}$, $w_{\max}$ are the maximum spectral density and temporal periodicity tested.

A response function with a large spread will be broadly tuned, and therefore have a large value of $\alpha_b$. Conversely, a sharply tuned response function, concentrated mostly around its center of mass, will have a comparatively small value of $\alpha_b$. As before, in order to examine the changes in breadth of tuning, we extracted the slope of the best linear fit to $\alpha_b$. Approximately half of the cell population studied (47%) broadened their tuning and the other half (53%) sharpened their tuning. Combined with the overall increase in center of mass, this result implies a gradual sharpening of the features to which neurons are tuned after the onset of a feature transient.

## Transient Evolution of Spectro-Temporal Tuning

When using sounds with rapidly changing spectro-temporal content, Shechter et al [24] show that the classical receptive field can be modified so that neural dynamics of the response to a sudden change in spectral profile can be modeled without the explicit introduction of a new timescale or new construct, as would happen if, for instance, we had uncovered the existence of two distinct and separate tunings, one onset and one sustained, and their corresponding STRFs. Even in earlier studies, we documented our inability to predict the response to sudden transitions in spectro-temporal content with the classical receptive field [23, 26]. The study extended the standard linear STRF model by introducing and measuring a lag-dependent receptive field. The new cortical model 1) enables us to quantitatively describe how tuning to the spectral envelope continuously evolves from the onset of the envelope to the steady-state tuning, and 2) will enable us to model how tuning evolves from the comparatively simpler subcortical representation to the cortical one (see below).

## Dynamic Filters

In classical terms of system modeling, we note that the goals of the auditory system are several and not compatible prima facie. In particular, the dual goals of sound *detection* and sound *identification* have opposite requirements: *detection* is most easily accomplished with filters that integrate power over as wide a bandwidth as possible, whereas *identification* is best accomplished through narrowly tuned filters. Therefore, it is reasonable that cortical cells might perform a continuously changing, dynamically adaptive filtering capable of accomplishing both goals of detection and identification. On the other hand, tuning to spectro-temporal content need not be dynamic; it is conceivable that one neural population would detect *changes* in the spectral profile, while a different distinct population would encode the *content* of the spectral envelope. Still other coding schemes are possible, of course. Our findings indicate that at the level of AI, at least, the same cells are coding for both the detection of change in spectro-temporal content and for the content itself.

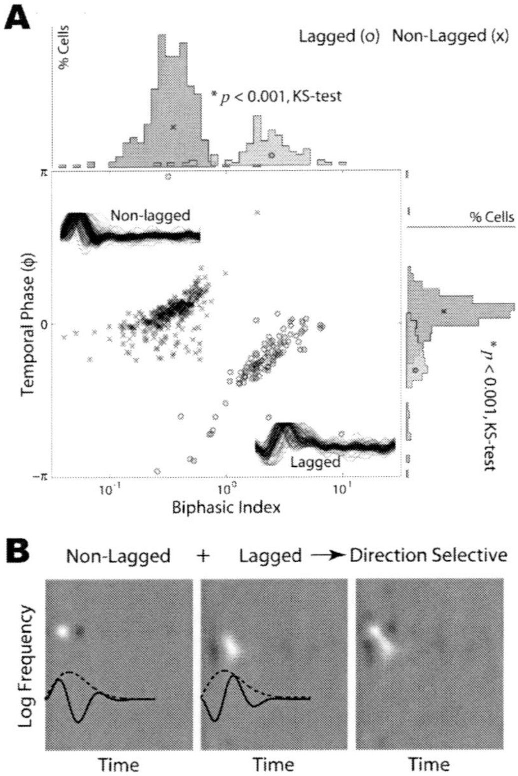


Figure 4. A. Distribution of temporal phase and biphasic index for a corpus of cells in inferior colliculus of the ferret. The STRF of each cell was characterized using auditory grating stimuli and its temporal profile was extracted. The temporal profile's phase is plotted as a function of its biphasic index, which measures the degree to which the temporal profile has a single peak or two (positive and negative) peaks. It is computed as the absolute magnitude ratio of the second peak to the first peak of the temporal response profile. The marginal distributions of temporal phase and biphasic index are shown. Two subpopulations of responses are readily distinguished, which are called 'lagged' and 'non-lagged', and are significantly distinct along each marginal (KS test, $P < 0.001$). Lagged cells are represented by 'o' and non- lagged cells are represented by 'x'. Note that the temporal phase is periodic with . The normalized STRF temporal profiles from each sub-population are inset. Lagged profiles have a characteristic inhibition first and delayed excitation, whereas non-lagged profiles first show excitation followed by a delayed inhibition. The time course of excitation and inhibition (as opposed to peak latency) are characteristic of each subpopulation. B. Direction selectivity emerges from lagged and non-lagged responses. A direction-selective STRF (right) can be created by adding non-lagged (left) and lagged (middle) separable STRFs. The temporal profiles (overlaid, solid line) of the non-lagged and lagged STRFs share the same envelope (overlaid, dotted line), but are phase-shifted with respect to each other.

## Models of Cortical Tuning

The model of spectral envelope feature extraction presented in this section augments the basic STRF model, taking into account the build-up of tuning from the onset of a feature transient. Simon et al [21] show that neurons in ferret AI are well described in the steady state by their STRF, but also have a distinctive property called *temporal symmetry*: Every temporal cross-section of the STRF (i.e., thinking of the STRF as a collection of linear, first-order Volterra kernels, the impulse response for each frequency band) is the same function of time, but for an overall scaling and Hilbert rotation (a shift of phase under a fixed envelope). Temporal symmetry is highly constraining regarding possible models of functional neural connectivity within and into AI. The simplest models of the thalamocortical functional connectivity are those in which the only constraint is that thalamic inputs to an AI cell have a best frequency to within half an octave of the AI cell. Such models are ruled out because they are incompatible with cortical temporal symmetry. Rather, temporally symmetric models predict that the thalamic inputs can be almost unrestricted in their spectral support, but must have the same low frequency temporal structure (e.g. approximately constant amplitude and phase linearity for a few tens of Hz). Simon et al [21] postulated a model to account for their observations predicts the existence of two populations of cells subcortically, called *lagged* and *non-lagged*.

These lagged cells have temporally phase shifted STRFs compared to canonical, non-lagged cells. This is not just a delayed response, but rather a change of phase of the oscillations of the temporal impulse functions under an envelope which is roughly the same for all cells. The effect of this change of phase would produce an initial inhibition followed by a delayed excitation. Physiological evidence for such lagged cells can readily be found in the literature: Shechter et al [22] reports on the lagged cells in ferret IC, and Mastronarde [27, 28] and Saul and Humphrey [29] showed the existence of lagged and non-lagged cells in cat LGN. Furthermore, Galazyuk et al [30] and Sullivan [31] find cells in bat IC which are inhibition first followed by excitation, which is characteristic of lagged response profiles (see Figure 4A). The existence of lagged responses might be induced by the existence of modulating cortico-collicular projections lim [22, 32, 33]. On the one hand, the existence of lagged cells was postulated to explain the presence of several properties observed in steady-state STRFs, and on the other, the staggered input of lagged cells and non-lagged cells into the cortical circuitry is likely to account for some of the aspects of the dynamics of tuning reported in this paper.

The integration of these classes of inputs – namely, the differences in the temporal characteristics of these lagged cells with respect to their non-lagged counterparts – provides the input needed to create directionally selective responses. Given two such classes, an integrating neuron could create a response for which the envelope is constant with respect to different spectral inputs, but of arbitrary scaling and phase-shift. The example in Figure 4B shows how a direction selective response can be created from the integration of these two classes of inputs. These comparatively simpler (separable) receptive fields in IC give rise to the more complex, temporally symmetric receptive fields observed in the cortex.

The majority of cortical cells display responses that are fully separable during the first 20 msec or so of the response. Quadrant separability (but not full separability), as well as temporal symmetry, emerges thereafter in AI. This output is likely sent back to the IC [32, 33] and may contribute to the emergence of the hypothesized lagged cells in IC. Lagged cells would provide additional input to AI cells, contributing to the dynamics of tuning we observed. This would form the basis for the cortical lag-dependent receptive field introduced in this study, which reaches a steady-state tuning that remains relatively stable over hundreds of milliseconds to several seconds [34] . These findings reinforce the idea that temporal symmetry without full separability is not an automatic property of the network, but rather arises from the contribution of several populations of cells.

This section has shown that neural tuning to spectro-temporal features is a dynamic process at the level of neurons in AI. At the same time, it shows that the dynamics involved in attaining a stable, steady-state tuning involves timescales of the order of 50ms or so. We now turn to the question of how stable the tuning represented by the STRF is over periods of many seconds.

# 3. Stability of Tuning over Long Timescales

In the previous section, we demonstrated that tuning in AI over short timescales is a dynamic process which emerges quickly over tens of milliseconds after the onset of a complex sound. Once that tuning has emerged, how stable is it? As mentioned several times, neurons are most typically characterized by their STRFs in their steady-state regime, when tuning is assumed to be stable. When using auditory gratings to probe the neural response, the typical range of spectral densities and temporal periodicities that must be spanned in order to sufficiently characterize the neuron is known. However, given the non-deterministic nature of neural responses, the stimulus duration needed to achieve a good estimate of the underlying probability density function governing neural firing is not *a priori* known. Given that auditory gratings are periodic, the duration of any sound can be extended until the characterization of the response for that stimulus is sufficiently stable.

Implementation of these sounds and other similar stimuli are of relatively long duration—generally seconds to minutes, and their spectro-temporal content is either fixed or changes slowly during the presentation. However, neurons in the central part of sensory pathways are thought to adapt in their responses to stimuli presented over extended periods of time. For instance, neurons in AI display a second order of adaptation, whereby the characteristics of their adaptation to the continuous presentation of alternating long-duration grating stimuli, that differ in their modulation depth, changes with each step-change in the modulation depth [35]. It is known that adaptation of neural output is not restricted to occur only in response to changes in the mean value of the input. For instance, neurons in the early visual pathway also adapt in response to changes in the variance (contrast) of input signals [36], and neurons in the auditory pathway adapt to changes in the kurtosis (a higher moment statistics of the modulation envelope, [37]. Adaptation has been shown to occur along different stations of the visual pathway, from the retina baccus [38] to primary visual cortex [39] and higher [40]. Computation of the STRF—and its subsequent usage in predicting responses—assumes a time-invariant system, in other words stationary response properties.

Evoked potentials typically contain multiple components, some lasting up to several seconds [41]. In order to test the assumption of the cell's steady-state receptive field being stationary throughout sound presentation we derived two receptive fields called early and late STRFs. These STRFs are computed from two distinct time windows of the response: one epoch closely following the onset of the auditory gratings (but after sufficient delay for tuning to emerge) and a second epoch a few seconds later, at which point the evoked potentials related to the sound onset have died out. Specifically, the early STRF is computed from responses to the first fourth of the stimulus (0.25 - 1.75 sec), which is then compared to the late STRF, computed from responses to the last fourth of the stimulus (4.5 - 6 sec). In this section, we report on the stability of the steady-state characterization of primary auditory cortical cells in response to sounds several seconds in duration.

## Response Reliability/SNR

A primary factor in the stability of neural tuning is the reliability of the response with respect to sound features. For example, if there is a change in reliability with which a certain feature is then translated into a neural response, the meaning of that response with respect to whether or not that feature was present in the sensory environment has also changed. In this sense, the neural tuning has changed, even though the exact features being encoded have not. Furthermore, if quality and reliability in the measurement of early vs. late STRF are different, comparison of the STRFs is not straightforward.

The signal-to-noise ratio described in [24, 34] measures the reliability of the STRF using a bootstrapping method. Briefly, for each auditory grating, it measures the reliability of the response to that grating as the average response power divided by the variance in that response. This gives the SNR for individual gratings, where the signal is the response itself and the noise is measured as the variance in that response. The overall SNR of the STRF is then computed as the power-weighted mean of these individual SNR measurements. There were no significant differences in SNR between early STRFs and late STRFs. This suggests that the reliability of the response, once it reaches its steady state value is stable over time. Furthermore, subsequent measures of the two conditions were directly comparable, as they would not be influenced by a change in response reliability (Figure 5A).

## The STRF is Stable in Its Steady State

As with response reliability, the steady-state tuning characteristics of neurons in AI are relatively stable over time. This stability was quantified by extracting descriptive measures of the STRF features for both early and late STRFs. These descriptive measures fell into three categories: magnitude, spectrum, and time.

Magnitude measures:

1. Peak spike rate (the maximal value of the STRF).
2. Total STRF power, defined as $P = \sum_x \sum_\tau |STRF(x,\tau)|^2$
3. Degree of inseparability $\alpha_{SVD}$ (defined in section 2).
4. Degree of directionality, defined as the difference in response power to up-going vs down-going gratings divided by the total response power $\alpha_d = \frac{P_{up} - P_{down}}{P_{up} + P_{down}}$. For example, if there is equal preference to up-going features and down-going features, $\alpha_d = 0$. Conversely, an absolute value of 1 implies the cell is responding only to up-

going or down-going features exclusively, where the sign of $\alpha_d$ indicates the directional preference.

5. Breadth of tuning $\alpha_b$ is a measure of the range of spectral density $\Omega$ and temporal periodicity $w$ to which the neuron responds. $\alpha_b$ is measured around the response center of mass (in terms of spectral density and temporal periodicity) as $\alpha_b = \sum_i \sum_j P(\Omega_i, w_j) \sqrt{\left(\frac{\Omega_i - \Omega_{CM}}{\Omega_{\max}}\right)^2 + \left(\frac{w_j - w_{CM}}{w_{\max}}\right)^2}$ (see Eq.4), where $P(\Omega_i, w_j)$ is the power of modulation in response to a grating of spectral density $\Omega_i$ and temporal periodicity $w_j$, $\Omega_{CM}, w_{CM}$, are the response center of mass for spectral density and temporal periodicity, respectively, and $\Omega_{\max}, w_{\max}$, are the maximum spectral density and temporal periodicity tested.

While the overall power in the STRF did not change significantly between the early and the late STRF, the peak value generally increased, with a sample mean increase of 2.8% ($p<0.02$). $\alpha_{SVD}$ and $\alpha_d$, which measure the degree of inseparability and the degree of direction selectivity, respectively, do not change significantly from earlier to later times in the response. $\alpha_b$, which measures how the response is spread around the tuning center of mass, also did not change significantly between the two epochs (Figure 5A).

*Spectral measures:*

1. Best frequency (the frequency at which the STRF attained its maximal value).
2. Bandwidth, defined as the width (in frequency) at 50% of the STRF maximum in the spectral cross-section containing the peak.
3. Spectral density center of mass $\Omega_{CM}$, computed as the response power weighted average of all spectral densities presented.
4. Spectral density bandwidth, defined as the width (in spectral density) at 75% of the maximal response.

Between the two analysis conditions, the BF of the STRF (the frequency at which the peak of the STRF occurred) did not change significantly. However, the bandwidth, which was measured at half the peak value along the spectral cross-section of the STRF corresponding to its latency, decreased by 5.2% ($p<0.02$) from the early STRF to the late STRF (corresponding to a narrower range of frequencies which elicit responses when modulated). Reflecting the change in bandwidth, the spectral density center of mass shifted to larger values by 3.3% ($p<0.02$). With the shift in center of mass, the spectral density bandwidth remained unchanged from early to late time periods in the response (Figure 5B).

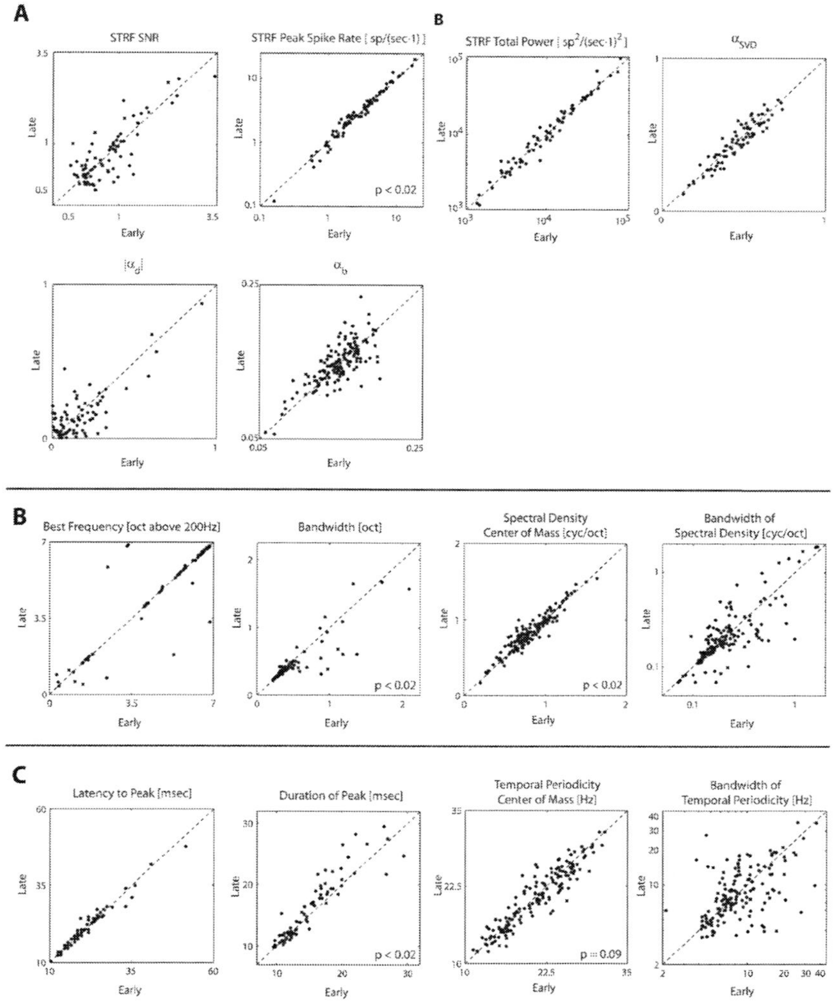


Figure 5. A. STRF magnitude measures. There was no significant difference in SNR between early and late STRFs. However, there was a significant difference between the peak magnitude of the early STRF when compared with the late STRF, with a mean increase of 2.8% across the entire population (P<0.02). The remainder of the magnitude measures showed no significant changes between the early and late STRFs: total power, the degree of inseparability $\alpha_{SVD}$ , the degree of direction selectivity $\alpha_d$ , and the sharpness of tuning $\alpha_b$ . B. There was no significant difference between the best frequency measured in the early STRF and that measured in the late STRF. The bandwidth of the excitatory feature decreased (with a mean decrease of 5.2%) from the early to late STRFs (p<0.02), and the spectral density center of mass increased with a mean of 3.3% (p<0.02). There were no significant differences between early and late STRFs in terms of the bandwidth of spectral density. C. Temporal measures. While the latency to the excitatory peak of the STRF did not change between early and late STRFs, there was a significant increase in the peak's duration by 4.8% (p<0.02). There was a 1% decreasing trend in the temporal periodicity center of mass which was approaching significance (P=0.09), but no significant differences between early and late STRFs in terms of bandwidth of temporal periodicity.

*Temporal measures:*

1. Peak latency (the time at which the STRF attained its maximal value).

2. Peak duration, defined as the width (in time) at 50% of the STRF maximum in the temporal cross-section containing the peak
3. Temporal periodicity center of mass $w_{CM}$, computed as the response power weighted average of all temporal periodicities presented.
4. Temporal periodicity bandwidth, defined as the width (in temporal periodicity) at 75% of the maximal response.

The latency to the peak of the STRF corresponds to the lag between the occurrence of modulation at the cells best frequency to the corresponding modulation in neural response it evokes or to the peak of its envelope. With increasing stimulus time (i.e., early vs. late), the latency did not change significantly. However, the duration of the excitatory feature (peak) increased by 4.8% ($p<0.02$), corresponding to a longer duration in which the cell responds to modulation at its best frequency. Analogously, the temporal periodicity center of mass shifted to smaller values by 1%; this trend, however, only approached significance ($p = 0.09$). The temporal periodicity bandwidth too did not change significantly (Figure 5C).

## Magnitude of Changes

The changes seen in the steady-state STRF during ongoing sound presentation are small in magnitude (e.g., 4.8% for duration, 5.2% for bandwidth). However, these changes are reliable in the population, and therefore constitute a significant effect. At the same time, many measures characterizing the response on average remain unchanged from earlier to later times during the stimulus presentation. This suggests that long duration sounds produce sufficiently stable responses for most applications of the STRF. This being said, it is important to note that the SNR-which is a measure of the reliability of observed responses-remains unchanged in the early and late epochs. This suggests that prolonged acquisition of data does not improve (but also does not deteriorate) results significantly. This also implies that the optimal number of sound presentations should be obtained from an on-line continuous estimation of the SNR reaching a stable value.

We also compare these early and late SNRs to the SNR measured from the entire duration of the stimulus. There is not a significant change between either early or late SNR to the full SNR, suggesting that responses are equally reliable at all times during the stimulus presentation. Since in electrophysiological experiments, stimulus presentation time is a valuable resource, this has strong implications. Shorter duration sounds should be sufficient for characterizing the response properties of neurons in primary auditory cortex; of course, this does not preclude from the use of longer durations either. Given that the STRF is used to characterize the steady-state properties of neurons, it is important to know how stable those steady-state properties are. Response analysis is generally started after the first period (250 msec) following the onset of each stimulus, during which time, the tuning is still stabilizing to the content of the stimulus. These results demonstrate the stability of tuning over several seconds, justifying the use of longer stimuli. In this manner, experimental time can be gained by the use of these longer sounds and minimizing the rejected response time during which neurons stabilize their tuning (in contrast to using multiple presentations of shorter stimuli).

### Plasticity vs. Adaptive Changes

The changes observed in the STRFs were in naïve listeners, with no behavioral paradigm. Previous literature has examined the dynamics of auditory cortical neurons [24, 42, 43], and in particular the changes in STRFs associated with listening task after training: specifically, Fritz et al [44] reported a temporal sharpening of the excitatory peak of the STRF and a commensurate increase in temporal periodicity center of mass, by measuring the response to a sequence of sounds made up of composite auditory gratings, interspersed with a pure tone target. These experiments are quite different since they show a change in STRF properties following several minutes of behavioral response, which resets itself between sound presentations. Note that the magnitude of the observed changes are opposite in direction between the plasticity experiments and the steady-state adaptation experiments. However, the observed effects (except for sign) are on the same order of magnitude with or without the introduction of a behavioral task during the sound presentation.

## 4. Complex Cells in AI: Phase Independent Responses

The neural encodings of sound discussed so far represent phase-dependent tunings; that is, the neural response to an auditory grating depends on the phase of the grating, or equivalently it depends on the precise location of the spectral peaks and spectral troughs as a function of time. We have seen that this tuning arises dynamically, and is relatively stable in the steady state. However, an underlying assumption of the STRF characterization is that the mean firing rate (averaged over any full period of the stimulus) remains constant across all stimulus conditions. In other words, the mean rate does not encode information about the different spectro-temporal modulations, but might instead depend on other parameters such as the mean level of the stimulus, the sound density, and temporal fine structure [23, 45, 46]. However, by integrating features from the auditory environment over a long timescale (with respect to the changing stimulus modulations), the auditory system could make use of a rate code encoding the presence of particular spectro-temporal modulations in the sound. Since this response would not follow the temporal dynamics of the stimulus, it would be independent of the specific phase of the stimulus.

This phase-independent contrast tuning is analogous to complex cell visual responses, in which the response to a grating stimulus does not depend on its spatial phase [47]. These complex cells cannot be characterized by the conventional reverse correlation techniques because they respond equally well to a grating stimulus in any given spatial phase. Instead, they must be characterized by the mean changes in firing rate in response to the different spatial gratings [48]. Similarly for the auditory system, a neuron which has a phase-independent contrast tuning responds to the mere presence of specific contrast features, irrespective of their exact placement along the spectral axis. Such feature extraction would be useful for generalization of a spectro-temporal structure (e.g, a formant ratio) from different sources or in varying conditions (e.g., different pitch). Alternatively, when analyzed in conjunction with the phase-locked response, a shift in the baseline firing rate could be used to enhance or ensure transmission of information contained in the phase-locked component of the response.

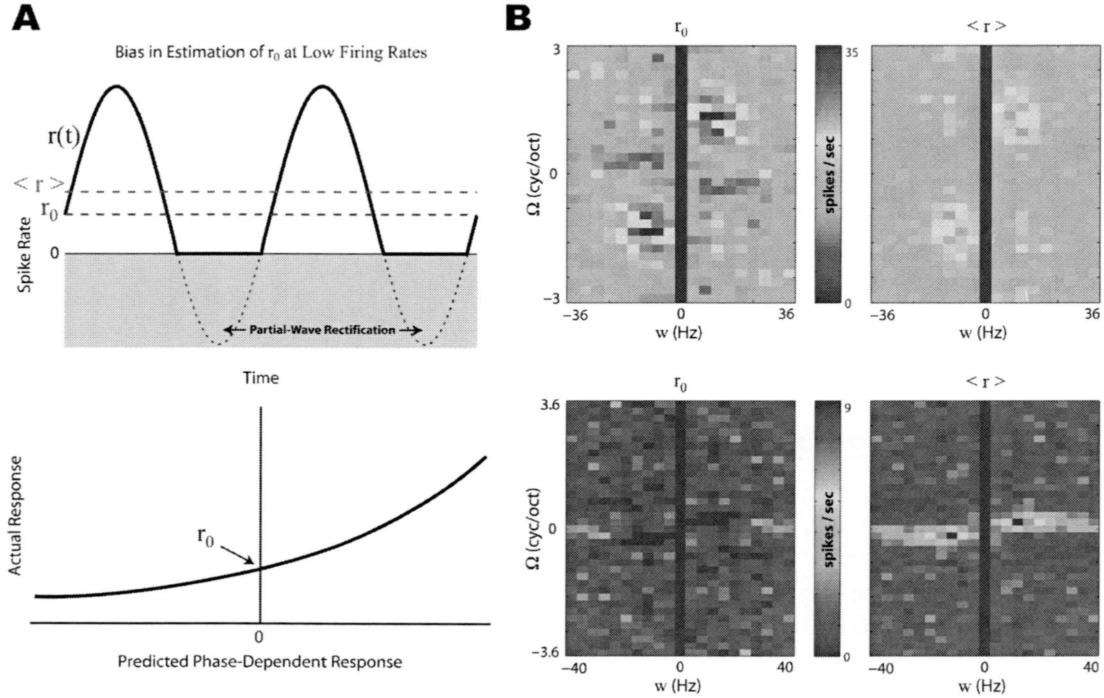


Figure 6. A. Given a neural response $r(t)$ consisting of a baseline firing rate ( $r_0$ ) which is modulated sinusoidally, the baseline rate can be computed as the mean amplitude. Top. However, with partial wave rectification, the mean amplitude $\langle r \rangle$ (red) overestimates the true baseline firing rate (blue). Bottom. Using a linear model, we predict the modulations in the neural response away from its baseline rate and compare it to the actual response. The baseline rate $r_0$ is measured as the neural response which occurs when the linear model predicts no modulation of the response. **B**. Measuring the baseline firing rate as the mean firing rate $\langle r \rangle$ (left column) results in estimation errors in the baseline firing rate. In some cases, measuring the mean firing rate obscures the $r_0$ response (top row), while in others, the mean firing rate measures artificial features which don't exist in $r_0$ (bottom row).

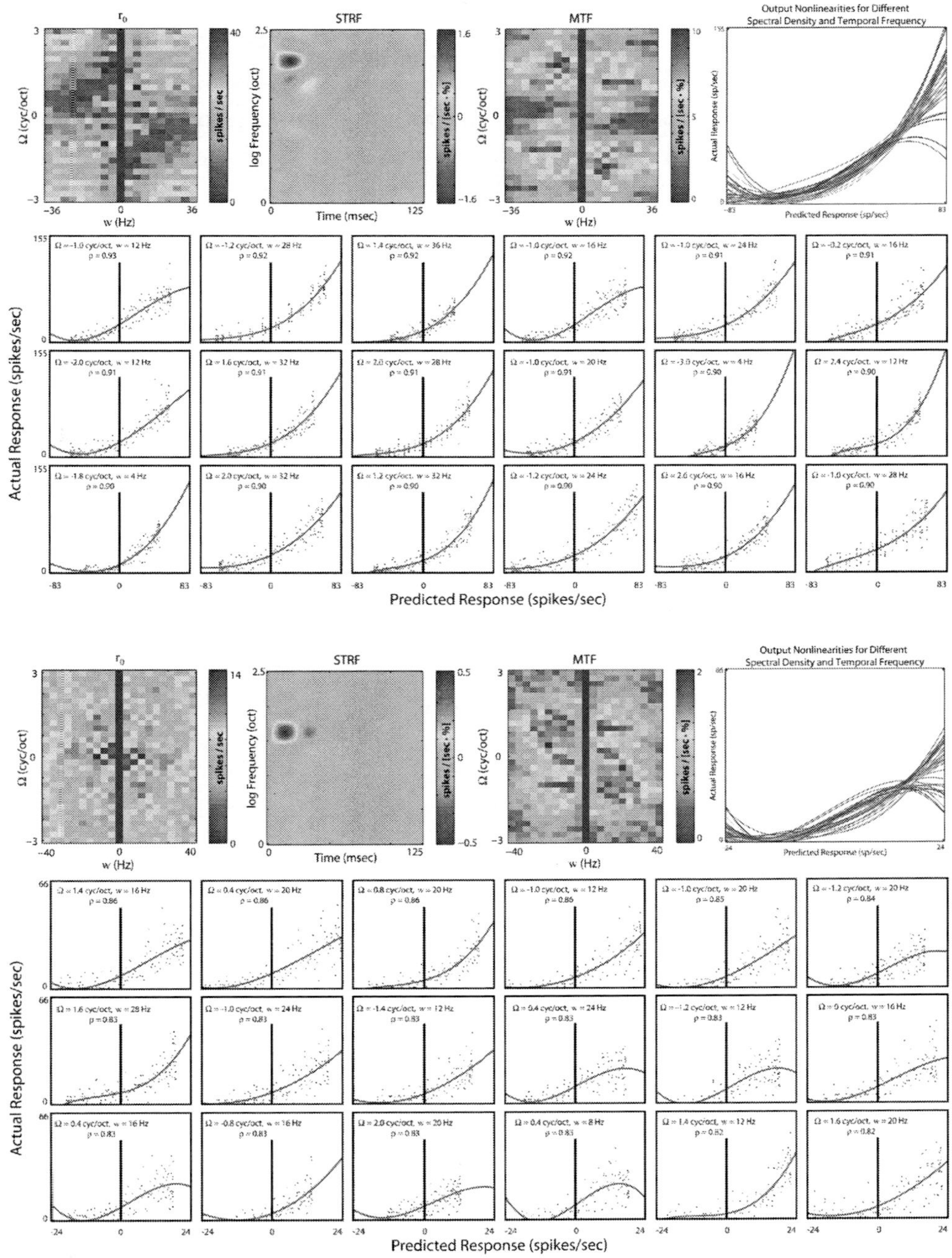


Figure 7. The phase-independent contrast response is measured for each spectral density and temporal periodicity presented in the auditory grating stimulus set. An output nonlinearity for each grating is computed by comparing the STRF predicted response to the actual response. $r_0$ is taken as the ordinate intersect of the output nonlinearity. Individual output nonlinearities are shown below for 18 auditory gratings, and all are overlaid (top right). The phase independent and phase dependent responses can be compared directly between $r_0$ and the MTF, respectively. For some cells, $r_0$ is inhibited for those stimuli to which the cell responds in a phase-dependent manner (top). In other cells, $r_0$ is enhanced for stimuli with a strong phase-dependent response (bottom).

An established measure of complex tuning is $f_1/f_0$ where $f_1$ and $f_0$ respectively refer to the first harmonic and DC (or average value) components of the Fourier transform of the response. This ratio measures the degree to which a neuron is phase locked to modulations in the stimulus relative to the degree to which the spiking rate is elevated irrespective of modulation phase [48, 49]. In order to use this metric to classify cells as simple or complex, their response must be either primarily phase-locked or primarily phase-independent [47-49]. While this is the case in V1, many cells in AI phase-lock reliably to stimulus modulations, making the standard measure of $f_1/f_0$ less than ideal for distinguishing phase-dependent from phase-independent tuning [14, 50]. In a recent study of phase-independent tuning in primary auditory cortex, [51] report that the distribution of $f_1/f_0$ is unimodal with a mean of 1. They find that for a large percentage of neurons, this ratio can be above 1 for some gratings and below 1 for others. The authors conclude that although significant nonlinearity exists in AI, there is no clear separation of cells based on simple and complex type responses.

However, the $f_0$ component of the response cannot be measured reliably in neurons that have low evoked firing rates and an appreciable response locked to stimulus modulations. The use of this approach in Ahmed et al. strongly biases their results (see Figure 6), which should be taken into account when interpreting their results. Trivial output nonlinearities, namely rectification at 0 spikes/sec, interfere with the measurement of the evoked firing rate (taken as the mean number of spikes per stimulus duration) during stimulus presentation. Any rectification induces an artificial elevation of the measured evoked rate and a decrease in the magnitude of the phase locked response (Figure 6). Despite the difficulty in measuring phase independent complexities in the response of AI neurons, it is plausible that such rate encodings of the sound environment co-exist with spike timing based schemes [48]. In the following, we explore phase-independent contrast tuning for cells in AI which also have reliable phase-locking responses.

## Measuring the Phase-Independent Contrast Response

The STRF measures modulations of the response away from a mean firing rate. Under ideal conditions, the phase-independent contrast response ($r_0$) can be measured by computing the mean firing rate ($f_0$) for the duration of the auditory grating stimulus. However, when the response rates are relatively low (as is often the case in AI), the response is subject to partial wave rectification due to the non-existence of negative spike counts. This will cause an over-estimation of $r_0$ ($f_0 > r_0$). A more robust estimate of $r_0$ can be obtained by determining the firing rate of the neuron when the phase-dependent component of the response is zero (Figure 6): using the STRF, we predict the response to each auditory grating stimulus. We find a polynomial fit between the predicted response and the actual response for every spectral density and temporal periodicity (third order polynomial was found sufficient). This polynomial fit is effectively an output nonlinearity function which depends on the stimulus. The zeroth order coefficient, where the fit intersects the ordinate, gives the correct sustained firing rate of the neuron in response to a grating of the same spatial density and temporal periodicity (i.e., $r_0$). In this manner, it is possible to measure the distinct phase dependent and independent responses which depend on the spectro-temporal statistics of the stimulus. In Figure 7, we show the individual nonlinearities for two different cells. Note that for cells without a reliable STRF but a reasonable rate of firing,, this measure of $r_0$ becomes equivalent to taking the mean rate during the entire stimulus presentation, since there is no modulation of the response by the stimulus spectro-temporal modulations and therefore no "crossing" of the zero spikes/second threshold.

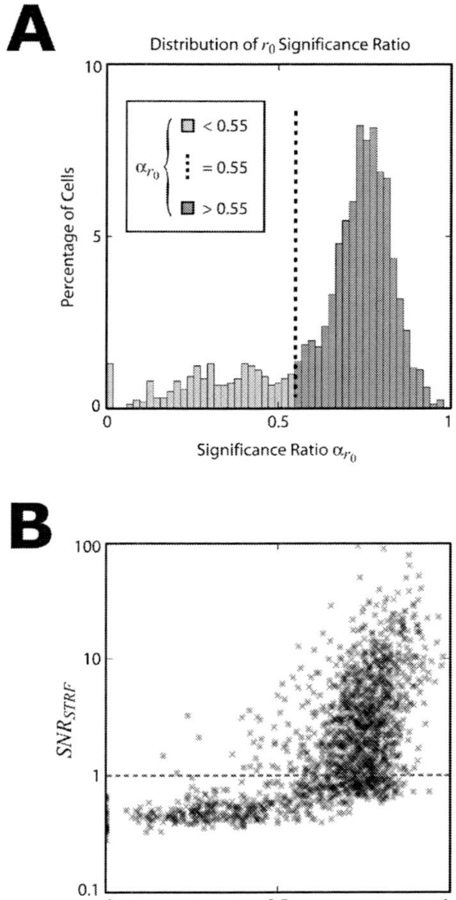


Figure 8. A. Distribution of $\alpha_{r_0}$. A significant phase independent response was defined as being modulated by changes in spectral density and temporal periodicity. For a given cell, the mean and standard deviation of $r_0$ was computed across spectral density and temporal periodicity. Of the points in $r_0$ which were at least 1 standard deviation away from its mean, $\alpha_{r_0}$ was computed as the fraction of points which were adjacent to other points that were also at least 1 standard deviation away from the mean. From this distribution, a critical value of $\alpha_{r_0} = 0.55$ was determined by visual inspection. 80% of cells had significant phase independent response determined by $\alpha_{r_0} > 0.55$. B. $SNR_{STRF}$ as a function of $\alpha_{r_0}$. Of the cells with significant $r_0$ tuning, 77% had significant STRF determined by $SNR_{STRF} > 1$.

Significance of the phase independent contrast tuning was defined on whether $r_0$ was modulated by changes in spectral density and temporal periodicity. For a given cell, we first found the mean and standard deviation of all values of $r_0$. Of the points in $r_0$ which were at least 1 standard deviation away from its mean, we determined the fraction of points which were adjacent to other points that were also at least 1 standard deviation away from the mean.

$$\alpha_{r_0} = \frac{\#\,\text{adjacent significant points}}{\#\,\text{significant points}} \tag{5.1}$$

Values of $\alpha_{r_0}$ near 1 imply significant phase independent responses, whereas values near 0 imply non-significant phase independent responses. We show the distribution of significance ratios $\alpha_{r_0}$ for the population of cells in Figure 8A. From this distribution, we set a critical value for $\alpha_{r_0}$ as 0.55—cells for which $\alpha_{r_0} > 0.55$ were classified as having significant phase-independent contrast response. The critical value was determined as a natural boundary from visual inspection of the $\alpha_{r_0}$ distribution. Based on this classification, 80% of cells had a phase-independent tuning which was significantly modulated by changes in spectral density and temporal periodicity of auditory gratings.

## Correlation of Phase-Independent and Phase-Dependent Responses

Of the cells which had a significantly modulated $r_0$ tuning, 77% also had significant phase dependent tuning, as determined by their STRF with $SNR_{STRF} > 1$. Figure 8B shows this SNR as a function of the $r_0$ tuning significance ratio. Since each point in $r_0$ corresponds to a specific spectral density $\Omega$ and temporal periodicity $w$, it follows that we should compare the phase-independent $r_0$ tuning to the phase-dependent tuning of that same grating (in terms of spectral density $\Omega$ and temporal periodicity $w$) as measured in the STRF.

From empirical observation, STRFs in AI were generally either low-pass or band-pass with higher response power at low spectral densities and temporal periodicities. However, many cells demonstrated an opposite effect in $r_0$: These responses were generally high-pass in that they display a reduced $r_0$ for low spectral densities and temporal periodicities and relatively higher overall firing rate for high spectral densities and temporal periodicities.

In order to compare phase-independent and phase-dependent responses, we computed the correlation coefficient between a template function (*T*) corresponding to a high-pass, distributed response and these two measures of the neural response as a function of spectral density $\Omega$ and temporal periodicity $w$: 1) the phase-independent response $r_0$ and 2) the magnitude of the grating responses $|MTF(\Omega, w)|$, where the MTF is the 2-dimensional Fourier transform of the STRF, such that:

$$T(\Omega, w) = \left|\frac{\Omega}{\Omega_{max}}\right| + \left|\frac{w}{w_{max}}\right|$$

The template T has higher values for high spectral density and temporal periodicity. Positive correlation values between T and the MTF or between T and $r_0$ indicate stronger responses at high spatial densities and temporal periodicities. Conversely, negative correlation values indicate stronger responses at low spatial densities and temporal periodicities.

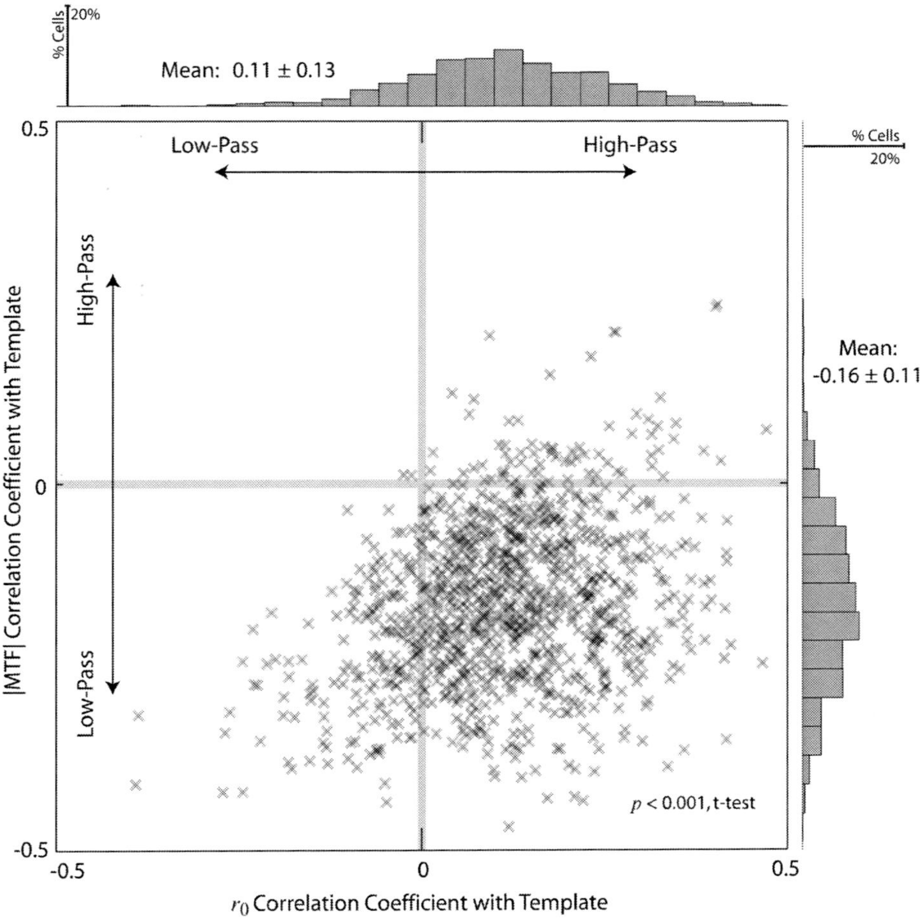


Figure 9. The localization of phase-dependent tuning and the phase-independent ($r_0$) tuning were compared by computing the coefficients of their correlation with a high-pass, decentralized template $T$. Correlation values greater than 0 indicate stronger responses to high spectral densities and high temporal periodicities (either as an increased average firing for $r_0$ or an increased phase-dependent tuning measured by the STRF). Conversely, correlation values less than 0 indicate stronger responses to low spectral densities and low temporal periodicities. The marginal distributions of correlation coefficients are depicted on their respective axes. These two distributions were significantly different ( $p < 0.001$, t-test). The majority of cells (75%) responded with increased baseline firing rates for high spectral densities and temporal periodicities, and increased phase dependent tuning at for low spectral densities and temporal periodicities.

Figure 9 shows the joint distribution of template correlation values for phase-dependent and phase-independent tuning and their marginals. The mean correlation value for the phase-independent tuning was $0.11 \pm 0.13$ and the mean correlation value for the phase-dependent tuning was $-0.16 \pm 0.11$. These two distributions were significantly different ( $p < 0.001$, t-test). These results match the empirical observations that phase-dependent responses were generally centralized to low spectral densities and temporal periodicities, whereas phase-independent responses were generally distributed to higher spectral densities and temporal periodicities. Of the cells with both significant phase-dependent and phase-independent tunings, 75% of cells showed this mismatched distribution of the response. The remaining cells showed the opposite effect where the these two tunings were either both centralized (at low $\Omega, w$) or both distributed (to high $\Omega, w$).

## Stationarity of the Mean Response in the STRF Model

Auditory gratings are constructed as a broadband noise carrier which is then modulated in spectrum and time according to the spectral density and temporal periodicity. The formulation of the STRF model attributes the baseline firing rate as a response to the underlying noise carrier; modulations in the firing rate away from that baseline rate are attributed to the modulations in the stimulus spectro-temporal envelope [11, 23, 45]. In other words, in this linear model, the baseline firing rate is assumed constant with respect to changing statistics *in the envelope*. While this is good as a first approximation, the results of this study show that $r_0$ *is* influenced by the spectro-temporal statistics of the modulation envelope. Furthermore, even for a single measurement of $r_0$, taking the mean firing rate during stimulus presentation will overestimate the true evoked firing rate due at the very least to the effects of partial wave rectification.

## "Complex" Type Cells in Primary Auditory Cortex

While much of the literature regarding simple and complex cells classifies cells as belonging exclusively to one type or the other, we find many cells which show both phase-dependent and phase-independent tuning simultaneously. Despite the prevalence of cells with concurrent phase dependent and independent tuning, we also find cells which have significant modulation of their $r_0$ tuning, but relatively unreliable phase-locking (as measured by low SNR, Figure 8B). These cells respond like the complex cells described in the visual literature. They show poor phase-locking to the stimulus modulation envelope, and as such, their STRF (if it exists) is relatively noisy. However, their structured $r_0$ tuning indicates a rate encoding of their preference for specific spatial densities and temporal periodicities. In Figure 10, we depict a number of example tunings of this type.

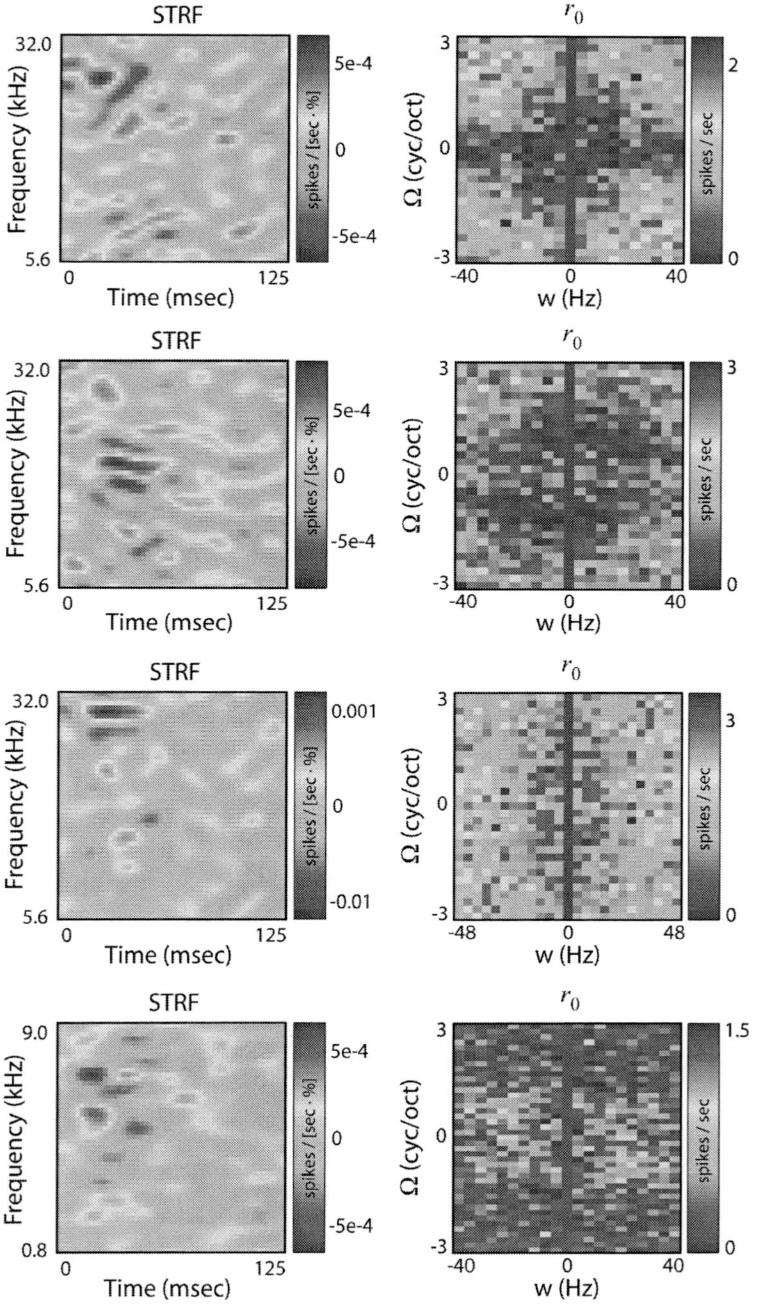


Figure 10. We find cells with significant phase independent tuning, but poor phase dependent tuning (in contrast to those cells which exhibited both phase independent and phase dependent tuning concurrently). These are analogous to complex cells of visual cortex that respond to a grating stimulus with a change in baseline firing rate irrespective of stimulus phase (i.e., their responses are not modulated with stimulus phase). We show STRF and $r_0$ characterizations for 4 example cells with complex responses. While these example cells show some phase specificity with some discernible features in their STRFs, they have a high degree of noise and low reliability. In this sense, these cells may not be complex in the strict sense, but have characteristics strongly resembling the complex response pattern.

### Functional Significance of Phase-Independent Tuning

Given that a large percentage of cells show both phase-dependent and phase-independent responses, we investigated how the two modalities related to each other. These two encoding schemes may be used to convey separate information, or alternatively, they may perform a cooperative role in conveying the same information. For the majority of cells (75%), the phase-independent tuning was inversely related to the phase-dependent tuning. In other words, for those stimulus modulations which elicited strong phase-locked responses, the baseline firing rate generally decreased. The converse was true for the remaining 25% of cells whereby strong phase-locking was correlated with an increase in baseline firing.

The different classes of tuning for $r_0$ (with respect to phase-locked tuning) may effectively serve to enhance the signal-to-noise in the neural output. The reduced baseline firing rate for well phase-locked modulations might suppress uncorrelated neural activity which does not convey information about the stimulus (modulations). Alternatively, an increase in baseline firing for well phase-locked stimulus modulations may raise the set point of neural firing in order to ensure transmission of information regarding the stimulus.

The phase-independent tuning represents an increase in the generality of responses. Whereas phase-dependent tuning measures responses to specific stimulus modulations under very specific constraints, changes in the overall firing rate indicate the mere presence of those stimulus modulations, irrespective of their exact placement on the spectral axis. This type of response could be the foundation for extracting sound input structure (such as vowels, or even consonant-vowel transitions) independent of the sound source.

## Conclusion

A lot of progress has been made in the last couple of decades to characterize primary cortical neurons in terms of naturalistic sounds with the use of primarily linear system methods. This has led to deep insight into the computations performed by the auditory system to detect, extract and identify particular sound streams in noisy and cluttered environments [52, 53]. While the linear methods that lead the characterization of neurons in terms of STRFs by multiple methods [13, 54, 55] are quite effective at describing neurons and predicting their response to new sounds, we need to better understand the nature of the full, non-linear, time-frequency representation used by the brain [56]. Most of the recent neurophysiological evidence points to the function of (primary) auditory cortex as generating a time-frequency representation, which is essential for segregating sources because of its robustness in noisy, cluttered environments with multiple, possibly moving components.

To summarize this chapters in just a few informal sentences, we found that at very short time-scales, comparable to the shortest timescales of running speech, auditory cortex neurons encode time-frequency content in a way that allows for the differentiation of any “consonant-vowel” or “vowel-vowel” transition. This differentiation in tuning to features often occurs at the shortest time scale we can use. At medium timescales of the order of tens to hundreds of milliseconds, important non-linearities can be uncovered. These non-linearities might be important in extracting the spectro-temporal envelope of a sound source in a noisy environment. In further work, we show that a careful analysis shows the existence of tuning to spectro-temporal content irrespective of its location on the tonotopic axis, similar to the complex cells of the visual pathway. This could lead to encoding of sound independently of the source, so that for instance the sound /ah/ will be encoded the same way whether spoken by a young person or an adult male. Finally, we found that over long timescales of the order of many seconds, receptive field are quite stable even in a passive listening situation though they display some systematic adaptation changes that are small but significant. In more details:

Evidence for a complex and well adapted time-frequency representation were presented throughout this chapter. When we considered spectro-temporal tuning over very short time-scales of the order of a few milliseconds, we found that tuning emerges almost instantaneously. For example, cortical cells were able to differentiate between envelopes modulated at 5Hz and 10Hz long before a full cycle had been presented. On the one hand, this is not surprising since the phonemic rate in most languages is of the order of 10Hz [57] - but it is remarkable that cells are essentially tuned as soon as one might expect them to be detecting and identifying features of sounds. This is a necessary requirement for an auditory processing system, as tuning to such features must emerge at least as fast as those features occur. In particular, models that would measure tuning purely based on Fourier analysis of the input would fail to accurately represent the complexity of the cortical representation. This cortical time-frequency representation achieves a better spectro-temporal resolution than woud be expected from a purely Fourier analysis.

In addition to the tuning dynamics being so remarkable at short timescales, the spectro-temporal tuning is comparatively stable over long timescales. This came as more of a surprise than the immediacy of short-term tuning, since background irrelevant sounds with unchanging spectro-temporal content are perceptually ignored or “adapted out” rather quickly (such as the sound of a computer fan in the background). However, if AI functions as a cortical front-end for further processing, such higher order changes in neural tuning might be detrimental. For down-stream use, the output of AI should likely be stable in what it represents. Adaptation of the background components of the auditory environment could easily be controlled from a higher order center, whose center of focus (a specific sound source, such as a speaker) might be directed by attention. In this way, having a stable, non-adapting tuning at the level of AI provides a good universal “front-end” for further processing, which then provides “higher processing centers” stable basis functions to further process the auditory scene. This can also enable the creation of an efficient and sparse encoding of the input. Alternatively, this might even allow for shifting the basis dynamically (through reciprocal/down/up/stream control) to suit the current needs of the system as the environment changes.

Building upon this idea, we found evidence for “complex cell” (phase-independent) responses in AI, which can provide a good basis for constructing a neural representation of sound independent of the source that produced them. This could thus serve as a stable basis function that allows for sparsification of the input, identifying spectro-temporal features irrespective of their placement along the tonotopic axis. Such an invariance relates directly to generalization across size-scaling of the sound source: in the case in speech, a change in the size of the speaker mostly results in a linear shift of the activity pattern generated along the tonotopic axis. However, it still remains to show that the output of these complex cells is used to provide such a source independent representation of sounds. Furthermore, one would need to show that complex cells can operate and provide a useful representation of the auditory environment on the timescales typical of natural sounds and speech.

Further research along the lines presented in this chapter is needed to truly understand the function of auditory cortex, especially in how it performs a noise-robust processing of the auditory scene. The performance of computer models in particularly challenging environments is not on par with the performance of humans in similar situations: this translates also to patients with hearing loss. While their deficit might generally be thought of in terms of a reduced sensitivity to sound, they typically also lack the ability of easily segregate sound sources in challenging environments. Understanding what features of the auditory scene are used for creating a noise-robust sensory representation could lead to the development of better speech processing algorithms and assistive listening devices.

A number of important directions to take in this vein of research stand out: In particular, how optimal is the time-frequency representation that emerges in AI in terms of its being advantageous to solving situations such as seen in the cocktail party effect (the ability to focus on a particular sound stream in a noisy environment)? How is tuning affected by attention or by the presence of multiple sources? Does the output of AI modify in a measurable way the neural activity in lower auditory centers, such as the inferior colliculus of the midbrain or the medial geniculate of the thalamus? Can the functional circuitry that leads to the results presented in this chapters be predicted from detailed models? We hope to address these questions in the near future.

## References

[1] Ferrier D. On the Localisation of the Functions of the Brain. *British medical journal*. 1874 Dec 19;2(729):766-7.

[2] Chi T, Gao Y, Guyton MC, Ru P, Shamma S. Spectro-temporal modulation transfer functions and speech intelligibility. *Journal of the Acoustical Society of America*. 1999 Nov;106(5):2719-32.

[3] Klein DJ, König P, Körding KP. Sparse spectrotemporal coding of sounds. *EURASIP Journal on Applied Signal Processing* 2003:659-67.

[4] Attias H, Schreiner CE. Low-order temporal statistics of natural sounds. *Advances in Neural Information Processing Systems*. 1997;9:27-33.

[5] Bieser A, Muller-Preuss P. Auditory responsive cortex in the squirrel monkey: neural responses to amplitude-modulated sounds. *Experimental Brain Research*. 1996;108(2): 273-84.

[6] Eggermont JJ. Between sound and perception: reviewing the search for a neural code. *Hear Res*. 2001 Jul;157(1-2):1-42.

[7] Kowalski N, Depireux DA, Shamma SA. Analysis of dynamic spectra in ferret primary auditory cortex. I. Characteristics of single-unit responses to moving ripple spectra. *Journal of Neurophysiology*. 1996;76(5):3503-23.

[8] Liang L, Lu T, Wang X. Neural representations of sinusoidal amplitude and frequency modulations in the primary auditory cortex of awake primates. *Journal of Neurophysiology*. 2002;87(5):2237-61.

[9] Schreiner CE, Urbas JV. Representation of amplitude modulation in the auditory cortex of the cat. II. Comparison between cortical fields. *Hear Res*. 1988 Jan;32(1):49-63.

[10] Schreiner CE, Urbas JV. Representation of amplitude modulation in the auditory cortex of the cat. I. The anterior auditory field (AAF). *Hear Res*. 1986;21(3):227-41.

[11] Marmarelis PZ, Marmarelis VZ. Analysis of physiological systems: The white-noise approach. New York: Plenum Press 1978.

[12] Eggermont JJ, Aertsen AM, Johannesma PI. Quantitative characterisation procedure for auditory neurons based on the spectro-temporal receptive field. *Hear Res*. 1983 May; 10(2):167-90.

[13] Escabi MA, Schreiner CE. Nonlinear spectrotemporal sound analysis by neurons in the auditory midbrain. *Journal of Neuroscience*. 2002 May 15;22(10):4114-31.

[14] Depireux DA, Simon JZ, Klein DJ, Shamma SA. Spectro-temporal response field characterization with dynamic ripples in ferret primary auditory cortex. *JNeurophys*. 2001;85(3):1220-34.

[15] Linden JF, Liu RC, Sahani M, Schreiner CE, Merzenich MM. Spectrotemporal structure of receptive fields in areas AI and AAF of mouse auditory cortex. *Journal of Neurophysiology*. 2003 Oct;90(4):2660-75.

[16] Schreiner CE, Calhoun BM. Spectral envelope coding in cat primary auditory cortex:Properties of ripple transfer functions. *Aud. Neurosci*. 1994;1:39-61.

[17] Shamma SA, Versnel H. Ripple analysis in ferret primary auditory cortex: II. Prediction of unit responses to arbitrary spectral profiles. *Aud. Neurosci*. 1995;1:255-70.

[18] Evans EF, Whitfield IC. Classification of Unit Responses in the Auditory Cortex of the Unanaesthetized and Unrestrained Cat. *The Journal of physiology*. 1964 Jun;171:476-93.

[19] Wang X, Lu T, Snider RK, Liang L. Sustained firing in auditory cortex evoked by preferred stimuli. *Nature*. 2005 May 19;435(7040):341-6.

[20] Bredfeldt CE, Ringach DL. Dynamics of spatial frequency tuning in macaque V1. *J. Neurosci*. 2002 Mar 1;22(5):1976-84.

[21] Simon JZ, Depireux DA, Klein DJ, Fritz JB, Shamma SA. Temporal symmetry in primary auditory cortex: implications for cortical connectivity. *Neural computation*. 2007 Mar;19(3):583-638.

[22] Shechter B, Marvit P, Depireux DA. Lagged cells in the inferior colliculus of the awake ferret. *The European journal of neuroscience*. 2010 Jan;31(1):42-8.

[23] Kowalski N, Depireux DA, Shamma SA. Analysis of dynamic spectra in ferret primary auditory cortex. II. Prediction of unit responses to arbitrary dynamic spectra. *Journal of Neurophysiology*. 1996;76(5):3524-34.

[24] Shechter B, Dobbins HD, Marvit P, Depireux DA. Dynamics of spectro-temporal tuning in primary auditory cortex of the awake ferret. *Hear Res*. 2009 Oct;256(1-2):118-30.

[25] Abdi H. Encyclopedia of Measurement and Statistics. In: Salkind NJ, ed. *Thousand Oaks (*CA): Sage 2007:907-12.

[26] Klein DJ, Simon JZ, Depireux DA, Shamma SA. Stimulus-invariant processing and spectrotemporal reverse correlation in primary auditory cortex. *J. Comput. Neurosci*. 2006 Apr;20(2):111-36.

[27] Mastronarde DN. Two classes of single-input X-cells in cat lateral geniculate nucleus. II. Retinal inputs and the generation of receptive-field properties. *J. Neurophysiol.* 1987 Feb;57(2):381-413.

[28] Mastronarde DN. Two classes of single-input X-cells in cat lateral geniculate nucleus. I. Receptive-field properties and classification of cells. *J. Neurophysiol.* 1987 Feb;57(2): 357-80.

[29] Saul AB, Humphrey AL. Spatial and temporal response properties of lagged and nonlagged cells in cat lateral geniculate nucleus. *Journal of Neurophysiology*. 1990 Jul;64(1):206-24.

[30] Galazyuk AV, Lin W, Llano D, Feng AS. Leading inhibition to neural oscillation is important for time-domain processing in the auditory midbrain. *Journal of Neurophysiology*. 2005 Jul;94(1):314-26.

[31] Sullivan WE, 3rd. Possible neural mechanisms of target distance coding in auditory system of the echolocating bat Myotis lucifugus. *J. Neurophysiol.* 1982 Oct;48(4):1033-47.

[32] Lim HH, Anderson DJ. Antidromic activation reveals tonotopically organized projections from primary auditory cortex to the central nucleus of the inferior colliculus in guinea pig. *J. Neurophysiol.* 2006 Dec 6.

[33] Bajo VM, Nodal FR, Bizley JK, Moore DR, King AJ. The Ferret Auditory Cortex: Descending Projections to the Inferior Colliculus. *Cereb. Cortex*. 2006 Mar 31.

[34] Shechter B, Depireux DA. Stability of spectro-temporal tuning over several seconds in primary auditory cortex of the awake ferret. *Neuroscience*. 2007;148(3):806-14.

[35] Shechter B, Depireux DA. Response adaptation to broadband sounds in primary auditory cortex of the awake ferret. *Hear Res*. 2006 Nov;221(1-2):91-103.

[36] Smirnakis SM, Berry MJ, Warland DK, Bialek W, Meister M. Adaptation of retinal processing to image contrast and spatial scale. *Nature*. 1997 Mar 6;386(6620):69-73.

[37] Kvale MN, Schreiner CE. Short-term adaptation of auditory receptive fields to dynamic stimuli. *Journal of Neurophysiology*. 2004 Feb;91(2):604-12.

[38] Baccus SA, Meister M. Fast and slow contrast adaptation in retinal circuitry. *Neuron*. 2002 Dec 5;36(5):909-19.

[39] Crowder NA, Price NS, Hietanen MA, Dreher B, Clifford CW, Ibbotson MR. Relationship between contrast adaptation and orientation tuning in V1 and V2 of cat visual cortex. *J. Neurophysiol.* 2006 Jan;95(1):271-83.

[40] Kohn A, Movshon JA. Adaptation changes the direction tuning of macaque MT neurons. *Nat. Neurosci*. 2004 Jul;7(7):764-72.

[41] Wang T, Ozdamar O, Bohorquez J, Shen Q, Cheour M. Wiener filter deconvolution of overlapping evoked potentials. *Journal of neuroscience methods*. 2006 Dec 15;158(2): 260-70.

[42] Irvine DR. Auditory cortical plasticity: Does it provide evidence for cognitive processing in the auditory cortex? *Hear Res*. 2007 Jan 16.

[43] Weinberger NM. Auditory associative memory and representational plasticity in the primary auditory cortex. *Hear Res*. 2007 Jan 17.

[44] Fritz J, Elhilali M, Shamma S. Active listening: task-dependent plasticity of spectrotemporal receptive fields in primary auditory cortex. *Hear Res*. 2005 Aug;206(1-2):159-76.

[45] Elhilali M, Fritz JB, Klein DJ, Simon JZ, Shamma SA. Dynamics of precise spike timing in primary auditory cortex. *Journal of Neuroscience*. 2004 Feb 4;24(5):1159-72.

[46] Norena AJ, Gourevitch B, Pienkowski M, Shaw G, Eggermont JJ. Increasing spectrotemporal sound density reveals an octave-based organization in cat primary auditory cortex. *J. Neurosci*. 2008 Sep 3;28(36):8885-96.

[47] Hubel DH, Wiesel TN. Receptive Fields and Functional Architecture in Two Nonstriate Visual Areas (18 and 19) of the Cat. *J. Neurophysiol*. 1965 Mar;28:229-89.

[48] Movshon JA, Thompson ID, Tolhurst DJ. Receptive field organization of complex cells in the cat's striate cortex. *The Journal of physiology*. 1978 Oct;283:79-99.

[49] Movshon JA, Thompson ID, Tolhurst DJ. Spatial summation in the receptive fields of simple cells in the cat's striate cortex. *The Journal of physiology*. 1978 Oct;283:53-77.

[50] Depireux DA, Ji YD, Powell EM, Shechter B. Changes in Inferior Colliculus Activity of the Rat Induced by Tinnitus Advances in tinntius assessment, treatment and neuroscience basis; 2007; Grand Island, NY; 2007. p. P3.

[51] Ahmed B, Garcia-Lazaro JA, Schnupp JW. Response linearity in primary auditory cortex of the ferret. *The Journal of physiology*. 2006 May 1;572(Pt 3):763-73.

[52] Shamma S. Neural and Functional Models of the Auditory Cortex. In: Arbib M, ed. *Handbook of Brain Theory and Neural Networks (2nd Edition)*. Boston, MA: Bradford Books, MIT Press 2003.

[53] Depireux DA, Varma S, Baras J, Srour N, Pham T. Vehicle Classification Using Acoustic Data Based on Biology Hearing Models and Multiscale Vector Quantization. Federated Lab00; 2000; College Park, MD; 2000.

[54] deCharms RC, Blake DT, Merzenich MM. Optimizing sound features for cortical neurons.[see comment]. *Science*. 1998;280(5368):1439-43.

[55] Valentine PA, Eggermont JJ. Stimulus dependence of spectro-temporal receptive fields in cat primary auditory cortex. *Hear Res*. 2004 Oct;196(1-2):119-33.

[56] Cohen L. Time-frequency analysis: theory and applications Upper Saddle River, NJ: Prentice-Hall 1995.

[57] Liberman AM, Cooper FS, Shankweiler DP, Studdert-Kennedy M. Perception of the speech code. *Psychol. Rev*. 1967 Nov;74(6):431-61.

In: Auditory Cortex: Anatomy, Functions and Disorders
Editor: Mounya Elhilali
ISBN 978-1-62100-685-5


*Chapter VI*

# Interstimulus Interval-Dependent Categorical Perception in Audition: Findings and a Hypothesis of the Role for the Primary Auditory Cortex

***Masashi Sakai****
Department of Physiology, Interdisciplinary Graduate School of Medicine and Engineering, University of Yamanashi, Yamanashi, Japan

## Abstract

Perception of plosive consonant-vowel syllables is "categorical" (ex., /da/–/ta/ phonemes). That is, as the interval from the consonant release to voicing onset (i.e., voice onset time [VOT]) is prolonged above a critical value (20-40 ms), perceived quality drastically alters from "voiced" (/da/) to "voiceless" (/ta/) with nothing in between. Such characteristic is obviously beneficial to increase variability of perceived phoneme categories with securing perceptual consistency within the same category. A growing body of evidence indicates that VOT-dependent categorical perception does not necessarily arise from a specific human speech mechanism but is rather based on general properties of the auditory system across species. Thus, neurophysiology analysis of animal brains is expected to provide valuable insights into neural processes underlying categorical perception of human phonemes. Here, I introduce several lines of evidence converging into the notion that VOT-dependent categorical perception is mediated by a subset of primary auditory cortex (AI) neurons with the capacity for stimulus locking. Stimulus-response characteristics of those neurons were well captured by our computational model which incorporates the temporal interplay of the excitatory and inhibitory post-synaptic potentials (EPSPs and IPSPs) in the AI along with short-term plasticity of thalamocortical synaptic connections.

* Corresponding author: Tel: +81-55-273-9486, Fax: +81-55-273-6731. E-mail: msakai@yamanashi.ac.jp.

# 1. Introduction

## 1.1. Examples of Two Perception Modes in Vision

"Continuous perception" and "categorical perception" are two major perception modes operating in the visual, auditory and somatosensory systems, whereby sensory signals are differentiated along a physical continuum(s) (reviewed by Harnad, 1987). First of all, as the most contrastive examples of such two perceptual modes, I introduce two color schemes.

Figure 1A schematizes the result of psychophysical experiment on "achromatic" color scheme (Festinger et al., 1971): a color series lacking hue but only brightness (including only black, gray and white). Physical magnitude of brightness, called luminance, varies along sRGB grayscale from 0 to 250 (abscissa). The corresponding perceived intensity, called *lightness*, gradually and smoothly elevates from 0 to 100 (in Cielab L*; ordinate). Such relationship is referred to as "continuous perception" and can be approximated by Weber-Fechner's law (Weber, 1834; Fechner, 1860):

$$R = k \log (S/S_0) \qquad \text{(equation \#1)}$$

where R is the perceived intensity, k is a constant fraction, S is the physical magnitude, and $S_0$ is the absolute threshold below which the stimulus is not perceived at all. This logarithmic relationship means that if the S varies in a geometric progression (i.e., multiplied by a fixed factor), the R changes in an arithmetic progression (i.e., in additive constant amounts). For example, in Figure 1A, if the luminance is tripled from ~50 to 150 along sRGB grayscale (i.e., 3 x 1), the lightness elevates from 40 to 80 in Ceilab L* (i.e., 1 + 1 = 2) (dotted lines). Stevens (1957) argued that the relationship between stimulus intensity (S) and sensation magnitude (R) can be more accurately describe by power functions:

$$R = kS^a \qquad \text{(equation \#2)}$$

where a is the power exponent whose value depends on the sensory modality and stimulus conditions. Whatever approximation is adopted, "continuous perception" is omnipresent perceptual experience and in audition it holds to number of dimensions such as *loudness* (Stevens, 1936), *pitch* (Stevens et al., 1937), *duration* (Michon, 1964) and so forth (reviewed by Gescheider, 1988).

Figure 1B illustrates the result of human psychophysical experiment on "chromatic" color scheme: a color that has *hue,* as like in rainbow (Gordon and Abramov, 1988; see legend for detail). In physics, chromatic colors differ only in wavelength which extends along a continuum (abscissa). Nonetheless, perceived colors change in an abrupt way into a number of "perceptual categories" labeled as violet, blue, green, yellow, red and so forth. For example, a pair of colors belonging to different categories (B2 [blue] and G1 [green], G2 [green] and Y [yellow], or Y and R1 [red]; all are separated with the same wavelength distance [ΔI], same as following) are more accurately and fast discriminated than the pairs belonging to the same category (B1 and B2 [blues], G1 and G2 [greens], R1 and R2 [reds]). Categorical perception is defined as such subjective experience to qualitatively differentiate a set of signals with equal-sized physical differences by compressing similarities or expanding differences depending on whether the signals belong to the same or different category, respectively.

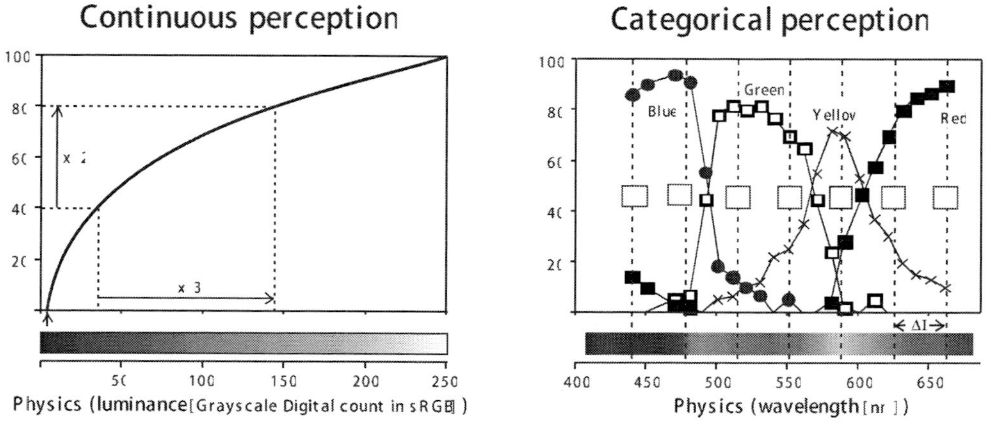


Figure 1. Example of continuous perception (A) and categorical perception (B) in vision. A: In achromatic colors, conversion from maximal black to maximal white along digital sRGB metric *(abscissa)* leads to gradual and quantitative change in perceived degrees of lightness indexed by CIE lightness metric, Cielab $L*$ (*ordinate*). B: *In* chromatic colors, a physical continuum of wavelength between 400 to 700 nm (*abscissa*) leads to perception of discreet color categories labeled as violet, blue (B1, B2), green (G1 , G2), yellow (Y), orange through red (R1, R2). The curves represent psychometric function reported by Gordon and Abramov (1988); observers stated percentages of their sensations (*ordinate*) for each wavelength using any combination of four hue term (blue, green, yellow and red) for a total of 100%. There is very little overlap between blue and yellow, or between green and red, indicating mutually exclusive perceptual quality within the pairs. See text for details.

## 1.2. Categorical Perception in Audition: Voice Onset Time (VOT) Dependence

In audition, one of the most intensively investigated cases of categorical perception is for English plosive, or oral stop, consonants such as /b/, /d/, /g/, /p/, /t/, /k/ (reviewed by Lieberman et al., 1967; Eimas, 1982; Kuhl, 1986). Categorical perception occurs when those consonants are presented in the context of consonant-vowel syllable (hereafter, plosive CV-syllable) such as /da/ and /ta/.

### *1.2.1. Physical Properties and Articulation Gesture of Plosive CV Syllables*

For better understanding of categorical perception of plosive CV-syllables, I provide a brief overview of their physical characteristics in relation to articulation gesture (based on Fant, 1960 and Stevens, 2000). The waveform (Figure 2A, upper trace) and spectrogram (lower trace) of /da/ and /ta/ have four major hallmarks, called (1) *closure*, (2) *release* (or *noise burst*), (3) *voicing* (or *vowel*), and (4) *voice onset time* (*VOT*).

*Closure* (Figure 2B-2) refers to the moment when the air flow, exhaled from the lungs, is completely occluded by the articulator such as alveolar ridge and tongue tip in this case. As a consequence, air pressure behind the closed articulator is progressively built up. *Release* (B-3) begins at the moment when the tongue tip is slightly lowered, creating a narrow crevice.

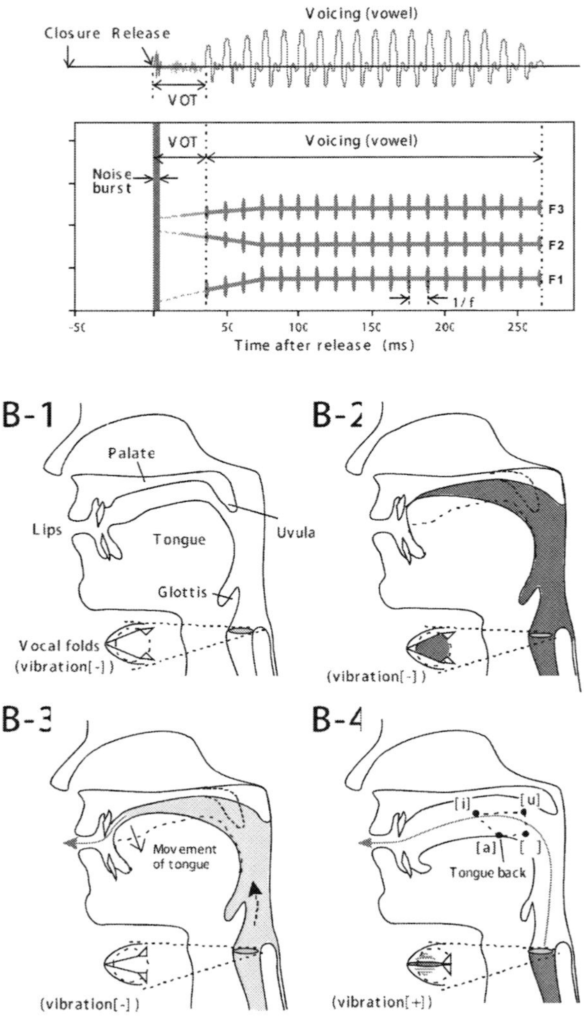


Figure 2. A: Schematized waveform (*upper*) and spectrogram (*lower*) of plosive consonant-vowel (CV) syllable. B: Midsaggital configuration of the vocal tract during steady state (-1) and articulation of the CV-syllable (-2 to -4) (the inset representing axial view of the vocal folds). The signal comprises several physical hallmarks that reflect distinct articulation processes namely *closure*, *release* (*noise burst*), *voicing* and *voice onset time (VOT)*. *Closure* (A, B-2): the airway closes so that no air can escape through the nose or mouth, raising pressure (marked with gray) behind the closure. The occlusion of the mouth is formed by a particular set of articulators – alveolar ridge and tongue tip in the present case (alveolar /d, t/). *Release* (A, B-3): downward movement of the tongue tip (solid arrow) creates a narrow crevice, through which air explosively passes with generating brief turbulence. Such turbulence produces audible *noise burst* (marked with blue) with its amplitude reaching the maximum within 1-2 ms. (Another minute turbulence noise is potentially generated by the glottis being in an open position [*aspiration noise*, broken arrow]). *Voicing* (A, B-4): the configuration of the glottis and the stiffness of the vocal folds are adjusted to permit continued vocal-folds vibration, which creates source sound of vowel (marked with red). As the sound passes through the vocal tract, particular frequency components are either enhanced or diminished. In spectral domain, the resultant acoustic energy comprises several bands, called "formants." The ratios of the center frequencies of the first three formants (F1, F2 and F3) play a prominent role in perception of the vowel. "*Voice onset time* (*VOT*)" (A), referred to as the interval between the onset of release and that of voicing, serves as a critical dimension in categorical perception of the plosive CV-syllables (see text).

Thought it, airflow explosively spouts out as turbulence, giving rise to audible *noise burst* whose amplitude reaches the peak within 1-2 ms after its onset. *Voicing* (B-4) is a product of the vibration of vocal-folds (marked with red; the vibration rate is referred to as "fundamental frequency [f0]"]). While the sound energy travels through the vocal tract, particular frequency components are either enhanced or diminished depending on resonance characteristics of local cavities such as larynx, pharynx, mouth and nose. In spectral domain, the resultant energy comprises several bands, named "formants" (F1, F2 and F3; Figure 2A, bottom). *VOT* corresponds to time difference between the onset of *release* and *voicing*. As will be further described below, *VOT* differs among naturally spoken /da/ and /ta/: in /da/, *voicing* starts almost simultaneously with *release* and continues throughout the syllable, thus *VOT* is close to zero; in /ta/, *voicing* does not start until well after *release*, thus *VOT* tends to be longer.

### 1.2.2. Early Studies on Categorical Perception of Plosive CV Syllables

Psychophysical studies on categorical perception of plosive CV syllables have conventionally taken advantage of using a speech synthesizer that can generate tokens of the syllables with variable VOT. Figure 3A exemplifies synthesized tokens of /da/ and /ta/ whose VOT was shifted from -10 to +60 ms with 10-ms steps; a negative value indicates *voicing* (marked with red line) precedes *release* (blue line).

Figure 3B schematically draws the mean performance of native English speakers in two versions of psychophysical experiments (i.e., labeling task and discrimination task) that were made using /da/-/ta/ tokens (based on Lisker and Abramson, 1970). In a labeling task, participants listened to one of the tokens and were asked to label it as either /da/ or /ta/. The solid curve represents the mean probability of labeling /da/ as a function of VOT (abscissa, bottom). The result indicates that a perceived quality jumps abruptly from /da/ to /ta/ with prolonging VOT, instead of changing gradually. The value of VOT at which this psychometric function crosses a chance level (=50 % correct) is termed "VOT boundary" (red line).

In a discrimination task, participants listened to a pair of tokens, say X and Y. X was followed by Y whose VOTs were separated together with a fixed distance of 20 ms (ex., -10 vs. 10 ms, 0 vs. 20 ms, 10 vs. 30 ms …; ref., abscissa, top). Then, the participants were asked to tell whether the tokens X and Y were the same or different. The broken curve represents the probability of telling "different" against the midst of each discrimination pair (ref., abscissa, top). The discrimination performance was high if the tokens were drawn from separate categories such as /da/ and /ta/ whereas was no better than chance (= 50 % correct) if the tokens were drawn from the same category.

According to Studalert-Kennedy et al. (1970), categorical perception is recognized in operation if (1) distinct labeling categories are separated with a sharp boundary instead of changing gradually (solid curve) and (2) equal-sized physical differences between stimuli perceptually expand or shrink depending on whether the stimuli belong to different categories or same one (broken curve) .

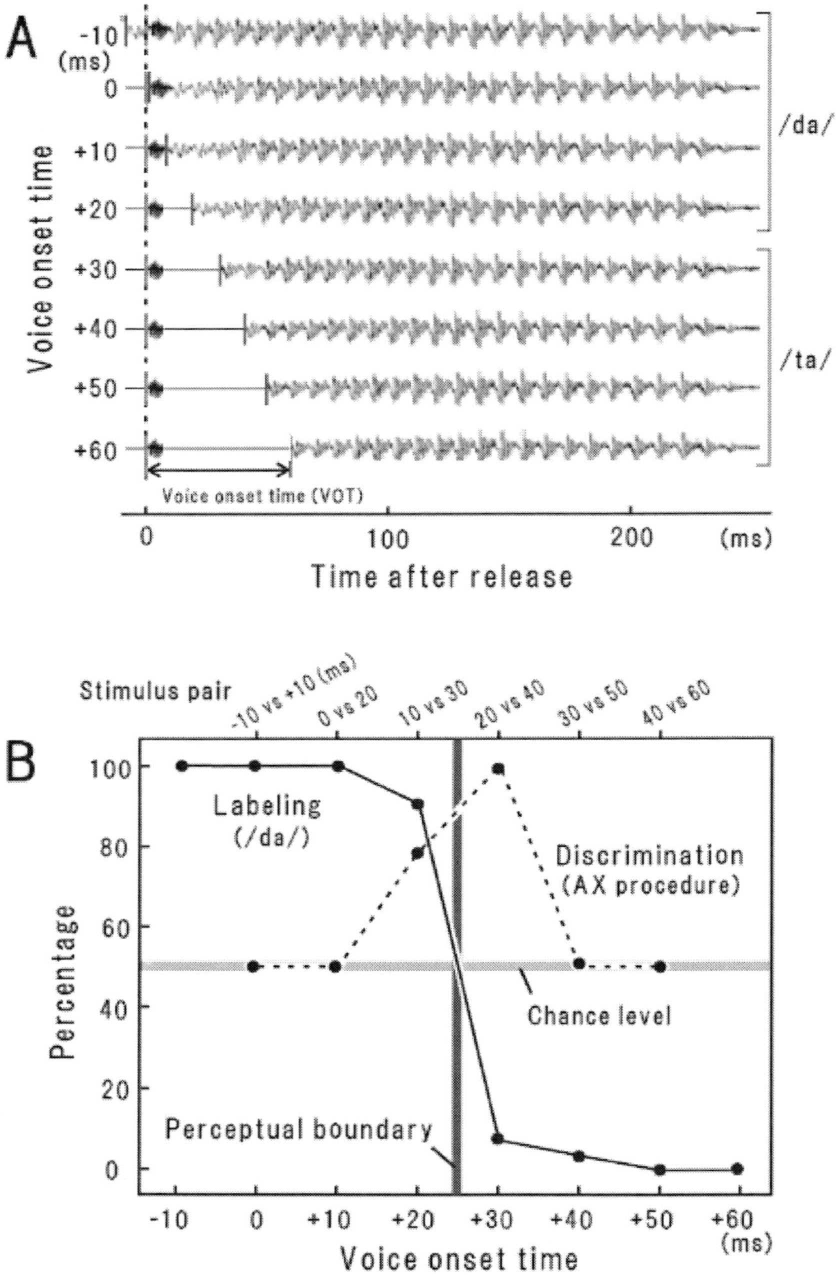


Modified from Lisker and Abramson, 1970.

Figure 3. Categorical perception of plosive CV-syllables depending on *voice onset time* (VOT). A: Waveforms of synthesized /da/-/ta/ tokens with variable VOT (-10 ms to +60 ms, shifted by 10-ms steps). A negative VOT means that the onset of *voicing* (red line) preceded *release* (blue line). B: The mean performance of native English speakers in two versions of psychophysical experiments using /da/-/ta/ tokens, such as identification (or labeling) task and discrimination task. For the identification task (solid curve), the *ordinate* gives the percentage of /da/ responses against the VOT (*abscissa*, bottom). The red line represents the "VOT boundary" where the identification function crosses the chance level (= 50% correct). For the discrimination task (broken curve), the *ordinate* gives the percentage of correct discrimination against the midst VOT within each discriminated pair (*abscissa*, top).

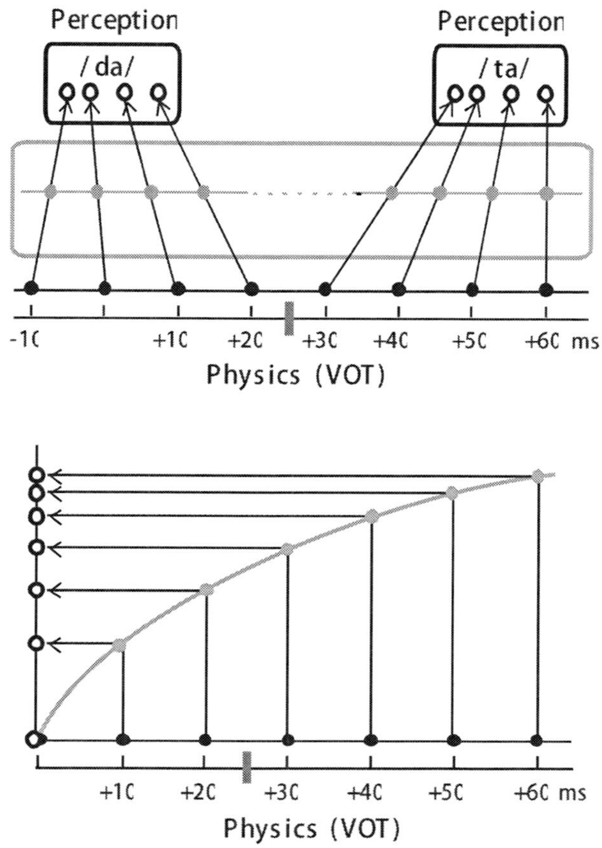


Figure 4. A: Schematics of the conversion process from physical continuum (VOT) into perceptual map (/da/ or /ta/). (Bottom) the sound signals demonstrated in Figure 3A (/da/-/ta/ tokens) were alighted along the VOT axis (the red line approximates the location of the VOT boundary). (Top) perceptual map was obtained from the psychophysics data (Figure 3B). (Middle) hypothesized neural processes whereby the VOT continuum is transformed into perceptual map. B: Weber-Fechner's law based prediction of perceptual distance among the /da/-/ta/ tokens (see text for details).

### *1.2.3. A Conceptual Model of VOT-Dependent Categorical Perception*

Figure 4A schematically draws the process to convert physical continuum (VOT) into perceptual space (/da/ or /ta/). The black circles (in bottom row) refer to the location of the /da/-/ta/ tokens along the VOT dimension. The white circles (top row) refer to perceived quality of those tokens which are categorized as /da/ or /ta/, nothing in between. The middle two rows depict hypothesized neural processes whereby the physical continuum is transformed into the perceptual map. In the initial stage (lower trace), VOTs are monotonically transduced into some electrochemical activities of the auditory system, namely *sensory analogs* (gray circles). In the next stage, the distance between the *sensory analogs* is compressed or expanded adapting to a category scheme (upper trace). This process appears to violate Weber-Fechner's law (Figure 4B) which predicts that (1) physical property (black circles) and perceived quality (white circles) are in continuous and monotonic relationship and (2) as the parameter value elevates along the physical axis, equal-sized physical differences become less discriminable in perception (see above for details). This issue inspired the claim that categorical perception of phonetic sounds requires a higher, special kind of mechanism beyond general auditory processing (Lieberman et al., 1961). The underlying neural processes are currently elusive. This is the main subject for the present article (see below).

# 2. Auditory Categorical Perception is not Exclusive to Speech Sounds

## 2.1. Variance of VOT Boundary among Place-of-articulation

In English, three sets of articulators are involved in the production of plosive CV-syllables (reviewed by Lieberman, 1984). One set of the articulators is upper and lower lips (Figure 5A, *left*) which leads to /b/ or /p/, holistically classified as "bilabials." The second (*middle*) is alveolar ridge and tongue tip leading to /d/ or /p/, classified as "alveolars." The third (*right*) is tongue blade and soft plate (or velum) leading to /g/ or /k/, classified as "velars."

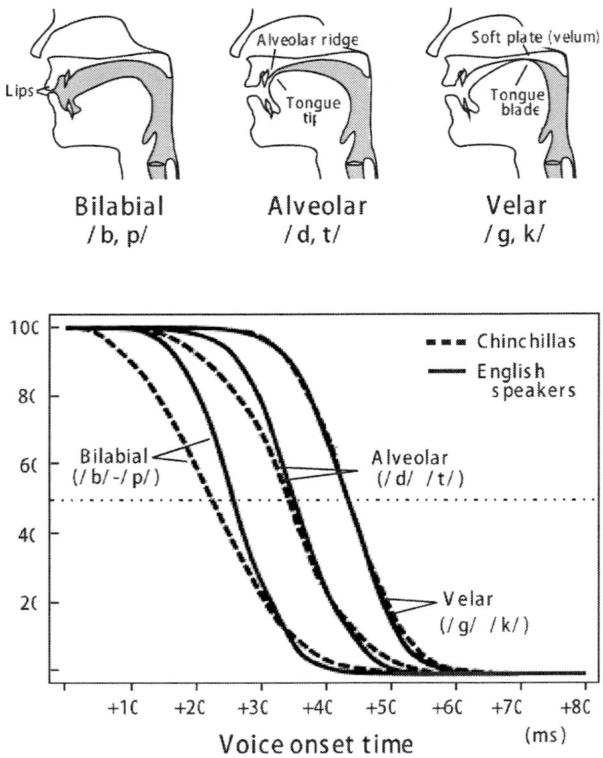


Modified from Kuhl and Miller, 1978.

Figure 5. A: Midsaggital configuration of the vocal tract at the moment of consonant release at distinct place-of-articulation (bilabials, alveolar and velar). B: Mean identification function obtained from humans (solid curves) and chinchillas (broken curve) for synthetic tokens of plosive CV-syllables with distinct place-of-articulation. For simplicity, raw data points were fitted to smooth curves.

The solid curves in Figure 5B depict the mean labeling-function for native English listeners to the three sets of syllables (Kuhl and Miller, 1978). The VOT boundary, at which this psychometric function crosses a chance level (50 % correct; dotted line), showed some variance among place-of-articulation: ~20 ms for bilabials, ~30 ms for alveolars, and ~40 ms for velars. Thus, the VOT boundary is not a fixed entity but shifts rightward with backward placement of the articulators (ref., Figure 5A).

This indicates that the phoneme boundary is not determined solely by VOT and may allow the following interpretation with two extremes. One extreme postulates the dominant role of "phonetic" processing, in that voiced-voiceless contrasts are differentiated by triggering "feature detectors" which are contemplated to represent distinctive and invariant features of individual phonemes (Eimas and Corbit, 1973; Blumstein and Stevens, 1979) or accessing to listener's "tacit knowledge of articulatory gestures" for producing individual phonemes known as "motor theory" (Lieberman et al., 1967). Another extreme emphasizes the involvement of "general auditory processing," whereby other acoustic variable(s) works in concert with VOT for voiced (/b, d, g/) vs. voiceless (/p, t, k/) distinction. Here I describe two independent lines of evidence that support the latter perspective: (1) animals, which conduct auditory processing but NOT phonetic processing, can also execute VOT-dependent categorical perception of CV syllables and (2) humans execute categorical perception of non-phonemic sounds.

## 2.2. Categorical Perception in Animals for Phonemic Sounds

Kuhl and colleague (Kuhl and Miller, 1975, 1978; Kuhl, 1981) employed a shock-avoidance procedure to train chinchillas to respond differently to the 0- and 80-ms VOT endpoints of a synthetic /da/-/ta/ tokens. On subsequent generalization trials, perceptual capacity of the animals was assessed by presenting a series of tokens with variable VOT (10-ms steps) and place-of-articulation. The labeling function of the animals (broken curves, Figure 5B) mirrored those of humans (solid curves) which were obtained using exactly the same sound signals. Of note, there were no significant across-species differences in the VOT boundary for each set of articulators. The peak of the animal's discrimination function was expectedly near the VOT boundary (Kuhl, 1981). These findings all meat the requisite for categorical perception that was proposed by Studalert-Kennedy et al. (1970) (see above). Similar results were also obtained from monkeys (Waters and Wilson, 1976; Kuhl and Padden, 1983) and birds (Dooling et al., 1989).

Taken together, it is likely that "non-linguistic" animals CAN categorically perceive phonemic sounds, un-warranting the perspective that categorical perception of phoneme sounds is mediated thoroughly by special phonetic processor.

## 2.3. Category Perception in Humans for Non-Phonetic Sounds

There is now very convincing evidence that humans execute categorical perception of non-phonetic sounds (Cutting and Rosner, 1974; Miller et al., 1976; Pisoni, 1977). In particular, Miller et al. (1976) employed "noise-buzz pairs" as a nonspeech analogue to plosive CV syllables: the preceding *noise* was regarded as *release*, succeeding *buzz* as *voicing*, and the inter-stimulus interval (ISI) as VOT (ref., Figure 2A). According to human listener's subjective experience, the preceding *noise* was clearly audible if the ISI was long enough (classified as "noise lead" category), but became nearly inaudible if the ISI was shortened below a critical value ("no-noise lead" category). The psychometric functions (data not shown) showed typical categorical-perception pattern: (1) the labeling function abruptly altered from "no-noise lead" category into "noise lead" category across the boundary at ~20 ms ISI and (2) discrimination scores were at chance level if the discrimination pair (same-different procedure) were drawn from an identical category, but heightened if the discrimination pair were drown from different categories.

A canonical example for temporal grain of human auditory processing is referred to as "temporal-order threshold" (Hirsh, 1959; Fraisse, 1984). According to Hirsh's definition (1959), this metric corresponds to the minimal ISI that must intervene between two signals for listeners to detect which of the two was presented first with 75% accuracy. Hirsh and colleague (Hirsh 1959; Hirsh and Sherrick, 1961) used pairs of various kinds of acoustic signals (ex., tone, band noise and click) of variable ISI: within a pair, a difference was made regarding to frequency (if those were tones), spectrum (if those were band noise), duration (if the pair consisted of both a brief and prolonged signal), laterality, etc. Under such circumstances, the listeners were asked which signal came first – tone or noise, higher or lower in pitch, from right or left, etc. The results indicated that the listeners could tell apart only if ISI was longer than 20 ms. This ISI value was virtually independent of frequency, bandwidth and laterality, suggesting that the temporal-order threshold is elaboration on central, receptor independent mechanisms.

The above mentioned three temporal metrics, such as VOT boundary, noise-buzz sequence boundary and temporal-order threshold, are comparable each other (~20 ms). This leads to widely accepted notion that all these metrics rely on common natural sensitivities of the auditory system.

## 2.4. Overview of Studies on Place-of-Articulation Mediated VOT-Boundary Shift

The question still remains as to what acoustic variable(s) is involved in the VOT boundary shift with place-of-articulation (see Figure 5B) and how. This issue is beyond the scope of the present article. Here, I will only briefly overview several acoustic variables that were reported to influence the VOT boundary.

Spectrogram of natural plosive CV-syllables has several characteristic features of place-of-articulation (reviewed by Liebermann et al., 1967; ref., Figure 2A). For example, starting frequency of the first formant (F1) transition is the highest for bilabials and the lowest for velars (Parker, 1988). Parametrical studies, using synthetic tokens in which starting frequency of the F1 transition and VOT were independently manipulated, demonstrated an inverse relationship between them (Summerfield and Haggard, 1977; Summerfield, 1982; Soli, 1983). This raises the possibility that starting frequency of the F1 transition is in a trading relationship with the VOT boundary. Similar relationship has been observed between the slope of F2 transition and VOT boundary, and between the direction of F2 transition and VOT boundary (Delattre et al., 1955; Lieberman et al., 1957).

Spectrogram of *noise burst* component also exhibit variance among place-of-articulation: the labials have diffuse falling spectrum, alveolars a diffuse rising spectrum, and velars a compact spectrum with most energy in the mid-frequency range (1000-3000 Hz) (Stevens, 2000). Blumstein and Stevens (1979), in the claim for the existence of phonetic feature-detectors, emphasized that gross spectral shape of this component, sampled at the time of *release* (within 26-msec time window), can serve as static "template" for specifying place-of-articulation.

In contrast, there are cogent arguments that not spectral information but temporal-envelop information predominantly contributes to intelligibility of plosive CV-syllables, and thus is mainly involved in place-of-articulation mediated VOT-boundary shift (reviewed by Rosen, 1992; Shannon, 2005). For example, Horst et al. (1999) demonstrated that such band noise whose temporal envelope was modulated with that of a plosive CV-syllable, providing greatly reduced spectral cue but preserved temporal cue to several cochlear channels, was sufficient for the listeners to correctly identify its original phoneme category (/b/, /d/, /g/, /p/, /t/, /k/). Specifically, the prolongation of F1 transition (Stevens and Klatt, 1974; Lisker, 1975; Summerfield and Haggard, 1977), which accompany backward placement of the articulators, has been shown to promote rightward shift of the VOT boundary.

Considerable efforts have been made in attempting to construct a collective scheme about mechanisms underlying place-of-articulation mediated VOT-boundary shift. This issue is, however, currently still highly speculative.

### 2.5. Summary

The above findings indicate that categorical perception is not unique to phonetic system but rather is based on general auditory processing.

## 3. Involvement of the AI for VOT-Dependent Categorical Perception

### 3.1. Case Reports for the Patients with Bilateral AI Legion: Pure Word Deafness

Humans with bilateral AI lesion were reported to show typical symptom, called "pure word deafness" (Kussmaul, 1877). The patients are, according to classical definition, impaired in only speech comprehension but maintain other basic language abilities such as reading, writing and speaking, or even normal in basic auditory capacity as assessed with pure-tone audiometry (Kussmaul, 1877; Lichtheim, 1885; Hemphill and Stengel, 1940). The patients typically complain: speech sounds are " like a great noise all the time ... you think you can catch it and it fades away ... like foreign folks speaking in the distance" (Klein and Harper, 1956) or speech sounds "resister" or "do not come up" (Saffran et al., 1976).

For the patients, normal utterance rate by other people appears too fast. If utterance rate is reduced, their speech comprehension was often improved (Albert and Bear, 1974). Lip-reading is usually very helpful for patients (Klein and Harper, 1956; Metz-Lutz and Dahl,

1984). One patient with lip-reading dependency said "if I go blind, I won't hear anything," nevertheless his lip-reading ability was greatly augmented when lip movement was actually accompanied with utterance (Auerbach et al., 1982). These observations imply that the deficit was caused, at least partially, by disorder of fine-grained temporal analysis which can be compensated by lip-reading to some extent.

Multiple studies have revealed that the degree of deficit of speech comprehension differ across phoneme types: (1) consonantal tasks such as /d/-/t/ distinction was considerably more impaired than vowel tasks such as /a/-/i/ distinction; (2) among consonantal tasks, discrimination of plosives (/b/, /d/, /g/ ...) was more heavily impaired than the other consonants such as fricative (/f/, /th/, /sh/...), nasal (/m/, /n/, /ng/...) or approximant (/l/, /r/, /y/...) (Saffran et al., 1976; Miceli, 1982; Stockert, 1982; Mendez and Geehan, 1988; Yaqub et al., 1988). The plosive consonants have temporal variance in the milliseconds to tens-of-milliseconds frame (ref, Figure 2A) whereas vowels and many other consonants are both longer in duration (tens to hundreds milliseconds) and less temporally punctuated (Stevens, 1980; Kurowski and Blumstein, 1987; Rosen, 1992). Therefore, the deficit is most manifested in a temporal grain over the milliseconds to tens-of-milliseconds range. Consistently, the patients are often spared in recognition of prosody and melody (Heilman et al., 1984; Yaqub, 1988), which are expressed over hundreds or thousands of milliseconds (Pickett, 1999).

There is longstanding uncertainty whether pure word deafness is a distinct disorder of brain function. For example, while a part of the patients indeed had deficit exclusively to speech sound (Metz-Luts and Dahl, 1984; Yaqub et al., 1988; Takahashi et al., 1992), not a few patients had deficit in non-speech perception such as prolongation of temporal-order threshold (see above), say from ~20 ms to 100 ms (Brugge, 1975; Brick et al., 1985). Another uncertainty regards the lateralization of brain function. Most patients, as mentioned above, suffered lesion on bilateral sides: after the first (unilateral) lesion, speech perception was typically intact excepting an initial period of disturbance; only after the second lesion (in the other hemisphere), the deficits become evident and permanent (Ulrich, 1978). According to Pöppel's survey (2001) on 42 patients with bilateral lesions, no clear difference was found regarding to severity and context of the deficits between left-before-right lesion group and right-before-left lesion group; on the other hand, there exists smaller but significant fraction of the patients (17 out of 59, or 29%) who drifted into permanent deficits only after unilateral lesion in the dominant hemisphere.

Thanks to accumulating body of psychophysical data and development of neuroimaging techniques (CT, PET, fMRI, MEG), it has been increasingly recognized that pure word deafness comprises largely two types (Auerbach et al., 1982; Pöppel, 2001; Price et al., 2005). The first type, namely "pre-phonemic type," typically accompanies temporal-resolving disorder of non-phonetic sounds, as manifested by prolongation of the temporal-order threshold (see above) (Auerbach et al., 1982; Tanaka et al., 1987; Buchtel and Stewart, 1989). Auerbach et al. (1982) reported that this type patient exhibited a normal labeling function for plosive CV-syllables but extreme difficulties in discrimination of VOT. He interpreted such symptom was primarily due to auditory dysfunction rather than linguistic dysfunction. The lesion in this type patients was commonly located in bilateral Heschl's gyrus (corresponding to Brodmann's area 41 and 42) which includes the AI (Chocholle et al., 1975; Auerbach et al., 1982; Mendez and Geehan, 1988). The widely accepted notion is that the "pre-phonemic type" results from disorder of the AI or its surroundings, which normally conduct fine-grained temporal analysis regardless of whether the signals are phonetic or non-phonetic (Phillips and Farmer, 1990; Griffiths et al., 1999; Poeppel, 2003).

The second type, namely "phonemic type," is often accompanied by a severely deteriorated labeling function for plosive CV-syllables (Saffran et al., 1976; Stefanatos et al., 2005). The patients suffer from unilateral (usually, left) lesion to posterior temporal lobe which includes Wernicke's area (corresponding to Brodmann's area 44) (Denes and Semenza, 1975; Saffran et al., 1976; Takahashi et al., 1992). Of note, Takahashi et al. (1992), by employing CT, PET and fMRI, found that the lesion widely extended to subcortical tissue in the left temporal lobe, crucially interrupted the ipsilateral auditory radiations as well as transcallosal projections from the contralateral side, thereby deafferenting Wernicke's area from incoming auditory information. This observation is consistent with the classical view based on autopsy studies (Lichtheim, 1885; Liepmann and Storch, 1902; Geschwind, 1965). Thus, "phonemic type" could be considered as a fragment of Wernicke's aphasia (Wernicke and Friedlander, 1883).

The above findings have important implications for functional architecture of human brain to fulfill VOT-dependent categorical perception: fine-grained temporal auditory processing is robustly bilateral, at least at the level of the AI; then subsequent computations of linguistic information are lateralized to the left with extending over higher auditory fields up to Wernicke's area.

### 3.2. Behavioral Studies in Animals with Ablation of Bilateral Auditory Cortex

Thus far, a number of behavioral studies have been conducted on cats, rats, ferrets and monkeys to estimate effects of ablation of bilateral auditory cortex (reviewed by Neff et al., 1975; Heffner and Heffner, 1990). It appears that ablation of bilateral auditory cortex as a whole does not usually produce sever audiometric hearing loss such as impairment of detection of tone onset (Kryter and Ades, 1943), intensity discrimination (Rosenzweig, 1946; Meyer and Woolsey, 1952) and frequency discrimination (Evarts, 1952; Butler et al., 1957; Cranford et al., 1976). In contrast, ablation of bilateral auditory cortex considerably hindered temporal tasks such as identifying the order of signals in cats (Diamond and Neff, 1957) and monkeys (Jerison and Neff, 1953), discrimination between 10- and 300-Hz trains of noise bursts in monkeys (Symmes, 1966), detection of amplitude-modulation (AM) rate below but not above ~30 Hz in rats (Grigoreva et al., 1988), and detecting temporal gaps between noise in rats (Ison et al., 1991) and ferrets (Kavanagh and Kelly, 1988).

Typically, Heffner and Heffner (1989) demonstrated that in monkeys, bilateral ablation of the primary and secondary auditory areas resulted in the permanent deficit in discriminating conspecific vocalizations without significant audiometric hearing loss. This is seemingly compatible with the symptoms for the patients suffering "pre-phonemic type" pure word deafness.

However, to my knowledge, such material behavioral studies have not yet been conducted to explicitly estimate effects of selective ablation of bilateral AI on the capacity for fine-grained temporal processing necessary for VOT-dependent categorical perception. Additional animal studies are needed to directly address this issue.

### 3.3. Summary

Case studies of patients with lesions restricted to the bilateral AI (i.e., "pre-phonemic type" pure word deafness) reported that (1) they were severally impaired in the VOT-dependent categorical perception of plosive CV syllables and (2) their temporal-order threshold was considerably elongated. These findings suggest that AI is critically involved in inter-stimulus interval (ISI) dependent differential perception regardless of whether the signals are phonetic or non-phonetic. Cortical ablation studies in animals, while still in infancy, provided compatible results.

## 4. Category-Like Responses of the AI

The above findings indicate that (1) basic neural mechanisms of VOT-dependent categorical perception in humans are shared with animals, and thus open to empirical investigation (section 2); (2) the AI is critically involved in fine-grained temporal analysis necessary for VOT-dependent categorical perception (section 3). The present section deals with a bulk of neurophysiology findings which may expand our understanding how the AI analyzes VOT.

### 4.1. Auditory Evoked Potentials

Sharma et al. (1999, 2000) recorded auditory evoked potentials (AEPs) in humans who were exposed to a series of /ga/-/ka/ tokens with variable VOT. The grand average of AEPs (over Fz, Cz and Pz scalp regions) exhibited two sorts of morphology change depending on VOT (examples: Figure 6A and B; summary: C). First, the latency of the N1 component, defined as a negative deflection with the peak(s) laying at ~100 ms after the consonant release, prolonged with the VOT increment (10-30 ms VOT [A]; 40-70 ms VOT [B]; summary [C as open bars]). Second, the number of peaks in the N1 component changed across phoneme category: only a single peak (N1) was evident for "voiced" /ga/ (A); additional peak (N1') preceded the N1 for "voiceless" /ka/ (B).

Then, in order to assess the involvement of the AI in /ga/-/ka/ distinction, the authors measured early component of mismatch negativity (MMN) in the "passive oddball condition," where an infrequent "deviant" auditory signal was presented in the sequence of repetitive "standard" signals (examples: Figure 6D and E; summary: F). MMN is found as downward deflection of AEPs evoked by the deviant signal as long as the subject can perceive the deviant signal as different from the standard signal (Näätänen and Winkler, 1999). The early component of MMN has been proved to arise from the AI (and/or its surroundings) regardless of whether the signals attract the subject's attention, and thus this component is recognized to signify pre-attentive auditory discrimination processes that operates primarily in the AI (Näätänen, 1992).

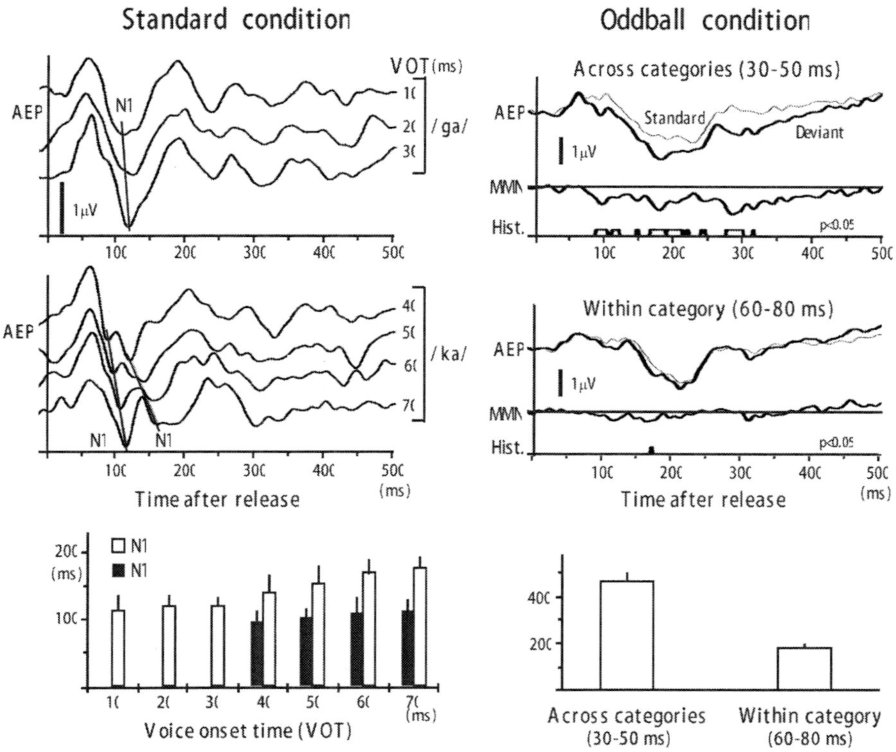


Adapted from Sharma and Dorman, 1999; Sharma et al., 2000.

Figure 6. Auditory evoked potentials (AEPs) in human brain produced by a series of synthetic plosive CV-syllables with variable VOT. A and B: Grand-average of AEPs (across Fz, Cz and Pz scalp regions) to the /ga/-/ka/ tokens. VOTs ≤ 30 ms (perceived as /ga/) produced a single negativity (*N1*) (A) whereas VOTs ≥ 40 ms (perceived as /ka/) produced two distinct negative components (*N1* and *N1'*) (B). C: The mean (plus SD) of the latency for the *N1* (open bar) and *N1'* (filled bar) as exemplified in A and B. D: Results in the "oddball condition" in which repetitive presentations of a "standard" signal were occasionally replaced with a "deviant" signal. VOT of those signals were either 30 or 50 ms. Because those values resided in different sides across the VOT boundary (~35 ms), the signals were called "across-category pair." (Top trace) The thick curve depicts AEP produced by the deviant signal when it was presented in the oddball condition. As a reference, the thin curve depicts AEP produced by the same stimulus as the deviant signal when it was presented alone (= standard condition). (Middle trace) The curve depicts "mismatch negativity (MMN)" which is obtained as the difference wave between the above two AEPs. (Bottom trace) The boxes indicate the region of a significant mismatch response ($p$<0.05, t-test). E: The result obtained similarly to D. The only difference was VOT of the signals (60 and 80 ms). Because both VOT values were of the same perceptual category (/ka/), the signals are called "between-category pair." F: The mean (plus SD) of the MMN area (ms * μV) calculated from D and E.

The measurement of MMN took the following four steps (ref., Figure 6D): (1) The mean AEPs to the deviant signal (30-ms VOT, perceived as "voiced" /ga/) were recorded (thick line, upper trace) in the oddball condition where 50-ms VOT (perceived as "voiceless" /ka/) was adopted as the standard signal; (2) as references, AEPs to the deviant signal (30-ms VOT) was recorded while it was presented alone (thin line, upper trace); (3) the difference between the above two AEPs (in the range of ~100-300 ms after consonant release) was calculated as the early component of MMN (middle trace); (4) the difference between the above two AEPs was statistically assessed every 10 ms (the region of a significant difference

[$p$<0.05, t-test] was indicated as the boxes; bottom trace). In this instance, where the two signals were drown from distinct categories (namely, "across-category pair"), NNM was statistically-significantly evident. However, it was not the case for another stimulus pair (60 and 80 ms VOT), which were drown from the same category /ka/ (namely "within-category pair"). Note that VOT difference was fixed 20 ms both in the across-category pair and within-category pair. The result was confirmed by across-subject comparison for the mean area of MMN (Figure 6F): the area was much larger for the across-category pair than the within-category pair. Collectively, it was suggested that the AI is critically involved in VOT-dependent categorical perception.

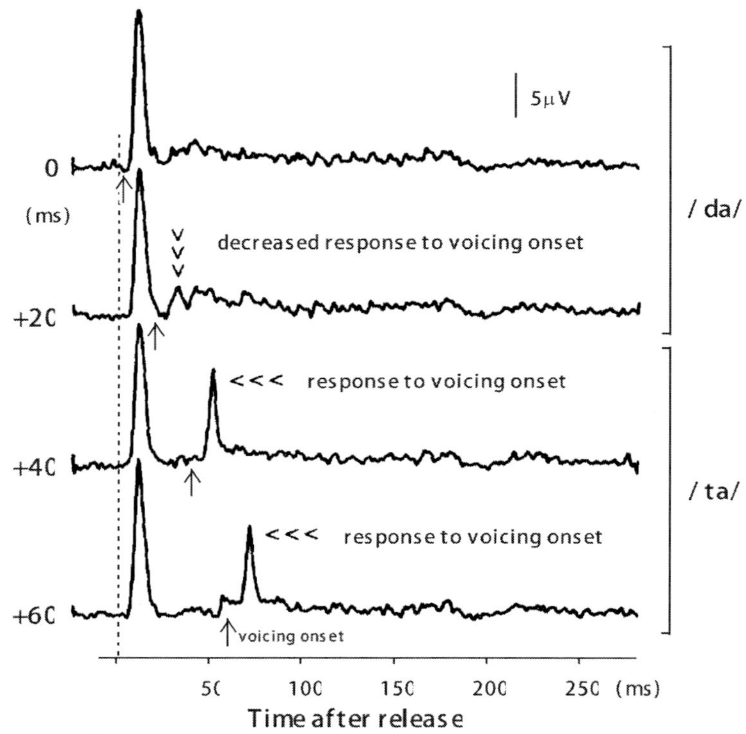


Adapted from Steinschneider et al., 1995.

Figure 7. Categorical-like responses of field potentials in the primary auditory cortex (AI) of the awake monkey. The stimuli adopted were /da/-/ta/ tokens with variable VOT. The consonant release (broken line) evoked robust transient response at any VOT. Such responses were followed by a period of reduced responsiveness. Accordingly, the voicing onset (arrow) with short VOTs (0 and 20 ms, leading to /da/ percept; upper two traces), hardly evoked robust responses. At longer VOTs (40 and 60 ms, leading to /ta/ percept; lower two traces), before which the reduced responsiveness had dissipated, the voicing onset could evoke robust responses (multiple arrow heads). These findings imply that distinct categories of the CV-syllables are differentiated represented the AI; /da/ is associated with namely "single-onset responses" whereas /ta/ with "double-onset responses."

## 4.2. Filed Potential

To more directly investigate neural mechanisms underlying VOT-dependent categorical perception, Steinschneider et al. (1995) inserted the electrode into the AI in awake monkeys and recorded field potentials (Figure 7). The electrode tips were placed in lower lamina III, which arbors efferent fibers to secondary auditory areas for further processing (Galaburda and Pandys, 1983). Thus, the evoked potentials expectedly reflect the outcome of intra-AI processing rather than sub-cortical activities. The sound signals delivered were /ta/-/da/ tokens with variable VOT (0, 20, 40 and 60 ms). If the VOT was long enough (40 and 60 ms [bottom two traces]), the field potential showed two distinctive local peaks (namely, "double on response"), implying that the AI represented both consonant release (vertical dotted line) and voicing onset (arrow) on component-to-component basis. When the VOT was shortened below 30 ms (upper two traces), the voicing onset hardly evoked the 2nd local peak. This feature is holistically referred to as "single on response." Since 30 ms corresponds to psychoacoustically determined VOT boundary, the authors inferred that the AI represents /ta/ and /da/ in a category-like manner: "voiceless" /ta/ is represented as "double on responses" whereas "voiced" /da/ as "single on response." Similar findings have been obtained for AI filed potentials in monkeys (Steinschneider et al., 1994, 1995, 2003), cats (Eggermont, 1995a,b, 1999), guinea pigs (McGee et al., 1996) and even in humans under epilepsy surgery (Liégeois-Chauvel et al., 1999; Steinschneider et al., 1999). Comparable activities have been also observed in MEG recordings in humans (Joliot et al., 1994; Ahissar et al., 2001).

## 4.3. Multi-Unit Activity

Eggermont and colleagues conducted a series of neurophysiology experiments on anesthetized cats (Eggermont, 1995a,b; Tomita et al., 2004) to obtain a multi-unit-level evidence for AI category-like responses. The sound signals adopted were /ba/-/pa/ tokens with variable VOT. Figure 8A and B are the result of Tomita et al. (2004). As shown in a rater dot display of discharges (Figure 8A, left panel), the AI vigorously responded to the consonant release with ~10-ms onset latency (abscissa) at any VOT examined (ordinate). Such robust onset responses were followed by a suppression period for several tens ms, where even spontaneous discharges scarcely took place (i.e., "post-activation suppression"). The voicing onset became to evoke robust responses only if it was presented with VOT $\geq$ 40 ms. In order to quantify VOT dependence of the responsiveness to voicing onset, evoked discharge rates were transformed into PSTH (5-ms bin width; middle panel), then the maximal discharge rates within a sliding 30-ms time window (bounded between two oblique lines) were plotted against the VOT (right panel). The data points looked somewhat binarily distributed so that those were fitted with a sigmoid function. Gross feature of this neurometric function curve resembled, while in an inverse manner, to the psychometric function curve for humans and chinchillas (Figure 5B, most left two curves). Therefore, it is plausible that stimulus-locking discharges of AI neurons contribute to VOT-dependent categorical perception. However, it should be mentioned that the quantitative difference between the neurometric function curve and psychometric function curves: the former (Figure 8A, right panel) had the midpoint at ~40-ms (marked by broken arrow), which was 15-ms longer than those for the latter (~25 ms; Figure 5B). Such difference, as discussed later, could be due to the effect anesthesia.

From the same recording locus as in Figure 8A, the authors continued recording while delivering sequences of two clicks with variable inter-stimulus intervals (Figure 8B; see inset in the right panel for stimulus configuration). Expectedly, similar temporal-response patterns were reproduced in that responsiveness to the trailing signal (i.e., 2nd click) exhibited sigmoid function with the midpoint at ~40-ms. This may indicate that category-like AI responses are mediated through "general" auditory processing rather than "specific" phonetic processing.

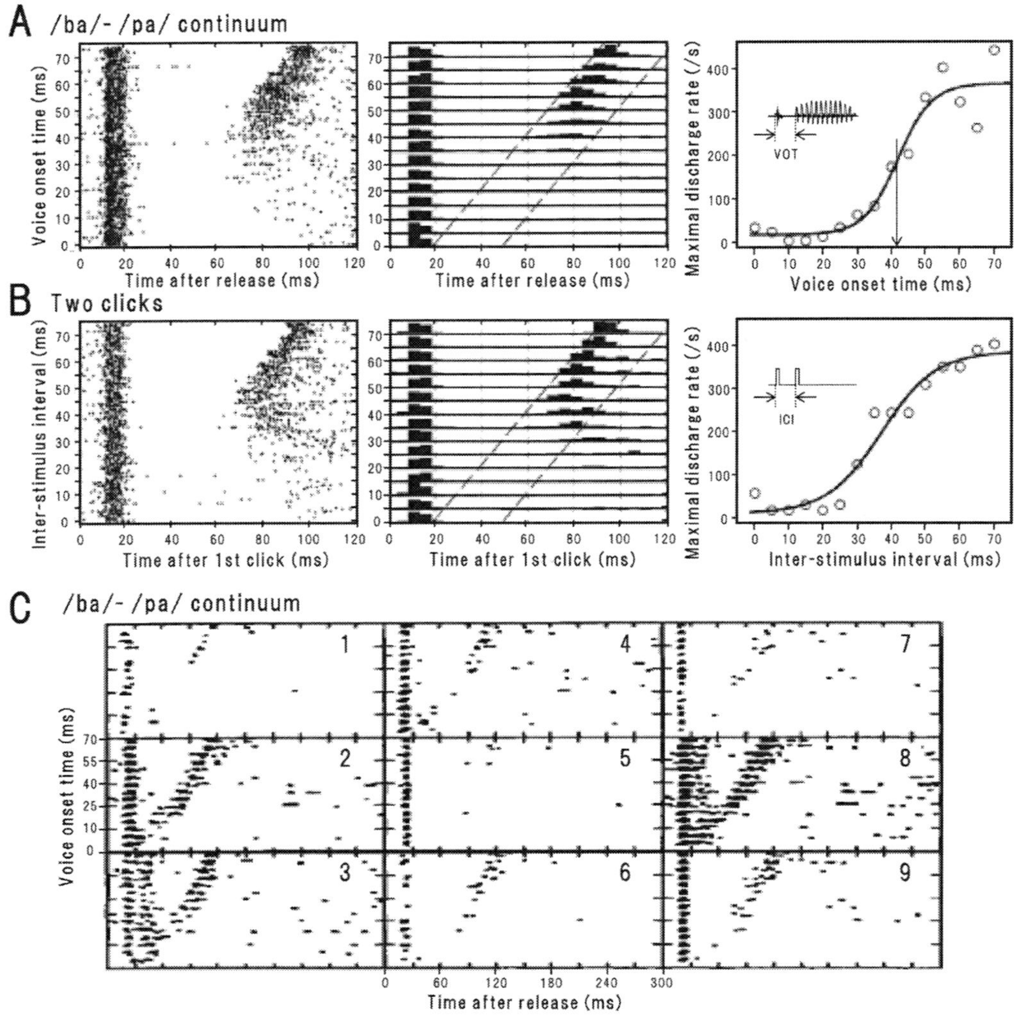


Adapted from Tomita et al., 2004 for A and B; Eggermont 1995a for C.

Figure 8. Category-like behavior of multi-unit activities in the anesthetized cat's AI. The sound signals were either /ba/-/pa/ tokens with variable VOT (A, C) or series of two clicks with variable inter-stimulus interval (B). A and B: Measuring made from the same recording site. Rater dot displays of discharges (left column) and peri-stimulus time histograms (PSTH; middle column) were organized vertically according to VOT (A) or inter-stimulus interval (B), and horizontally time after the preceding signal (= consonant release in A; 1st click in B). The maximal discharge rate within a shifting 30-ms time window (bordered between two oblique lines) in PSTH was plotted against VOT or inter-stimulus interval (right column). The data points were fitted with a sigmoid curve. C: Rater dot displays of discharges for seven single-unit activities (1-7) and two multi-unit activities (8, 9). The multi-unit activities (8) were sorted into four single-unit activities (1-4); another multi-unit activities (9) into three single-unit activities (5-7).

Figures 8C-8 display multi-unit activities in another anesthetized cat that was exposed to the /ba/-/pa/ continuum (Eggermont, 1995a). These activities were sorted into four single-unit activities (1-4). Each unit had, more or less, had a stimulus-locking capacity to both consonant release and voicing onset. However, not a small difference was notified across units with respect to the minimal VOT which gave rise to stimulus-locking responses to the voicing onset: it was ~60 ms in (1), but it was as short as ~10 ms in (2). An across-unit difference was also found in another set of single-unit activities (5-7) which were sorted from another multi-unit activity (9). Specifically, the unit in (5) responded almost exclusively to the consonant release, but the unit in (6) responded to both components with degraded responsiveness to the consonant release. Such across-unit differences should be kept in mind if one aims to investigate biological processes underlying AI category-like responses at the level of single neuron (see below).

## 4.4. Single-Unit Activity

While the field potential, multi unit, and neuroimaging recording techniques are useful in mapping the summated, net responses of the neural cluster, it reveals little about the individual neurons that may have divergent stimulus-response characteristics (Phillips and Irvine, 1979). To this end, Sakai et al. (2009a,b) applied single-unit recording techniques to the cat's AI and studied inter-stimulus dependent responses. The animals were kept alert during recording session to exclude plausible influence of anesthetics (Franks and Lieb, 1994; Zurita et al., 1994) as well as state of vigilance (Edeline et al., 2001).

First delivered were click signals rather than the plosive CV-syllables because we intended to investigate "general" auditory processing for category-like responses as much as possible. The experimental procedures, namely "click train paradigm" are as follows: (1) a single recording session comprised 180-360 trials (10-20 min), (2) each trial was made up of a 500-ms-long stimulus period and a 2.5- to 3.5-s-long silent period, (3) during each stimulus period, rectangular pulses (1-ms duration) were delivered in a train fashion with variable inter-stimulus intervals (ISI) ranging 2-480 ms and (4) the overall stimulus intensity was arranged at 30-80 dB SPL by 10 dB steps.

The units that exhibited vigorous excitatory responses were classified largely into 2 classes depending on whether they had the stimulus-locking capacity (synchronization units: n = 72) or not (non-synchronization units: n = 44) (Table).

**Table. Variables (milliseconds; mean ± S.D.) of stimulus-locking responses**

| Unit type | *N* | Click trains | | | /da/-/ta/ tokens |
|---|---|---|---|---|---|
| | | Longer limit ($\alpha$-$\beta$ border) | Best ISI | Shorter limit ($\beta$-$\gamma$ border) | VOT boundary |
| Synchronization (band-pass) | 46 | 174 ± 112 ms | 71.4 ± 19.6 ms | 30.6 ± 25.9 ms | 41.7 ± 34.1 ms |
| Synchronization (low-pass) | 26 | — | 80.6 ± 23.8 ms | 33.1 ± 28.7 ms | |
| Non-synchronization | 25 | — | — | — | |

See Figure 9 and text for classification of units.

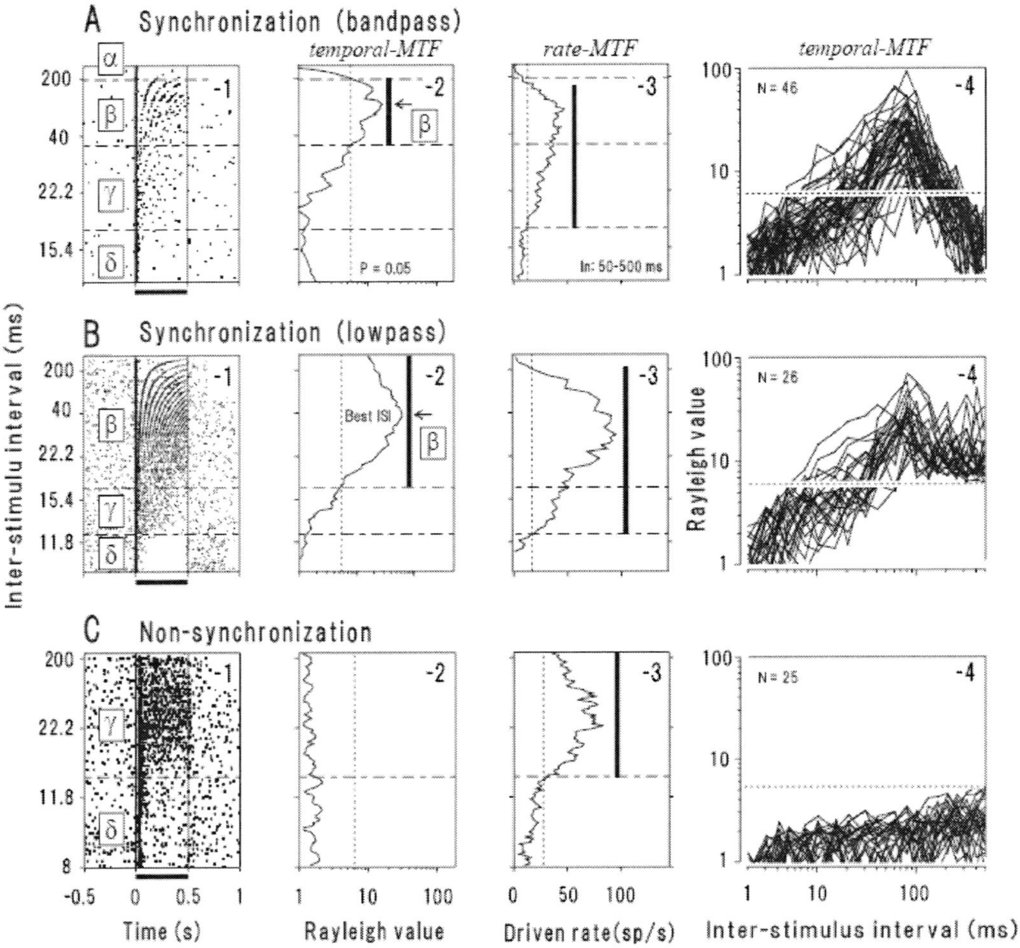


Figure 9. Examples of 3 single-unit activities in awake cat's AI in the click-train paradigm. If the given unit robustly responded to a single click, it was allotted further analysis by employing the click train paradigm (see below), and then they were classified into 3 types (A-C). Examples of each type were demonstrated in the 1st-3rd column, and pooled data in 4th column. 1st column: Raster display of discharges before, during (horizontal bar, below *abscissa*) and after 0.5-s long click trains with variable inter-stimulus intervals (ISI; *ordinate*). 2nd column: The degree of stimulus locking was quantified referring to "temporal modulation transfer function (temporal-MTF)" where Z value of vector strength was plotted as a function of the ISI. The ISI that gave the maximal Z value was denominated as best ISI (arrow). The unit showing statistically-significant stimulus locking ($P < 0.05$, Rayleigh statistics; dotted line) was classified as "synchronization unit" (A and B), and the reminder as "non-synchronization unit" (C). The "synchronization units" were divided into two subtypes according to the shape of the temporal-MTF such as "bandpass subtype" (A) and "lowpass subtype" (B). 3rd column: The amount of evoked discharges was quantified referring to "rate modulation transfer function (rate-MTF)" where the driven rate measured 50-500 ms after the onset of the train was plotted as a function of the ISI. 4th column: Pooled data of temporal-MTF for each type units (in the same format as B). (Modified from Sakai et al., 2009a). For convenience of latter analysis, we specify the following four response region. *Region $\alpha$,* where only onset responses are evident; *Region $\beta$,* stimulus locking takes place (vertical bar in A-2); *Region $\gamma$,* discharges are intermittently elicited without stimulus locking; *Region $\delta$,* onset responses are evident.

Figure 9A-1 is a raster dot display of discharges for a representative synchronization unit (the stimulus period is marked as horizontal bar at the bottom). According to our criterion, this unit had 4 qualitatively distinct response regions (α-δ). Specifically, in region α (ISI ≥ 200 ms), only the onset response was evident. In region β (ISI: 38-200 ms), "stimulus-locking responses" to individual clicks was evident, in that temporal modulation transfer function (temporal-MTF, A-2), defined as Z value of a vector strength (Goldberg and Brown, 1969), exceeded the statistically significant level ($P < 0.05$, Rayleigh statistic; vertical dotted line). By comparing the temporal-MTFs that were obtained at different SPLs, we defined the value of the SPL and ISI to produce the largest Z value as the "best SPL" and "best ISI" (arrow), respectively. The following data were obtained at the best SPL, unless otherwise specified. In region γ (ISI: 16-38 ms, A-1), discharges occurred intermittently during the stimulus period without stimulus locking (A-2). The driven rate measured 50-500 ms after the onset of the train (rate modulation transfer function: rate-MTF, A-3) exceeded the threshold for excitation (vertical dotted line). In region δ (ISI ≤ 16 ms, A-1), the onset response entailed an unresponsive (or suppressive) period. Region β was flanked by regions α and γ, looking as "bandpass" shaped (A-2). Forty-six synchronization units exhibited bandpass temporal-MTF (pooled data in A-4).

The remaining 26 synchronization units, as exemplified in Figures 9B, had 3 response regions (β-δ). Since region β of this subset was bordered with only region γ (B-1), the temporal-MTF was regarded as "lowpass" shaped (B-2; pooled data in B-4). Regardless of temporal-MTF shape, the border between regions β and γ (hereafter, β–γ border), in other words, the shorter ISI limit for stimulus locking, was at on average ~30 ms (Table). This value is in line with the previous AI single-unit studies on un-anesthetized animals (Maruyama et al., 1979; Bieser and Müller-Preuss, 1996; Miller et al., 2001; Lu et al., 2001; Liang et al., 2002), but rather shorter than that (40-200 ms) measured under barbiturate-anesthesia (Brosch and Schreiner, 1997; Reale and Brugge, 2000; Nakamoto et al., 2006). Such difference, as will be discussed later, probably reflects the fact that barbiturate enhances $GABA_A$-mediated post-synaptic inhibitory potentials (Franks and Lieb, 1994).

Figures 9C display responses of a non-synchronization unit. A part of them were considered to summate the impact of consecutive acoustic signals over a time window (up to ~160 ms; Sakai et al., 2009b). The synchronization units, however, will not be further analyzed since the main interest here is to elucidate fine-grained temporal processing necessary for VOT-dependent categorical perception.

We conducted the click-train paradigm at various stimulus intensities and found that the stimulus-locking capacity for individual synchronization units was substantially invariant to stimulus intensity over at least 20-dB SPL ranges. For example, the shorter limiting ISI for stimulus locking (= β-γ border, Figure 9A-2; Table) did not statistically-significantly differed between at the best SPL and 20-dB below it (Sakai et al., 2009a,b; data not shown here). This is in accordance with the relative level-invariance for temporal-order threshold (Hirsh, 1959) and VOT boundary for the plosive CV-syllables (Ehret, 1987).

A part of the synchronization units (all were bandpass type; n = 14) were delivered with the /da/-/ta/ tokens of variable VOT (Figure 3A). The result (not shown) resembled to Figure 8A: the midpoint of the neurometric function was on average 41.7 ± 34.1 ms (Table). This value is roughly equivalent to the shorter ISI limit for stimulus locking to the click trains.

Above all, it is likely that stimulus-locking responses of AI neurons have a relevance to perceived quality of successive signals regardless of whether the signals are non-phonetic (discreteness vs. continuousness) or phonetic (voiced vs. voiceless).

### 4.5. Comparison between Auditory Thalamus (Medial Geniculate Body: MGB) and AI for Stimulus-Locking Responses

To date, click trains and sinusoidally amplitude-modulated (AM) tones have been most commonly employed for exploring how periodic auditory information is processed and represented along the neuroaxis of the auditory system. While these two signals are not totally equivalent, they do capture closely related aspects of the neural process (Joris et al., 2003). Thus, in this section, I combine neurophysiology data that were obtained by those signals.

An accumulating body of single-unit data in anesthetized animals converges to the notion that as one ascends the auditory system, temporal-coding capacity for periodic auditory information progressively declines. Specifically, the maximal repetition rate (or minimal ISI) of acoustic signals for eliciting stimulus-locking responses is about 1000-2500 Hz (0.4-1 ms in ISI) in the auditory nerve (Palmer, 1982; Joris and Yin, 1992), 600-1500 Hz (0.6-1.6 ms) in most of the cochlear nucleus (Møller, 1974; Rhode and Smith, 1986; Frisina et al., 1990), 500-1000 Hz (1-2 ms) in the superior olivary complex (Batra et al., 1997; Joris and Yin., 1998), 200-500 Hz (2-5 ms) in the inferior colliculus (Rees and Møller, 1987; Krishna and Semple, 2000), hundred to several hundreds Hz (3-10 ms) in the medial geniculate body (MGB) (Rouiller et al., 1981; Miller et al., 2002), and 10-20 Hz (50-100 ms) in the AI (Brosch and Schreiner, 1997; Reale and Brugge, 2000; Nakamoto et al., 2006). Similar general tendency was preserved, with reservation of some quantitative differences, for single-unit data in un-anesthetized animals (auditory nerve: Parham et al., 1996; cochlear nucleus: Kim et al., 1990; superior olivary complex: Kuwada and Batra, 1999; inferior colliculus: Condon et al., 1996 and Müller-Preuss et al., 1994; MGB: Creutzfeldt et al., 1980 and Preuss and Müller-Preuss, 1990; AI: Wang et al., 2003 and Sakai et al., 2009a,b).

The degradation of temporal-coding capacity along the auditory neuroaxis is widely considered to reflect a transformation of a "temporally-coded" periodicity of the signal at lower levels into "rate-coded" information at higher levels (reviewed by Langner, 1997). For example, the auditory nerves and neurons in the most cochlear nuclei are rather poorly tuned in discharge rate to periodicity of the signal (Rhode and Smith, 1986; Joris and Yin, 1992). In contrast, at the level of the inferior colliculus, rate-coding appears to be favored over temporal-coding, particularly for higher repetition rates: most neurons do not exhibit stimulus-locking responses at the repetition rate $\geq$ ~400 Hz ($\leq$ 2.5 ms in ISI), but do systematically alter their discharge rate as a function of repetition rate (Møller and Rees, 1986; Langner and Schreiner, 1988). This tendency is further manifested at the level of the AI in un-anesthetized animals: single units appeared to comprise largely two subsets, one subset conducting temporal code at the repetition rate $\leq$ ~30 Hz ($\geq$ 30 ms in ISI) while another subset conducting only rate code at the repetition rate above several tens Hz (Maruyama et al., 1979; Bieser and Müller-Preuss, 1996; Lu et al., 2001; Liang et al., 2002; Sakai et al., 2009a,b).

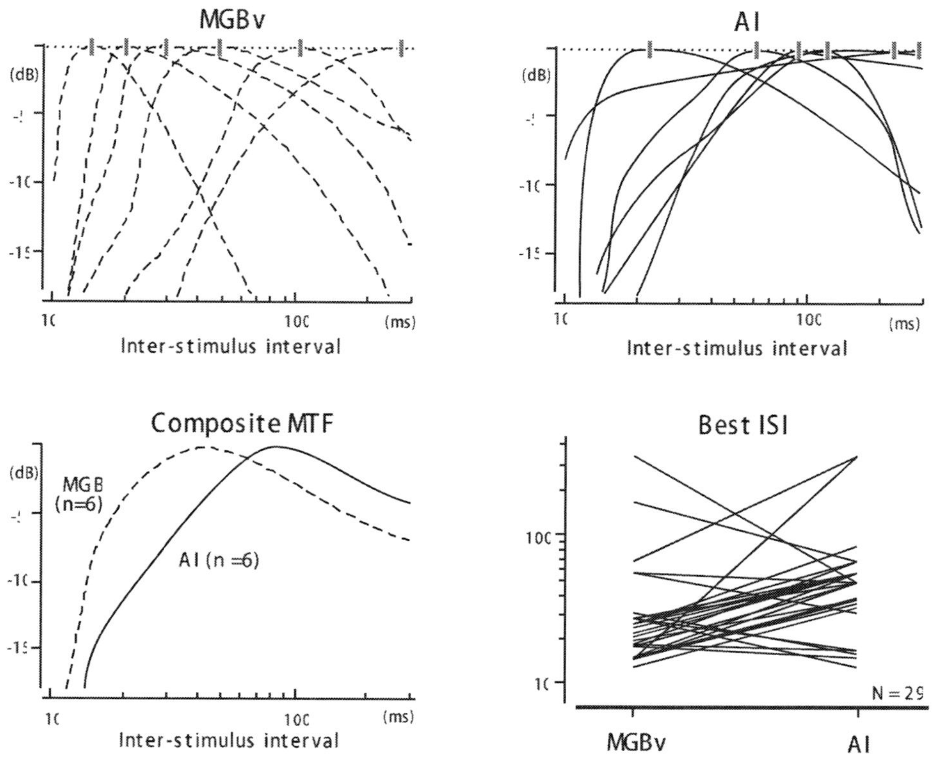


Adapted from Miller et al., 2001 and 2002.

Figure 10. Comparison of temporal-MTF between functionally connected single neurons in the auditory thalamus (ventral division of the medial geniculate body [MGBv]) and AI. A and B: Temporal-MTFs of representative single units in the MGBv and AI, respectively. The magnitude of stimulus locking was normalized to that observed at the best ISI (marked with blue bar; ref., Figure 9A-2) in individual units. C: Composite temporal-MTF for the MGBv (broken curve, obtained from A) and AI (solid curve, from B). The latter deviated rightward than the former, reflecting degenerated stimulus-locking capacity. D: Comparison of the best ISI between functionally connected pairs of single units, one is located in the MGBv and another in the AI. No rank correlation was revealed (P >0.2, Spearman rank correlation); MGBv units with longer (shorter) best ISI did not preferentially connect with AI units with longer (shorter) best ISI. This suggests that prolongation of the best ISI from the MGBv to AI (see C) cannot be simply attributed to a degradation of temporal resolution due to intrinsic membrane properties or synaptic delay but is rather due to more elaborated intra-cortical processing.

Accordingly, one would reasonably speculate that stimulus locking of the synchronization units (ex., Figure 9A) is merely rudiment of sub-cortical activities, and thus the contribution of intra-AI processing in itself is only minor. However, this conjecture is rebutted by the report of Miller et al. (2001) who simultaneously recorded pairs of functionally connected single units, one located in the ventral division of the MGB and another in the AI. Functional connectivity was confirmed if a cross-correlogram between their activities possessed a clear peak within 1–5 ms lag time (the MGB unit leading the AI unit) under both spontaneous and stimulus-driven conditions. Of note, no rank relationship was found for the best ISI (ref., arrow in Figure 9A-2): MGB units with longer (shorter) best ISI did not preferentially connect to AI units with longer (shorter) best ISI (Figure 10D). Similar result had been obtained from another set of single-unit study (Creutzfeldt et al., 1980). Therefore, degradation of temporal-coding capacity from the MGB to AI (see above) cannot be attributed simply to passive phenomenon that is related to intrinsic membrane properties or synaptic delay. Some elaborated intra-AI mechanisms may operate to refine temporal behavior of AI neurons (this issue will be discussed in detail below).

### 4.6. Summary

A subset of AI neurons (i.e., synchronization units) generated discharges time-locked to temporal envelop of phonetic and non-phonetic signals. The shorter limiting ISI of such responses was on average ~30 ms with level tolerance consistently to the perceptual boundary for VOT-dependent categorical perception of plosive CV syllables as well as temporal-order threshold.

## 5. Synaptic Mechanisms Underlying Temporal Behavior of AI Neurons

I devised a numerical model in an attempt to understand the neural mechanisms that underlie AI category-like responses (see above). The model comprises two versions: 4-receptor version (section 5.1) and full version (section 5.2). In each section, I firstly demonstrate key response features of our synchronization units. Second, by introducing in vitro data of other researchers, I discuss the neural elements that would be responsible for the responses the synchronization unit. Then, by employing plausible neural elements, I conduct simulation study in order to capture temporal behavior of the synchronization units.

### 5.1. Temporal Interplay between Excitation and Inhibition

#### *5.1.1. In Vivo Findings*

As demonstrated above (Figure 8A, most left), it is likely that "post-activation suppression" is involved in AI category-like responses. To examine this conjecture, we conducted an additional experiment on 35 single units (non-synchronization units, n = 8; synchronization units with bandpass temporal-MTF, n = 14; synchronization units with lowpass temporal-MTF, n = 13) that showed an appreciable amount of spontaneous discharge rate for detecting suppression.

In this recording session (namely, "single-click paradigm"), a single acoustic pulse (1-ms duration, at the best SPL) was presented 10-20 times at intervals of 4.0-5.5 s. The discharge occurrence was examined with dot raster plots (Figure 11, upper row) and post-latency time histogram (bottom row; bin width = 10 ms; the mean of the spontaneous firing rate was normalized as zero). The threshold for "excitation" was set at +2*SD of the spontaneous firing rate (dotted line, upper), and that for "suppression" at -2*SD of the spontaneous firing rate (dotted line, lower). We recognized 4 temporal patterns: (1) excitation (marked with red) alone ("E-alone"; 1st column); (2) excitation and following suppression (i.e., "post-activation suppression" [marked with blue]) ("E-S sequence"; 2nd column); (3) excitation, suppression then excitation ("E-S-E sequence"; 3rd column); (4) excitation, suppression, excitation then suppression ("E-S-E-S sequence"; last column).

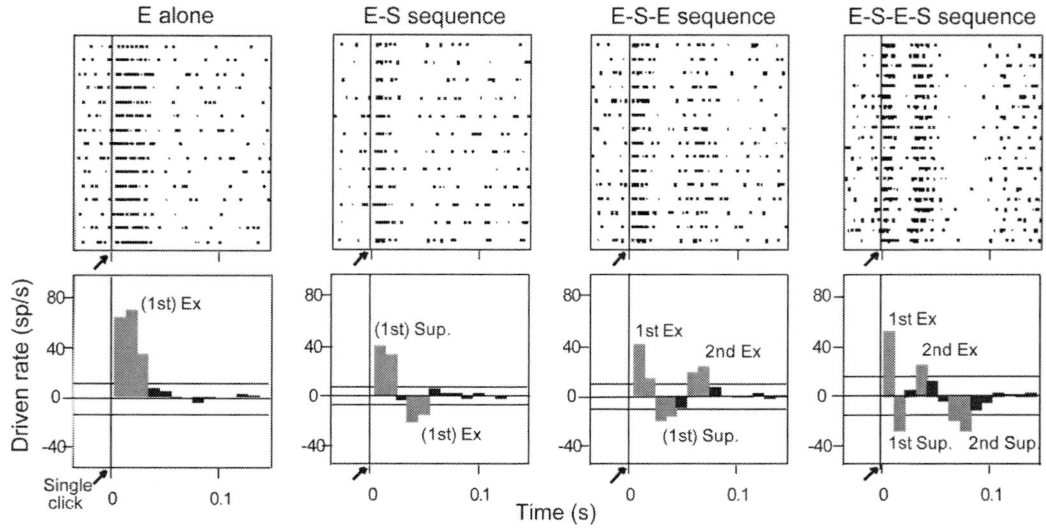


Modified from Sakai et al., 2009a.

Figure 11. Temporal interplay between excitation and suppression in awake cat's AI. Temporal response patterns of 4 representative units (1st column: non-synchronization type; others: synchronization type) triggered by a single click (arrow). Spike occurrence was examined with raster dot plots (upper panels) and PSTH (10-ms bin width; lower panels). The threshold for excitation (E) and suppression (S) was set at plus/minus 2*SD of the mean of spontaneous discharge rate (dotted line), respectively. The qualitatively distinct responses were aligned in the following sequence: only excitation (E; 1st column); excitation followed by suppression ("E-S sequence"; 2nd column); "E-S-E sequence" (3rd column); "E-S-E-S sequence" (last column).

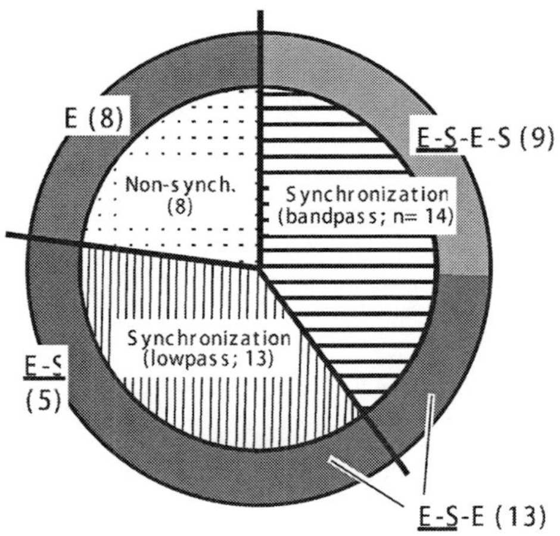


Modified from Sakai et al., 2009a.

Figure 12. Comparison of the results in Figure 9 (click trains) and Figure 11 (single click). The subjects were 35 single units that showed an appreciable amount of spontaneous discharges for detecting suppression. Note (1) all non-synchronization units had only single excitatory period (E-alone); (2) all synchronization units had the 1st excitation and 1st suppression (post-activation suppression; underlined). This implies the critical role for temporal interplay of excitation and suppression in stimulus-locking responses.

As summarized in Figure 12, all non-synchronization units showed "E-alone" pattern whereas all synchronization units showed the remaining patterns. Because all the remaining patterns by definition involve "post-activation suppression" (1st suppression subsequent to the 1st excitation; underlined), such neural process may be responsible for stimulus locking to a train of clicks. Among the synchronization units, the 2nd suppression (marked with asterisk) was present in 9 out of 14 units with bandpass temporal-MTF, whereas it was absent in all the units with lowpass temporal-MTF. Fisher's exact test revealed a significant effect of the 2nd suppression on the shape of the temporal-MTF ($P < 0.001$). This implies that the 2nd suppression constrains the shape of the temporal-MTF (bandpass vs. lowpass).

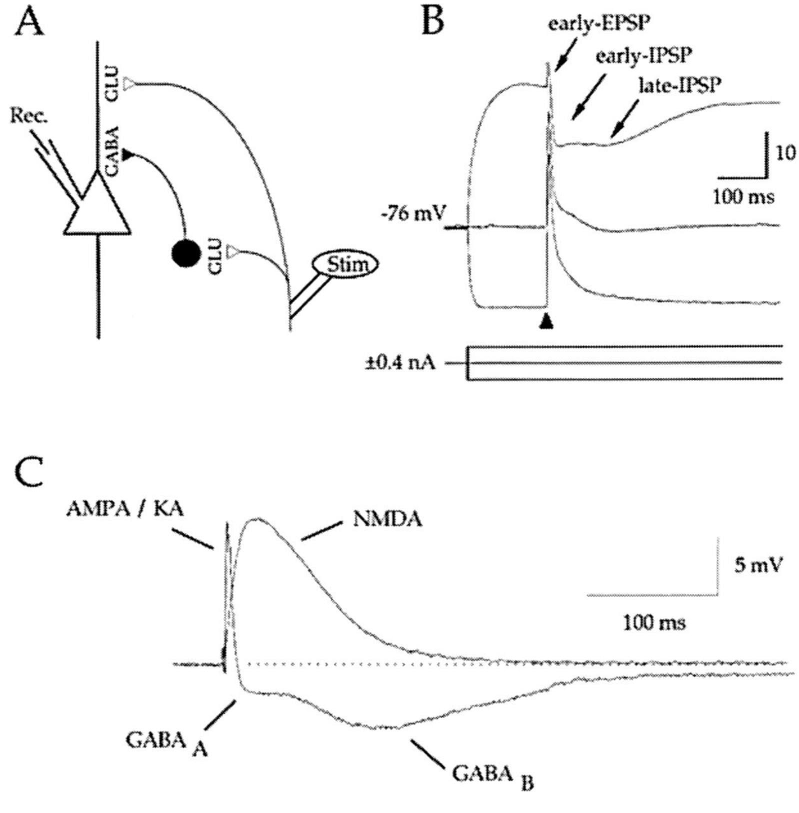


Adapted from Metherate, 1998.

Figure 13. Excitatory and inhibitory post synaptic potentials (EPSP and IPSP, respectively) in slice preparation from rat's AI. A: Schematic of a hypothetical local circuit in the AI. Electrical stimulation was given to the layer VI, and whole-cell recording was made from layer III pyramidal neuron. B: Single pulse stimulation (triangle) elicited an early-EPSP followed by early IPSP and late IPSP (upper trace). Stimulation during membrane depolarization and hyperpolarization (lower trace) demonstrates different reversal potentials for each component. C: Pharmacological manipulations indicate that the above mentioned three components are mediated by AMPA/KA, $GABA_A$, and $GABA_B$ receptors. A fourth potential, the NMDA receptor-mediated late-EPSP, is usually masked by early IPSP and late IPSP. The full late-EPSP was observed after pharmacologically eliminating those IPSP components.

### 5.1.2. In Vitro Findings

de Ribaupierre and colleagues (de Ribaupierre et al., 1972) reported in AI single unit study that stimulus locking was greatly related to the temporal interplay of depolarization and hyperpolization. Compelling evidence indicates that depolarization and hyperpolization of AI neurons are chiefly based on excitatory post-synaptic potentials (EPSPs) and inhibitory post-synaptic potentials (IPSPs), respectively (Cox et al., 1992; Metherate and Ashe, 1994; Ojima and Murakami, 2002; Wehr and Zador, 2005). Of note, Cox and colleagues (1992), by employing patch-clamp technique on slice preparations from rat's AI, measured post-synaptic potentials at the soma of a pyramidal neurons that were evoked by electrical stimulation to thalamocortical afferent fibers (Figure 13A). They observed at maximum 4 components in the following order: a fast-EPSP, fast-IPSP, slow-EPSP then slow-IPSP (Figure 13B; see legend for details). Pharmacological experiments in combination with current injection procedure proved those components were mediated chiefly by AMPA-, $GABA_A$-, NMDA- and $GABA_B$-receptors, respectively (Figure 13C; schematized in Figure 14A).

### 5.1.3. Model Idea

The above findings inspire a hypothesis of intra-AI mechanisms to regulate temporal behavior of the synchronization unit. For simplicity, consider the case in which an AI neuron receives two successive brief afferent signals (Figure 14B; similar time scale holding to Figure 14A-C). If the interval between the 1st signal (filled arrow, Figure 14B-1) and 2nd signal (open arrow) is short enough that the 2nd signal arrives during the existence of the 1st-signal-elicited fast-EPSP (ref., Figure 14A; same as followings), the 2nd signal may readily evoke discharges. However, the discharge clusters evoked by each signal are seemingly somewhat contiguous so that stimulus locking, if any, would be unequivocal. Accordingly, the predicted temporal-MTF (Figure 14C, schematically drown) may show a little upward deflection (colored with red, left). Second, if the 2nd signal arrives during the 1st-signal-elicited fast-IPSP (Figure 14B-2) or slow-IPSP (B-3), it may hardly evoke discharges and so for stimulus-locking responses. Accordingly the predicted temporal-MTF (Figure 14C) may show two downward deflections (colored with blue). Third, when the 2nd signal arrives during the 1st-signal-elicited slow-EPSP (Figure 14B-4), it may readily evoke discharges. The discharge clusters evoked by the 1st and 2nd signal would be separated by virtue of the fast-IPSP resulting in clear stimulus-locking responses. Accordingly, the predicted temporal-MTF (Figure 14C) is expected to have a prominent upward deflection at several tens millisecond in ISI (red, right).

Of note, the total body of the predicted temporal-MTF (colored curve), excepting short ISI portion, markedly resembled to both (1) temporal-MTF to click trains that was averaged for the bandpass-type synchronization units (black solid curve, attached with region name [α-δ]; based on Figure 9A-4). This leads to the hypothesis that temporal-coding capacity of the AI neuron is constrained by temporal interplay of EPSPs and IPSPs and (2) neurometric function for multi-unit activities responding to two-click sequences (broken curve; same as in Figure 8B, right panel [Tomita et al., 2004]).

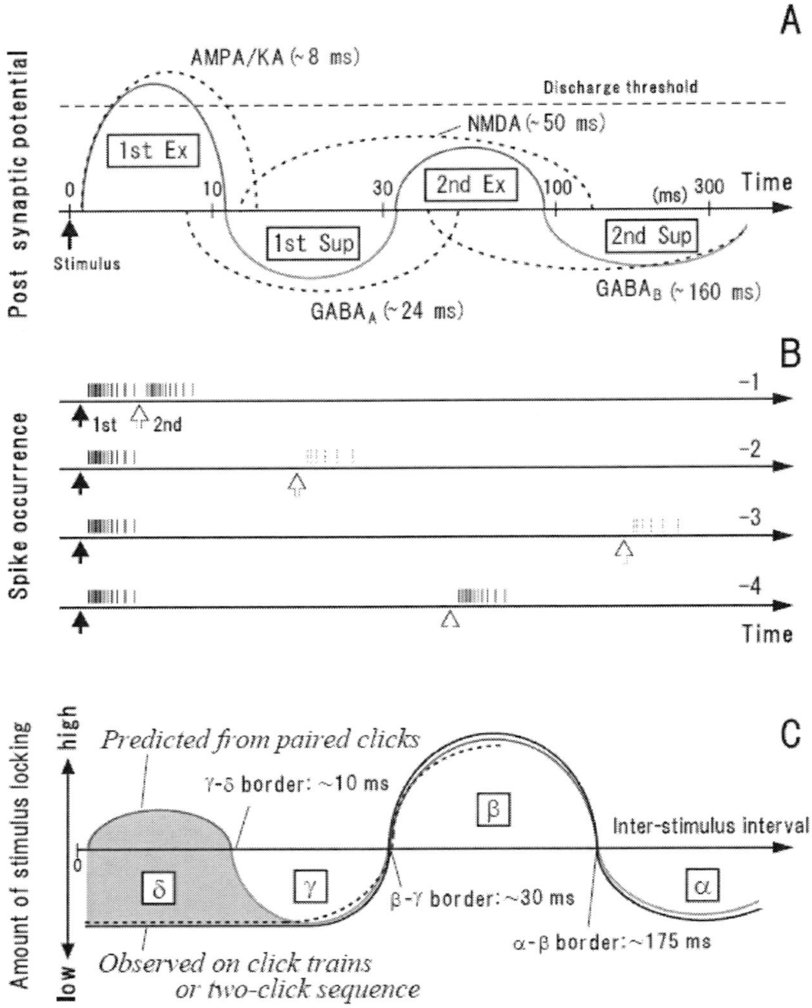


Modified from Sakai et al., 2009a.

Figure 14. Prediction of the temporal-MTF based on the vitro study. A: Scheme for a sequence of EPSP and IPSP components (dotted curves) at the soma of pyramidal neuron in the AI (based on in vitro study by Cox et al., 1992 and Metherate, 1998). The time course of those components was approximated referring to the afferent stimulation (arrow) with numerals within parentheses depicting latency-to-peak. Temporal interaction between those components is expected to produce four phases (solid curves): 1st excitation (red), 1st suppression (blue), 2nd excitation (red), then 2nd suppression (blue). Identical time scale is applied to A-C. B: Prediction of discharges evoked by paired stimuli (1st: filled arrow; 2nd: open arrow) with various inter-stimulus intervals. When the 2nd stimulus is given during the presence of the 1st excitation (ref., A), it would readily evoke discharges (-1). However, the discharge clusters evoked by the 1st and 2nd stimulus may merge together so that stimulus locking would be ambiguous. When the 2nd stimulus is given during the 1st suppression (-2) or 2nd suppression (-3), it would hardly evoke discharges, and consequently, little or no stimulus locking responses. When the 2nd stimulus is given during the 2nd excitation (-4), it would readily evoke discharges. The discharge clusters evoked by the 1st and 2nd stimulus could be separated together by virtue of the 1st suppression. C: Scheme for the temporal-MTF predicted from A and B (colored with red and blue) and temporal-MTF observed in the click train paradigm (solid, black; ref., Figure 9A-4) and neurometric function to two-click sequence for unit-unit activities (broken, black; same as in Figure 8B, right). Regions α–δ correspond to those in Figure 9A-1. Note the resemblance between the three curves, excepting at short ISIs (the difference is highlighted with gray).

### *5.1.4. Simulation Results (4-Recepor Version)*

To numerically examine the above hypothesis, Sakai et al. (2009a) conducted a simulation study. The model was made on such AI neuron that was embedded in the local circuitry as schematized in Figure 13A, with receiving afferent input via various combinations of AMPA, $GABA_A$, NMDA and/or $GABA_B$ receptors. The external input was modeled as 1-ms-long repetitive square-wave pulses with fixed amplitude. Each panel in Figure 15A shows simulated membrane potentials responding at 70-ms ISI. Because this value corresponded to the mean of the best ISI for bandpass-type synchronization units (Table), our expectance was of typical "region β" (ex., Figure 9A-1). If only AMPA receptors were incorporated into the model (Figure 15A-1), each signal evoked discharges. However, robust onset responses, which always accompanied to the onset of the stimulus train, was

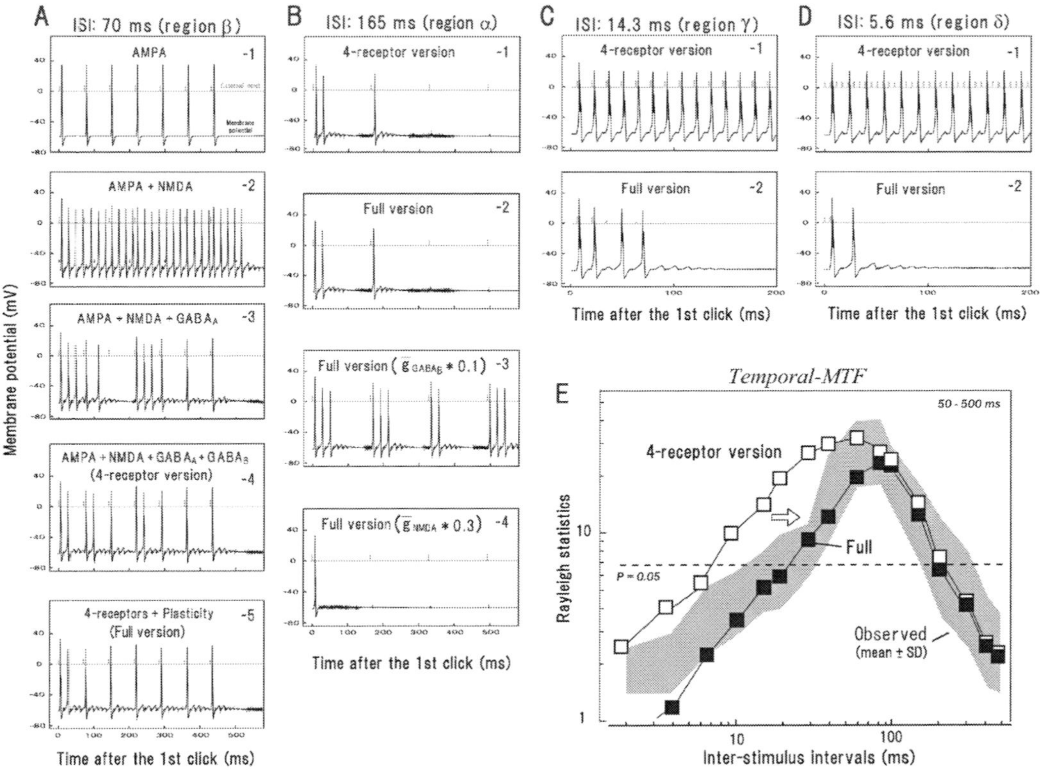


Modified from Sakai et al., 20009a.

Figure 15. A neurocomputational model for the membrane potentials at the soma of a single pyramidal neuron in the AI. The neuron was hypothesized to be involved in the local circuitry as illustrated in Figure 13A. Thalamocortical afferent signal was modeled as 1-ms-long repetitive square-wave pulses (initial amplitude: 12.5 $\mu Acm^{-2}$) (blue line). The simulation was made on various combinations of the receptors (AMPA, $GABA_A$, NMDA and/or $GABA_B$ receptors) with/without short-term plasticity (frequency-dependent depression [FDD] and paired-pulse facilitation [PPF]) of thalamocortical synaptic connections. A-D: Membrane potentials calculated at inter-stimulus interval (ISI) of 70 ms (region β; A), 165 ms (region α; B), 14.3 ms (region γ; C) and 5.6 ms (region δ; D). E: The temporal MTF calculated in different conditions. For comparison, gray sphere demarcates the mean ± SD of the data in Figure 9A-4.

If NMDA receptors were added into the model (A-2), then dischargers took place all through the stimulus train; however, stimulus locking was unclear. If $GABA_A$ receptors were added to the model (A-3), then the neuron re-gained the stimulus-locking capacity. While this feature, more or less, looked alike the physiological observation in region β (Figure 9A-1), the former differed from the latter in that: (1) the 3rd stimulus failed evoking discharges and (2) the discharge clusters evoked by the 4th and 5th stimulus merged together. Such discrepancies were diminished if $GABA_B$ receptors were further incorporated into the model (Figure 15A-4; namely "4-receptor version"). This version model generally well captured physiologically observed responses at relatively long ISIs. For example, at 165-ms ISI, the predicted discharge pattern (Figure 15B-1) resembled to that in "region α" (Figure 9A-1) where only onset responses were prominent.

The power of 4-receptor version model declined with shortening of the ISI. For example at 14.3-ms ISI, at which typical "region γ" pattern was expected (ref., Figure 9A-1), the model predicted succinct stimulus-locking discharges to each stimulus (Figure 15C-1). At 5.6-ms ISI, where typical "region δ" pattern was expected (ref., Figure 9A-1), the model predicted "skipping" of discharges every three stimuli (Figure 15D-1) which had never been actually observed.

The predicted temporal-MTF (open squares, Figure 15E) expanded leftward as compared to the physiological data (gray sphere: mean ± SD for bandpass-type synchronization units [based on Figure 9A-4]). Such disparity may indicate the involvement of other neural element(s) in modulating temporal behavior of the synchronization neurons, whose relative contribution increases at shorter ISI (or higher repetition rate).

## 5.2. Involvement of Short-Term Plasticity

It is widely accepted that repetitive stimulation exerts accumulation effects on responsiveness of auditory neurons especially those in the auditory cortex (reviewed by Amitai, 2001; Zucker and Regehr, 2002). It is, thus, possible that such accumulation effects do exert influence on the synchronization unit. We examined this possibility on the pooled data that was obtained using the click-train paradigm (same units as in section 4.4.). In the following two sections, we paid special attention to regions β and δ, where the causative relationship between a given stimulus and discharges can be clearly identified.

### *5.2.1. In Vivo Findings*

Figure 16A (upper trace) displays the number of discharges (#discharges; bin width = 5 ms) for a representative synchronization unit (identical unit as in Figure 9A) that were evoked at the best ISI (92 ms). For simplicity, we uniformly adopted the best ISI of individual units to examine typical "region β" response. #Discharges in each discharge cluster in this unit (Figure 16B, open circles) progressively decreased as a progression of the stimulus train, indicating that the impact of successive clicks were accumulated to reduce the responsiveness to the following signals. This was confirmed by the population data (Figure 16C, open circles) where #discharges evoked by each click was normalized to that evoked by the 1st click (hereafter, control level; broken line). The accumulation effect disappeared by 3.6 s after the termination of the trains at any ISIs (Sakai et al., 2009a; data not shown here). The observed features were all consistent with so-called "frequency-dependent depression" (Galarreta and Hestrin, 1998).

Figure 16A (lower trace) displays #discharges in region δ for the same synchronization unit. For simplicity, we uniformly adopted the ISI value at 0.9 multiples of the γ-δ border (15.6-ms in this instance) to analyze typical "region δ" response. The onset response was ~30

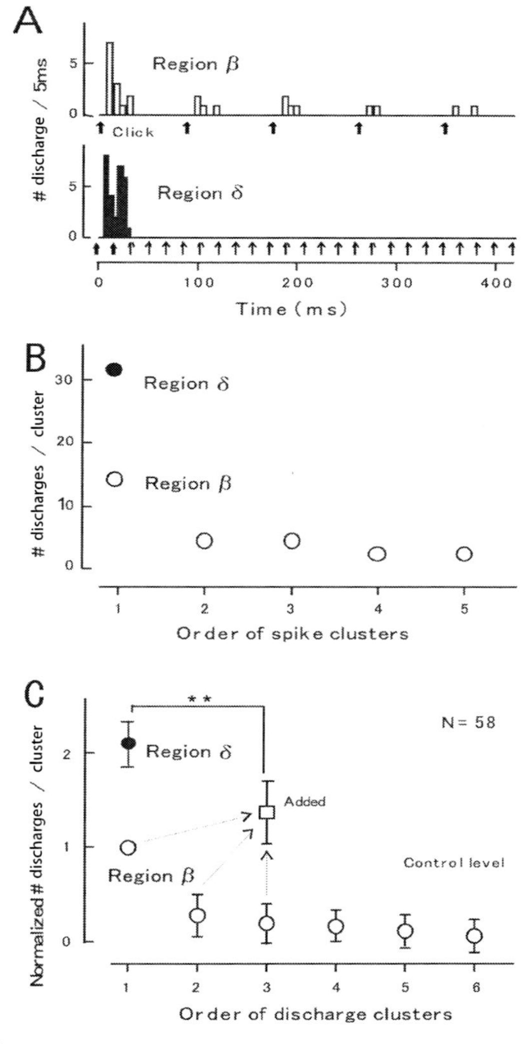


Modified from Sakai et al., 2009a.

Figure 16. Short-term plasticity of responsiveness in region β (at the best ISI) and region δ (at 0.9 multiples of the γ-δ border) for the synchronization units (identical unit as in Figure 9A). A and B: Examples of PSTH (5-ms bin width; A) and the number of discharges involved in each discharge cluster (B). C: Population data (mean ± SD) for B (the number of discharges was normalized to that involved in the 1st discharge cluster [= control level]). In region β, the number of discharges declined with the progression of the click train, consistently with "frequency-dependent depression." The number of discharges involved in the onset response in region δ (filled circle), which is contributed to by on average 2.4 ± 0.7 clicks (see text), is larger than the total amount of discharges involved in the initial three discharge clusters in region β (**P < 0.01, paired t-test). This suggests that when several consecutive clicks fall within a few tenths of millisecond (in region δ), there is a synergy of impact, resulting in "paired-pulse facilitation."

ms in duration, into which 2 clicks fell (bold arrows) indicating that discharge clusters evoked by the 1st and 2nd click merged together. The onset response included 31 discharges (Figure 16B, filled circle). This number was much larger than the total amount of #discharges which were evoked by the 1st and 2nd click in region $\beta$ (broken circle).

This finding was confirmed by population data: (1) the onset response in region $\delta$ was on average $36.8 \pm 18.1$ ms in duration, into which $2.4 \pm 0.7$ clicks fell; (2) the normalized #discharges involved in the onset response was on average $2.1 \pm 0.3$ (Figure 16C, filled circle); (3) this value was significantly larger than the total amount of the normalized #discharges which were evoked by the initial 3 clicks in region $\beta$ ($P < 0.01$, paired t-test). These findings suggest that when several consecutive clicks fall within a few tenths of millisecond, there is a synergy of impact. This phenomenon is consistent with "paired-pulse facilitation" (Kamiya and Zucker, 1994).

Collectively, it was suggested that responsiveness of the synchronization units subjects to short-term plasticity such as "frequency-dependent depression" and "paired-pulse facilitation."

### *5.2.2. In Vitro Findings*

There is very convincing evidence that short-term plasticity, such as frequency-dependent depression and paired-pulse facilitation, is omnipresent across the central nervous system of mammals including the AI (reviewed by Zucker and Regehr, 2002). While a number of biophysical processes are likely to underlie such phenomena, the most prominent ones appear to reside at presynaptic terminals including temporal exhaustion of readily releasable neurotransmitter pool for frequency-dependent depression (Galarreta and Hestrin, 1998) and a residual elevation in intracellular calcium concentration for paired-pulse facilitation (Kretz et al., 1982; Kamiya and Zucker, 1994). This implies that our numerical model will gain more prediction power if the amplitude of external input was incorporated with short-term plasticity (Figure 13A, plasticity [+]) instead of being fixed (plasticity [-]).

The relevant information can be typically obtained from the study of Varela et al. (1997) who recorded excitatory post-synaptic currents (EPSCs) of pyramidal neuron in slice preparations from the primary visual cortex in rats. Peak amplitude of EPSCs ($A_0$, $A_1$, $A_2$ ...) was recorded from layer II/III pyramidal neuron while electrical stimulus was delivered to layer IV in a train fashion (Figure 17A). The vertical lines in Figures 17B-D represent the amplitude of $A_1$, $A_2$, $A_3$ ... (averaged over 10 trials) and the dotted horizontal does line the amplitude of $A_0$ when the stimulus was repeated at 4 Hz (250 ms in ISI; B), 5 Hz (200 ms; C) or 10 Hz (100 ms; D). As a whole, the response amplitude was once facilitated immediately after the initiation of the stimulus train then gradually declined for a while.

In order to capture dynamic properties of the responsiveness, the authors adopted a three component model which contained a single facilitation factor (F) and two depression factors ($D_1$ [fast and robust] and $D_2$ [slow and minute]):

$$A_n = A_0*F*D_1*D_2 \ (n = 1, 2, 3 \ldots)$$

where $\tau_F*dF/dt = 1- F$, $\tau_{D1}*dD_1/dt = 1- D_1$, and $\tau_{D2}*dD_2/dt = 1- D_2$.

The parameter values in the equations were modified to best fit the data. The relationship of the parameters values to $\Delta t$ was shown in Figure 17E. Then, in turn, the best fitted results were plotted as dots in Figures 17B-D. The biological correlates to individual parameters in the above equations were not specified. Nonetheless, the model well captured the net effect of short-term plasticity.

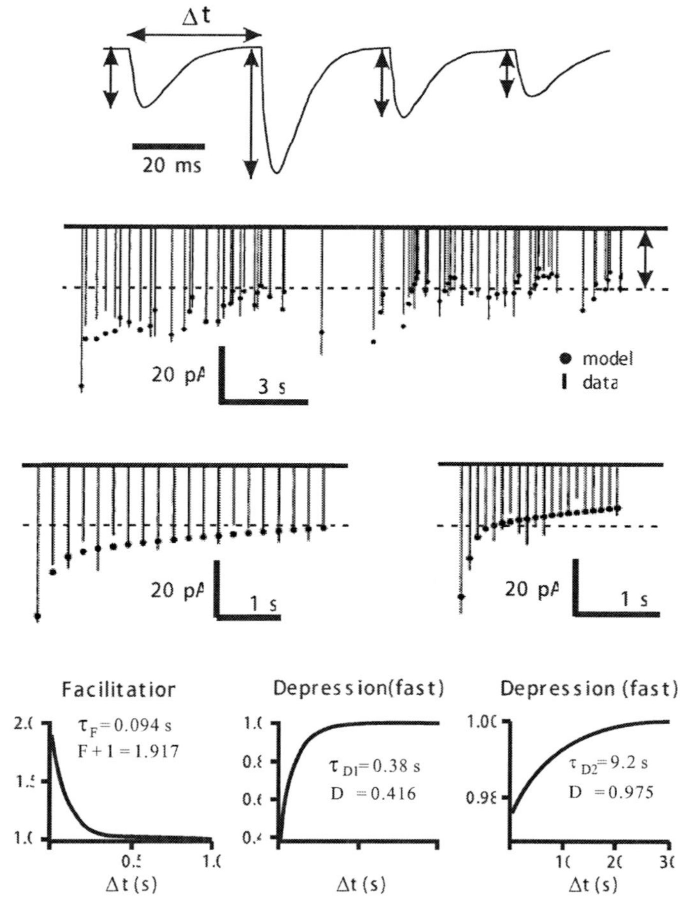


Modified from Varela et al., 1997.

Figure 17. Short-term plasticity of excitatory post-synaptic currents (EPSCs) of layer II/III pyramidal neuron in slice preparation from rat's primary visual cortex. A: Scheme of raw data. Peak amplitude of EPSCs ($A_0$, $A_1$, $A_2$ ...) was measured while low amplitude electrical stimulus train was delivered to layer IV with an interval of $\Delta t$. B-D: Average amplitude of $A_1$, $A_2$, $A_3$ ... (line; over 10 repetitions) evoked by the stimulus train of 4 Hz (poison distribution: B), 5 Hz (constant rate: C), 10 Hz (ibid: D). Dotted line depicts $A_0$ as a reference. Dots are the best fitted to the three component model which contains a single facilitation factor (F) and two depression factor ($D_1$ and $D_2$): $A_n = A_0{*}F{*}D_1{*}D_2$ (n = 1, 2, 3 ...) where $\tau_F{*}dF/dt = 1- F$, $\tau_{D1}{*}dD_1/dt = 1- D_1$, $\tau_{D2}{*}dD_2/dt = 1- D_2$. E: The amplitude and time course of F, $D_1$ and $D_2$.

### *5.2.3. Simulation Results (Full Version)*

We implemented short-term plasticity to external inputs of the 4-receptor version model. To do this, we adopted Varela et al's (1997) equations (see above) (depression factor D2 was deleted because it was negligibly small in practice). The parameter values of their equations were arranged to best fit to our data (Figure 16C). Hereafter, this version model will be referred to as "full version" (Sakai et al., 2009a).

In region β, the full version model (Figure 15A-5) predicted similar responses to those simulated by 4-receptor version (A-4). This was also the case when the comparison was made on responses in region α (cf., B-2 to B-1). In general, both versions well captured temporal behavior of synchronization units at relatively long ISIs (> ~60 ms).

At shorter ISIs, two versions of the model made highly contrastive predictions. For example, in region γ, the 4-receptor version predicted unrealistically-magnificent stimulus locking (C-1); the full version predicted only modest stimulus locking only at the beginning of the stimulus train (C-2) consistently to physiological observations (Figure 9A-1). In region δ, the 4-receptor version predicted "skipping" of stimulus-locking responses to every several stimuli (Figure 15D-1); the full version did not predict such unrealistic feature but only onset responses (D-2) consistently to physiological observations (Figure 9A-1).

As a whole, the full version model, comparing to the 4-receptor version, predicted less potent stimulus locking at short ISIs leading rightward shift of the rising limb of the temporal-MTF curve (filled squares, Figure 15E). The resultant temporal-MTF curve well fitted to the physiologically observed one for the bandpass-type synchronization units (gray sphere). This makes it likely that temporal behavior of the synchronization units are also mediated through short-term plasticity of thalamocortical synaptic connections.

It should be mentioned that the 4-receptor version model, in its original form, is not applicable to lowpass type synchronization units, which by definition maintain stimulus-locking capacity at long ISIs (Figure 9B-2). Given that the 2nd suppression was present exclusively in the bandpass type synchronization units (marked with asterisk, Figure 12), it is possible that the 2nd suppression hinders the capacity for stimulus locking at long ISIs, and thus configures the shape of temporal-MTF. If so, manipulation of activities of the $GABA_B$ receptors or NMDA receptors may alter stimulus-locking capacity at long ISIs because, as described above, the 2nd suppression is likely to be mediated chiefly by $GABA_B$-receptor mediated IPSP and NMDA-receptor mediated EPSP (Figure 14A). In the model, when the conductance of the $GABA_B$-receptors ($_{GABAB}$) (originally 1.0 nS, according to Otis and Mody [1992]) was reduced by factor of 0.1, responsiveness to the initial several stimuli elevated, enhancing low-pass effect (Figure 15B-3; cf., B-2). Contrariwise, when the conductance of the NMDA-receptors ($g_{NMDA}$) (originally 0.38 nS, according to Jonas and Spruston [1994]) was reduced by factor of 0.3, responsiveness to the 2nd and latter stimuli degraded, enhancing low-cut effect (B-4). Manipulation of the conductance of the AMPA or $GABA_A$ receptors did not greatly affect responsiveness at long ISIs (data not shown). Collectively, it was suggested that the shape of the temporal-MTF (bandpass vs. lowpass) is configured based on the balance between $GABA_B$-receptor mediated IPSP and NMDA-receptor mediated EPSP.

### *5.2.4. Discussion*

Having high predictability of neurophysiological data, our computation model raises the possibility that stimulus-locking capacity of AI neurons are mediated chiefly through temporal interplay of EPSPs and IPSPs along with short-term plasticity of thalamocortical synaptic connections. Under this scheme, the shorter ISI limit for stimulus locking (i.e., β–γ border, Figure 9A-1), the presumed neural correlate to the VOT boundary as well as temporal-order threshold (see above), corresponded to the time point of transition from the 1st suppression to the 2nd excitation (Figure 14A).

The mean of the shorter ISI limit for stimulus locking that was measured in the present single unit study (~30 ms, Table) is compatible to the neurophysiological data that was obtained from un-anesthetized animals (Maruyama et al., 1979; Bieser and Müller-Preuss, 1996; Miller et al., 2001; Lu et al., 2001; Liang et al., 2002; Sakai et al., 2009a,b) but rather shorter than the data (40-200 ms) obtained from anesthetized animals (Brosch and Schreiner, 1997; Reale and Brugge, 2000; Nakamoto et al., 2006). Some anesthetics, such as pentobarbital, are known to potentate $GABA_A$-receptor mediated IPSPs (Franks and Lieb, 1994). This may enhance the 1st suppression and consequently diminish the 2nd excitation, especially in its early phase. As a consequence, the transition point between the two components would shift afterward, prolonging the shorter ISI limit for stimulus locking.

A question remains why the majority of the synchronization units (bandpass type) exhibited "low-cut" effects in temporal filtering (Table). Our computational model attributes such property to the 2nd suppression which dominates at ~100-300 ms after the stimulus onset (Figure 14A). 100-300 ms (or repetition rate of 3-10 Hz) fits to both (1) duration of most syllables (Hoequist, 1983; ex., Figure 2A) and (2) utterance rate on which intelligibility of speech sounds predominantly relies (Houtgast and Steeneken, 1985; Greenberg and Arai, 2004). Drullman et al. (1994) found that intelligibility of speech sounds was considerably hindered when the waveform envelop was artificially lowpass filtered below 4 Hz (250 ms in ISI) and suggested that such effect was mainly due to blurring the temporal contrast between successive syllables. Within commonly encountered reverberant environments, reverberant sounds are intermingled with the original signals so that (1) temporal-modulation depth is reduced and (2) distribution of temporal-modulation rate shifts down to 1-2 Hz (Houtgast and Steeneken, 1985). Such effects hinder intelligibility of speech sounds especially at 2-6 Hz in temporal-modulation rate. Therefore, it is possible that "low-cut" effect in bandpass-type synchronization units is of great use to improve intelligibility of speech sounds by mean of assorting syllables along temporal domain with buffering against reverberation.

### 5.3. Summary

Temporal behavior of synchronization units in the AI, including the shorter ISI limit for stimulus locking, were well captured by our computational model which incorporated (i)AMPA-receptor-mediated EPSP, (ii)$GABA_A$-receptor-mediated IPSP, (iii)NMDA-receptor-mediated EPSP, (iv)$GABA_B$-receptor-mediated IPSP and (v)short-term plasticity of thalamocortical synaptic connections.

## Conclusion

Accumulating body of psychophysical, clinical and neurophysiological evidence indicate that VOT-dependent categorical perception of plosive CV syllables does NOT arise from a specific speech mechanism as previously believed, but is based on general auditory processing of inter-stimulus intervals (ISIs), especially in the AI. Specifically, a subset of AI neurons (i.e., synchronization units) showed a capacity to generate discharges time-locked to temporal envelop regardless of whether the signals are phonetic or non-phonetic. The shorter limiting ISI of such responses (~30 ms) as well as its level tolerance was compatible with various ISI-dependent categorical perception including VOT-dependent categorical perception of plosive CV syllables. Stimulus-response features of the synchronization units were well captured by our computational model, indicating that such perceptual phenomenon are mediated thought temporal interplay of EPSPs and IPSPs in the AI neuron along with short-term plasticity of thalamocortical synaptic connections.

## References

Abramson, A.S., and Lisker, L. (1970). Discriminability along the voicing continuum: cross language tests. In *Proceedings of the 6th International Congress of Phonetic Sciences* (pp. 569-573). Prague, Czech Republic: Academia Press.

Ahissar, E., Nagarajan, S., Ahissar, M., Protopapas, A., Mahncke, H. and Merzenich, M.M. (2001). Speech comprehension is correlated with temporal response patterns recorded from auditory cortex. *Proc. Natl. Acad. Sci. USA 98,* 13367-13372.

Albert, M.L. and Bear, D. (1974). Time to understand. A case study of word deafness with reference to the role of time in auditory comprehension. *Brain 97,* 373-384.

Amitai, Y. (2001). Thalamocortical synaptic connections: efficacy, modulation, inhibition and plasticity. *Rev. Neurosci. 12,* 159-173.

Auerbach, S., Allard, T., Naeser, M., Alexander, M. and Albert, M. (1982). Pure Word Deafness: analysis of a case with bilateral lesions and a defect at the prephonemic level. *Brain 105,* 271-300.

Batra, R., Kuwada, S. and Fitzpatrick, D.C. (1997). Sensitivity to interaural temporal disparities of low- and high-frequency neurons in the superior olivary complex. II. Coincidence detection. *J. Neurophysiol. 78,* 1237-1247.

Bieser, A. and Müller-Preuss, P. (1996). Auditory responsive cortex in the squirrel monkey: neural responses to amplitude-modulated sounds. *Exp. Brain Res. 108,* 273-284.

Blumstein, S.E. and Stevens, K.N. (1979). Acoustic invariance in speech production: evidence from measurements of the spectral characteristics of stop consonants. *J. Acoust. Soc. Am. 66,* 1001-1017.

Brick, J.F., Forst J.L., Schoshe, Jr S.S., Gutmann, L. and Crosby, T.W. (1985). Pure word deafness: CT localization of the pathology. *Neurology 35,* 441-442.

Brosch, M. and Schreiner, C.E. (1997). Time course of forward masking tuning curves in cat primary auditory cortex. *J. Neurophysiol. 77,* 923-943.

Brugge, I.F. (1975). Progress in neuroanatomy and neurophysiology of auditory cortex. In D. B. Tower (Ed.), *The Nervous System. Vol. 3. Human Communication and Its Disorders* (pp. 97-111). New York: Raven Press.

Buchtel, H.A. and Stewart, J.D. (1989). Auditory agnosia: apperceptive or associative disorder? *Brain and Language 37,* 12-25.

Butler, R.A., Diamond, I.T. and Neff, W.D. (1957). Role of auditory cortex in discrimination of changes of frequency. *J. Neurophysiol. 20,* 108-120.

Chocholle, R., Chedru, F., Botte, M.C., Chain, F. and Lhermitte, F. (1975). Psychoacoustic study of a case of "cortical deafness". *Neuropsychologia 13,* 163-172.

Condon, C.J., White, K.R. and Feng, A.S. (1996). Neurons with different temporal firing patterns in the inferior colliculus of the little brown bat differentially process sinusoidal amplitude-modulated signals. *J. Comp. Physiol. A Sens. Neural. Behav. Physiol. 178,* 147-157.

Covey, E., Kauer, J.A. and Casseday, J.H. (1996). Whole-cell patch-clamp recording reveals subthreshold sound-evoked postsynaptic currents in the inferior colliculus of awake bats. *J. Neurosci. 16,* 3009-3018.

Cox, C.L., Metherate, R., Weinberger, N.M. and Ashe, J.H. (1992). Synaptic potentials and effects of amino acid antagonists in the auditory cortex. *Brain Res. Bull. 28,* 401-410.

Cranford, J.L., Igarashi, M. and Stramler, J.H. (1976). Effect of auditory neocortex ablation on pitch perception in the cat. *J. Neurophysiol. 39,* 143-152.

Creutzfeldt, O.D., Hellweg, F.C. and Schreiner, C.E. (1980). Thalamocortical transformation of responses to complex auditory stimuli. *Exp. Brain Res. 39,* 87-104.

Cutting, J.E. and Rosner, B.S. (1974). Categorical boundaries in speech and music. *Percept. Psychophys. 16,* 564-570.

de Ribaupierre, F., Goldstein, M.H. Jr. and Yeni-Komshian, G. (1972). Intracellular study of the cat's primary auditory cortex. *Brain Res. 48,* 185-204.

Delattre, P.C., Lieberman, A.M. and Cooper, F.S. (1955). Acoustic loci and transitional cues for consonants. *J. Acoust. Soc. Am. 27,* 769-773.

Denes, G. and Semenza, D. (1975). Auditory modality-specific anomia: evidence from a case of pure word deafness. *Cortex 11,* 410-411

Destexhe, A., Mainen, Z.F., and Sejnowski, T.J. (1998). Kinetic models of synaptic transmission. In C. Koch, and I. Segev (Eds.), *Methods in Neuronal Modeling* (pp.1-25). Cambridge, MA: MIT Press.

Destexhe, A. and Sejnowski, T.J. (1995). G-protein activation kinetics and spill-over of GABA may account for differences between inhibitory responses in the hippocampus and thalamus. *Proc. Natl. Acad. Sci. USA 92,* 9515-9519.

Divenyi, P.L. and Sachs, R.M. (1978). Discrimination of time intervals bounded by tone bursts. *Perception and Psychophysics 24,* 429-436.

Divenyi, P.L. and Danner, W.F. (1977). Discrimination of time intervals marked by brief acoustic pulses of various intensities and spectra. *Perception and Psychophysics 21,* 125-142.

Dobrunz, L.E. and Stevens, C.F. (1997). Heterogeneity of release probability, facilitation, and depletion at central synapses. *Neuron 18,* 995-1008.

Dooling, R.J., Okanoya, K. and Brown, S.D. (1989). Speech perception by budgerigars (Melopsittacus undulatus): the voiced-voiceless distinction. *Percept. Psychophys. 46,* 65-71.

Drullman, R., Festen, J.M. and Plomp, R. (1994). Effect of temporal envelope smearing on speech reception. *J. Acoust. Soc. Am. 95,* 1053–1064.

Edeline, J.M., Dutrieux, G., Manunta, Y. and Hennevin, E. (2001). Diversity of receptive field changes in auditory cortex during natural sleep. *Eur. J. Neurosci. 14,* 1865-1880.

Eggermont, J.J. (1999). Neural correlates of gap detection in three auditory cortical fields in the cat. *J. Neurophysiol. 81,* 2570-2581.

Eggermont, J.J. (1995a). Representation of a voice onset time continuum in primary auditory cortex of the cat. *J. Acoust. Soc. Am. 98,* 911-920.
Eggermont, J.J. (1995b). Neural correlates of gap detection and auditory fusion in cat auditory cortex. *NeuroReport 6,* 1645-1648.
Ehret, G. (1987). Categorical perception of sound signals: facts and hypotheses from animal studies. In S. Harnad (Ed.), *Categorical Perception* (pp. 301-331). Cambridge, UK: Cambridge University Press.
Eimas, P.D. (1982). Speech perception: a view of the initial state and perceptual mechanisms. In J. Mehler, M. Garret, and E. Walker (Eds.), *Perspectives in mental representation* (pp. 339–360). Hills-dale, NJ: Erlbaum Press.
Evarts, E.N. (1952). Effect of auditory cortex ablation on frequency discrimination in monkey. *J. Neurophysiol. 15,* 443-448.
Fant, G. *Acoustic theory of speech production.* Hague, Netherlands: Mouton Press; 1960.
Fechner, GT. *Elemente der Psychophysik.* Leipzig, Germany: Breitkopf und Härtel Press; 1860 (Reprinted, Bristol, UK: Thoemmes Press; 1999).
Festinger, L., Allyn, M.R. and White, C.W. (1971). The perception of color with achromatic stimulation. *Vision Res. 11,* 591-612.
Fraisse, P. (1984). Perception and estimation of time. *Annu. Rev. Psychol. 35,* 1-36.
Franks, N.P. and Lieb, W.R. (1994). Molecular and cellular mechanisms of general anaesthesia. *Nature 367,* 607-613.
Frisina, R.D., Smith, R.L. and Chamberlain, S.C. (1990). Encoding of amplitude modulation in the gerbil cochlear nucleus: I. A hierarchy of enhancement. *Hearing Res. 44,* 99-122.
Galarreta, M. and Hestrin, S. (1998). Frequency-dependent synaptic depression and the balance of excitation and inhibition in the neocortex. *Nat. Neurosci. 1,* 587–594.
Gescheider, G.A. (1988). Psychophysical scaling. *Annu. Rev. Psychol. 39,* 169-200.
Geschwind, N. (1965). Disconnection syndromes in animals and man. *Brain 88,* 237-294.
Goldberg, J.M. and Brown, P.B. (1969). Response of binaural neurons of dog superior olivary complex to dichotic tonal stimuli: some physiological mechanisms of sound localization. *J. Neurophysiol. 22,* 613-636.
Golomb, D., Shedmi, A., Curtu, R. and Ermentrout, G.B. (2006). Persistent synchronized bursting activity in cortical tissues with low magnesium concentration: a modeling study. *J. Neurophysiol. 95,* 1049-1067.
Gordon, J. and Abramov, I. (1988). Scaling procedures for specifying color appearance. *Color Res. and Application 13,* 149-152.
Greenberg, S. and Arai, T. (2004). What are the essential cues for understanding spoken language? *IEICE Trans Inf. and Syst. E87-D,* 1059-1070.
Griffiths, T.D., Rees, A. and Green, G. (1999). Disorders of human complex sound processing. *Neurocase 5,* 365-378.
Grigoreva, T.I., Figurina, I.I. and Vasilev, A.G. (1988). Role of the medial geniculate body in the production of conditioned reflexes to amplitude-modulated stimuli in rats. *Zh. Vyssh Nervn. Deyat 37,* 265-271.
Grothe, B. (2003). New roles for synaptic inhibition in sound localization. *Nat. Rev. Neurosci. 4,* 540-550.
Harnad, S. *Categorical Perception: the Groundwork of Cognition.* Cambridge, UK: Cambridge University Press; 1987.

Hashimoto, K. and Sasaki, K. (1982). On the relationship between the shape and position of the tongue for vowels. *J. Phonetics 10,* 291-299.

Heffner, H.E., and Heffner, R.S. (1990). Role of primate auditory cortex in hearing. In W.C. Stebbins, and M.A. Berkley (Eds.), *Comparative Perception II* (pp. 279-310). New York: Wiley Press.

Heffner, H.E. and Heffner, R.S. (1989). Effect of restricted cortical lesions on absolute thresholds and aphasia-like deficits in Japanese macaques. *Behav Neurosci 103,* 158-169.

Heilman, K.M., Bowers, D., Speedie, L. and Coslett, H.B. (1984). *Comprehension of affective and nonaffective prosody. Neurology 34,* 917-921.

Hemphill, R.E. and Stengel, E. (1940). A study on pure word-deafness. *J. Neurol. Psychiatry 3,* 251-262.

Hirsh, I.J. (1959). Auditory perception of temporal order. *J. Acoust. Soc. Am. 31,* 759–767.

Hirsh, I.J. and Sherrick, C.E. (1961). Perceived order in different sense modalities. *J. Exp. Psychol. 26,* 423-432.

Hodgkin, A. and Huxley, A. (1952). A quantitative description of membrane current and its application to conduction and excitation in nerve. *J. Physiol. 117,* 500-544.

Hoequist, Jr C. (1983). Syllable duration in stress-, syllable- and mora-timed languages. *Phonetica 40,* 203-237.

Horst, R., Leeuw, A.R. and Dreschler, W.A. (1999). Importance of temporal-envelope cues in consonant recognition. *J. Acoust. Soc. Am. 105,* 1801-1809.

Houtgast, T. and Steeneken, H. (1985). A review of the MTF concept in room acoustics and its use for estimating speech intelligibility in auditoria. *J. Acoust. Soc. Am. 77,* 1069–1077.

Ison, J.R., O'Connor, K., Bowen, G.P. and Bocirnea, A. (1991). Temporal resolution of gaps in noise by the rat is lost with functional decortication. *Behav. Neurosci. 105,* 33-40.

Joliot, M., Ribary, U. and Llinas, R. (1994). Human oscillatory brain activity near 40 Hz coexists with cognitive temporal binding. *Proc. Natl. Acad. Sci. USA 91,* 11748-11751.

Jonas, P. and Spruston, N. (1994). Mechanisms shaping glutamate-mediated excitatory postsynaptic currents in the CNS. *Curr. Opin. Neurobiol. 4,* 366–372.

Joris, P.X., Schreiner, C.E. and Rees, A. (2004). Neural processing of amplitude-modulated sounds. *Physiol. Rev. 84,* 541-577.

Joris, P.X. and Yin, T.C. (1998). Envelope coding in the lateral superior olive. III. Comparison with afferent pathways. *J. Neurophysiol. 79,* 253-269.

Joris, P.X. and Yin, T.C. (1992). Responses to amplitude-modulated tones in the auditory nerve of the cat. *J. Acoust. Soc. Am. 91,* 215-232.

Kamiya, H. and Zucker, R.S. (1994). Residual $Ca^{2+}$ and short-term synaptic plasticity. *Nature 371,* 603–606.

Kim, D.O., Sirianni, J.G. and Chang, S.O. (1990). Responses of DCN-PVCN neurons and auditory nerve fibers in unanesthetized cats to AM and pure tones: analysis with autocorrelation/power-spectrum. *Hear Res. 45,* 95-113.

Klein, R. and Harper, J. (1956). The problem of agnosia in light of a case of pure word deafness. *J. Ment. Sci. 102,* 112-120.

Kretz, R., Shapiro, E. and Kandel, E.R. (1982). Post-tetanic potentiation at an identified synapse in aplysia is correlated with a Ca2+-activated K+ current in the presynaptic neuron: evidence for Ca2+ accumulation. *Proc. Natl. Acad. Sci. USA 79,* 5430–5434.

Krishna, B.S. and Semple, M.N. (2000). Auditory temporal processing: responses to sinusoidally amplitude-modulated tones in the inferior colliculus. *J. Neurophysiol. 84,* 255-273.

Kryter, K.D. and Ades, H.W. (1943). Studies of the function of higher acoustic nervous centers in the cat. *Am. J. Psychol. 56,* 501-536.

Kuhl, P.K. (1986). Theoretical contributions of tests on animals to the special-mechanisms debate in speech. *Exp. Biol. 45,* 233-265.

Kuhl, P.K. and Padden, D.M. (1983). Enhanced discriminability at the phonetic boundaries for the place feature in macaques. *J. Acoust. Soc. Am. 73,* 1003-1010.

Kuhl, P.K. (1981). Discrimination of speech by nonhuman animals: basic auditory sensitivities conducive to the perception of speech-sound categories. *J. Acoust. Soc. Am. 70,* 340-349.

Kuhl, P.K. and Miller, J.D. (1978). Speech perception by the chinchilla: identification function for synthetic VOT stimuli. *J. Acoust. Soc. Am. 63,* 905-917.

Kuhl, P.K. and Miller, J.D. (1975). Speech perception by the chinchilla: voiced-voiceless distinction in alveolar plosive consonants. *Science 190,* 69-72.

Kurowski, K. and Blumstein, S.E. (1987). Acoustic properties for place of articulation in nasal consonants. *J. Acoust. Soc. Am. 81,* 1917-1927.

Kussmaul, A. (1877). Disturbances of speech. In H. von Ziemssen (Ed.), *Cyclopedia of the Practice of Medicine* (pp. 581-875). New York: William Wood Press.

Kuwada, S. and Batra, R. (1999). Coding of sound envelopes by inhibitory rebound in neurons of the superior olivary complex in the unanesthetized rabbit. *J. Neurosci. 19,* 2273-2287.

Langner, G. (1997). Neural processing and representation of periodicity pitch. *Acta Otolaryngology Suppl. 532,* 68-76.

Langner, G. and Schreiner, C. (1988). Periodicity Coding in the Inferior Colliculus of the Cat. *J. Neurophysiol. 60,* 1805-1822.

Lichtheim, L. (1885). On aphasia. *Brain 7,* 433-484.

Lieberman, P. *The Biology and Evolution of Language*. Cambridge, MA: Harvard University Press; 1984.

Lieberman, A.M., Isenberg, D. and Rakerd, B. (1981). Duplex perception of cues for stop consonants: evidence for a phonetic mode. *Percept. Psychophys. 30,* 133-143.

Lieberman, A.M., Cooper, F.S., Shankweiler, D.P. and Studdert-Kennedy, M. (1967). Perception of the speech code. *Psychological Review 74,* 431-461.

Lieberman, A.M., Harris, K.S., Kinney, J.A. and Lane, H.L. (1961). The discrimination of relative onset time of the components of certain speech and nonspeech patterns. *J. Exp. Psychol. 61,* 378-388.

Lieberman, A.M., Harris, K.S., Hoffman, H.S. and Griffith, B.C. (1957). The discrimination of speech sounds within and across phoneme boundaries. *J. Exp. Psychol. 54,* 358-368.

Liégeois-Chauvel, C., de Graaf, J.B., Laguitton, V. and Chauvel, P. (1999). Specialization of left auditory cortex for speech perception in man depends on temporal coding. *Cereb. Cortex 9,* 484-496.

Liepmann, H. and Storch, E. (1902). Der mikroskopische Gehirnbefund bei dem Fall Gorstelle. *Monatsschrift fur Psychiatrie und Neurologie 11,* 115-120.

Lisker, L. (1975). Is it VOT or a first-formant transition detector? *J. Acoust. Soc. Am. 57,* 1547-1551.

Lisker, L., and Abramson, A.S. (1970). The voicing dimension: some experiments in comparative phonetics. In Proceedings of the 6th International Congress of Phonetic Sciences (pp. 563-567). Prague, Czech Republic: Academia Press.

Lu, T., Liang, L. and Wang, X. (2001). Temporal and rate representations of time-varying signals in the auditory cortex of awake primates. *Nat. Neurosci. 4,* 1131-1138.

Maruyama, N., Saitoh, K. and Kudoh, M. (1979). Unit responses of the cat's auditory cortex to synthesized formant. *Proc. Japan Acad. B 55,* 413-417.

Massaro, D.W. and Oden, D.W. (1980). Evaluation and integration of acoustic features in speech perception. *J. Acoust. Soc. Am. 67,* 996-1013.

McGee, T., Kraus, N., King, C. and Nicol, T. (1996). Acoustic elements of speechlike stimuli are reflected in surface recorded responses over the guinea pig temporal lobe. *J. Acoust. Soc. Am. 99,* 3606-3614.

Mendez, M.F. and Geehan, G.R. Jr. (1988). Cortical auditory disorders: clinical and psychoacoustic features. *J. Neurology, Neurosurgery, and Psychiatry 51*, 1-9.

Metherate, R. (1998). Synaptic mechanisms in auditory cortex function. *Front Biosci.* 3, 494-501.

Metherate, R. and Ashe, J.H. (1994). Facilitation of an NMDA receptor-mediated EPSP by paired-pulse stimulation in rat neocortex via depression of GABAergic IPSPs. *J. Physiol. 481,* 331-348.

Metz-Lutz, M.N. and Dahl, E. (1984). Analysis of word comprehension in a case of pure word deafness. *Brain and Language 23,* 13-25.

Meyer, D.R. and Woolsey, C.N. (1952). The effect of localized cortical destruction upon auditory discriminative conditioning in the cat. *J. Neurophysiol. 15,* 149-162.

Miceli, G. (1982). The processing of speech sounds in a patient with cortical auditory disorder. *Neuropsychologia 20,* 5-20.

Michon, J.A. (1964). Studies on subjective duration I: differential sensitivity in the perception of repeated temporal intervals. *Acta Psychologica 22,* 441-450.

Miller, J.D., Wier, C.C., Pastore, R.E., Kelly, W.J. and Dooling, R.J. (1976). Discrimination and labeling of noise-buzz sequences with varying noise-lead times: an example of categorical perception. *J. Acoust. Soc. Am. 60,* 410-417.

Miller, L.M., Escabi, M.A., Read, H.L. and Schreiner, C.E. (2002). Spectrotemporal receptive fields in the lemniscal auditory thalamus and cortex. *J. Neurophysiol. 87,* 516-527.

Miller, L.M., Escabi, M.A., Read, H.L. and Schreiner, C.E. (2001). Functional convergence of response properties in the auditory thalamocortical system. *Neuron 32,* 151-160.

Møller, A.R. (1974). Responses of units in the cochlear nucleus to sinusoidally amplitude-modulated tones. *Exp. Neurol. 45,* 105-117.

Müller-Preuss, P., Flachskamm, C. and Bieser, A. (1994). Neural encoding of amplitude modulation within the auditory midbrain of squirrel monkeys. *Hearing Res. 80,* 197-208.

Näätänen, R. and Winkler, I. (1999). The concept of auditory stimulus representation in cognitive neuroscience. *Psychol. Bull. 125,* 826-859.

Näätänen, R. *Attention and Brain Function*. New York: Lawrence Erlbaum Press; 1992.

Nakamoto, K.T., Zhang, J. and Kitzes, L.M. (2006). Temporal nonlinearity during recovery from sequential inhibition by neurons in the cat primary auditory cortex. *J. Neurophysiol. 95,* 1897-1907.

Neff, W.D., Diamond, D.M., and Casseday, J.H. (1975). Behavioral studies of auditory discrimination. In W.D. Keidel, and W.D. Neff (Eds.), *Handbook of Sensory Physiology* (pp. 307-400). New York: Springer Press.

Ojima, H. and Murakami, K. (2002). Intracellular characterization of suppressive responses in supragranular pyramidal neurons of cat primary auditory cortex in vivo. *Cereb. Cortex. 12,* 1079–1091.

Oswald, A.M., Schiff, M.L. and Reyes, A.D. (2006). Synaptic mechanisms underlying auditory processing. *Curr. Opin. Neurobiol. 16,* 371-376.

Otis, T.S. and Mody, I. (1992). Differential activation of GABAA and GABAB receptors by spontaneously released transmitter. *J. Neurophysiol. 67,* 227-235.

Palmer, A.R. (1982). Encoding of rapid amplitude fluctuations by cochlear nerve fibers in the guinea pig. *Arch. Otorhinolaryngol. 236,* 197-202.

Parham, K., Zhao, H.B. and Kim, D.O. (1996). Responses of auditory nerve fibers of the unanesthetized decerebrate cat to click pairs as simulated echoes. *J. Neurophysiol. 76,* 17-29.

Parker, E.M. (1988). Auditory constraints on the perception of voice-onset time: the influence of lower tone frequency on judgments of tone-onset simultaneity. *J. Acoust. Soc. Am. 83,* 1597-1607.

Phillips, D.P. and *Farmer,* M.E. (*1990*). *Acquired word deafness* and the temporal grain of sound representation in the primary auditory cortex. *Behav. Brain Res. 40,* 85-94.

Phillips, D.P. and Irvine, D.R. (1979). Methodological considerations in mapping auditory cortex: binaural columns in AI of cat. *Brain Res. 161,* 342-346.

Pickett, J.M. (1999). Prosodic and tonal features. In J.M. Pickett (Ed.), *The Acoustics of Speech Communication: fundamentals, Speech Perception Theory, and Technology* (pp. 75-98). Boston, MA: Allyn and Bacon Press.

Pisoni, D.B. (1977). Identification and discrimination of the relative onset time of two component tones: implications for voicing perception in stops. *J. Acoust. Soc. Am. 61,* 1352-1361.

Poeppel, D. (2003). The analysis of speech in different temporal integration windows: cerebral lateralization as "asymmetric sampling in time." *Speech Communication 41,* 245-255.

Pöppel, E. (2001). Pure word deafness and the bilateral processing of the speech code. *Cognitive Science 25,* 679-693.

Preuss, A. and Müller-Preuss, P. (1990). Processing of amplitude modulated sounds in the medial geniculate body of the squirrel monkey. *Exp. Brain Res. 79,* 201–211.

Price, C., Thierry, G. and Griffiths, T. (2005). Speech-specific auditory processing: where is it? *Trends in Cognitive Science 9,* 271-276.

Reale, R.A. and Brugge, J.F. (2000). Directional sensitivity of neurons in the primary auditory (AI) cortex of the cat to successive sounds ordered in time and space. *J. Neurophysiol. 84*, 435-450.

Rhode, W.S. and Smith, P.H. (1986). Encoding timing and intensity in the ventral cochlear nucleus of the cat. *J. Neurophysiol. 56,* 261-286.

Rosen, S. (1992). Temporal information in speech: acoustic, auditory and linguistic aspects. *Philos. Trans. R. Soc. Lond. B. Biol. Sci. 336,* 367-373.

Rosenzweig, M. (1946). Discrimination of auditory intensities in the cat. *Am. J. Psychol. 59,* 127-136.

Rouiller, E., de Ribaupierre, Y., Toros-Morel, A. and de Ribaupierre, F. (1981). Neural coding of repetitive clicks in the medial geniculate body of cat. *Hear Res. 5,* 81-100.

Saffran, E.M., Marin, S.M. and Yeni-Komshian, G.H. (1976). An analysis of speech perception in word deafness. *Brain and Language 3,* 209-228.

Sakai, M., Chimoto, S., and Sato, Y. (2009a). Neural mechanisms of interstimulus interval-dependent responses in the primary auditory cortex of awake cats. *BMC Neuroscience* [10], 10.

Sakai, M., Chimoto, S., Qin, L. and Sato, Y. (2009b). Differential representation of spectral and temporal information by primary auditory cortex neurons in awake cats: relevance to auditory scene analysis. *Brain Res. 1265,* 80-92.

Sakai, M. and Sato, Y. Circular sensitivity to the temporal-envelope period of the primary auditory cortex (AI) neuron in awake cats (submitted).

Shannon, R.V. (2005). Speech and music have different requirements for spectral resolution. *Int. Rev. Neurobiol. 70,* 121-134.

Sharma, A., Marsh, C. and Dorman, M.F. (2000). Relationship between N1 evoked potential morphology and perception of voice-onset-time. *J. Acoust. Soc. Am. 108,* 3030-3035.

Sharma, A. and Dorman, M.F. (1999). Cortical auditory evoked potential correlates of categorical perception of voice-onset time. *J. Acoust. Soc. Am. 106,* 1078-1083.

Shevell, SK. *The science of color.* Oxford, UK: Elsevier; 2003.

Stefanatos, G.A., Gershkoff, A. and Madigan, S. (2005). On pure word deafness, temporal processing, and the left hemisphere. *J. Int. Neuropsychol. Soc. 11,* 456-470.

Steinschneider, M., Fishman, Y.I. and Arezzo, J.C. (2003). Representation of the voice onset time (VOT) speech parameter in population responses within primary auditory cortex of the awake monkey. *J. Acoust. Soc. Am. 114,* 307-321.

Steinschneider, M., Volkov, IO., Noh, M.D., Garell, P.C. and Howard, M.A. (1999). Temporal encoding of the voice onset time (VOT) phonetic parameter by field potentials recorded directly from human auditory cortex. *J. Neurophysiol. 82,* 2346-2357.

Steinschneider, M. Schroeder, C.E., Arezzo, J.C. and Vaughan, H.G. Jr. (1995). Physiologic correlates of the voice onset time (VOT) boundary in primary auditory cortex (A1) of the awake monkey: temporal response patterns. *Brain Lang. 48,* 326-340.

Steinschneider, M., Schroeder, C., Arezzo, J.C. and Vaughan, H.G. Jr. (1994). Speech-evoked activity in primary cortex: effects of voice onset time. *Electroenceph. Clin. Neurophysiol. 92,* 30–43.

Stevens, KN. *Acoustic phonetics. Current studies in linguistics.* Cambridge, MA: MIT Press; 2000.

Stevens, K.N. (1980). Acoustic correlates of some phonetic categories. *J. Acoust. Soc. Am. 68,* 836-842.

Stevens, K.N. and Klatt, D.H. (1974). Role of formant transitions in the voiced–voiceless distinction for stops. *J. Acoust. Soc. Am. 55,* 653-659.

Stevens, S. (1957). On the psychophysical law. *Psychological Review 64,* 153–181.

Stevens, S., Volkman, J. and Newman, E. (1937). A scale for the measurement of the psychological magnitude pitch. *J. Acoust. Soc. Am.* 8,185-190.

Stevens, S. (1936). A scale for the measurement of the psychological magnitude: loudness. *Psychological Review 43,* 405-416.

Stockert, T.R. (1982). On the structure of word deafness and mechanisms underlying the fluctuation of disturbances of higher cortical functions. *Brain Lang. 16,* 133-146.

Studalert-Kennedy, M., Lieberman, A.M., Harris, K.S. and Cooper, F.S. (1970). Theoretical notes. Motor theory of speech perception: a reply to Lane's critical review. *Psychol. Rev. 77,* 234-249.

Summerfield, Q. (1982). Differences between spectral dependencies in auditory and phonetic temporal processing: relevance to the perception of voicing in initial stops. *J. Acoust. Soc. Am. 72,* 51-61.

Summerfield, Q. and Haggard, M. (1977). On the dissociation of spectral and temporal cues to the voicing distinction in initial stop consonants. *J. Acoust. Soc. Am. 62,* 435-448.

Symmes, D. (1966). Discrimination of intermittent noise by macaques following lesions of the temporal lobe. *Exp. Neurol. 16,* 201-214.

Takahashi, N., Kawumura, M., Shinotou, H., Hirayama, K., Kaga, K. and Shindo, M. (1992). Pure word deafness due to left hemisphere damage. *Cortex 28,* 295-303.

Tanaka, Y., Yamadori, A. and Mori, E. (1987). Pure word deafness following bilateral lesions: a psychophysical analysis. *Brain 110,* 381-403.

Tomita, M., Norena, A. and Eggermont, J.J. (2004). Effects of an acute acoustic trauma on the representation of a voice onset time continuum in cat primary auditory cortex. *Hearing Res. 193,* 39-50.

Ulrich, G. (1978). Interhemispheric functional relationships in auditory agnosia: an analysis of the preconditions and a conceptual mod. *Brain and Language 5,* 286-300.

Varela, J.A., Sen, K., Gibson, J., Fost, J., Abbott, L.F. and Nelson, S.B. (1997). A quantitative description of short-term plasticity at excitatory synapses in layer 2/3 of rat primary visual cortex. *J. Neurosci. 17,* 7926-7940.

Waters, R.S. and Wilson, W.A. (1976). Speech perception by rhesus monkeys: the voicing distinction in synthesized labial and velar stop consonants. *Percept. Psychophy. 19,* 285-289.

Weber, EH. *De pulsu, resorptione, auditu et tactu. Annotationes anatomicae et physiologicae.* Lipsiae, Germany: Koehler Press; 1834.

Wehr, M. and Zador, A.M. (2005). Synaptic mechanisms of forward suppression in rat auditory cortex. *Neuron 47,* 437-445.

Wernicke, C. and Friedlander, C. (1883). Ein Fall von Taubheit in Folge von doppelseitiger Laesionen des Schlafenlappens. *Fortschr Med.* 1, 177-185.

Yaqub, B.A., Gascon, O., AI-Nosha, M. and Whitaker, H. (1988). Pure word deafness (acquired verbal auditory agnosia) in an Arabic speaking patient. *Brain 111,* 457-466.

Young, E.D. (2007). Neural representation of spectral and temporal information in speech. *Philos. Trans. R. Soc. Lond. B. Biol. Sci. 363,* 923-945.

Zucker, R.S. and Regehr, W.G. (2002). Short-term synaptic plasticity. *Annu. Rev. Physiol. 64,* 355-405.

Zurita, P., Villa, A.E., de Ribaupierre, Y., de Ribaupierre, F. and Rouiller, E.M. (1994). Changes of single unit activity in the cat's auditory thalamus and cortex associated to different anesthetic conditions. *Neurosci. Res. 19,* 303-316.

In: Auditory Cortex: Anatomy, Functions and Disorders
Editor: Mounya Elhilali
ISBN 978-1-62100-685-5


*Chapter VII*

# Cortical Activity during Postural Audio-Biofeedback: A Study Based on Quantitative EEG

***Marco Pirini, Martini Mancini and Lorenzo Chiari****
DEIS - Department of Electronics, Computer Science, and Systems - Università di Bologna, Italy

## Abstract

The control of postural sway depends on the dynamic integration of multisensory information in the Central Nervous System. Augmentation of sensory information, such as during auditory biofeedback (ABF) of the trunk acceleration, has been shown to improve postural control. We evaluated, by means of quantitative electro-encephalography (EEG), which are the basic processes in the brain involved in the perception and cognition of auditory signals used for ABF.

ABF and Fake ABF (FAKE) auditory stimulations were delivered to 10 healthy naive subjects during quiet standing postural tasks, with eyes open and closed. Trunk acceleration and 19-channels EEG were recorded at the same time. Advanced, state-of-the-art EEG analysis and source modeling methods were employed to assess the possibly differential, functional activation and localization of EEG spectral features (power in the $\alpha$, $\beta$, and $\gamma$ bands) between the FAKE and the ABF conditions, for both the eyes open and the eyes closed tasks.

Subjects gained advantage by ABF in reducing their postural sway, as measured by a reduction of the root mean square of trunk acceleration during the ABF compared to the FAKE condition. EEG outcomes support the idea that ABF for postural control heavily modulates (increases) the cortical activation in healthy subjects. Population-wise cortical localization analysis (based on the sLORETA method) performed on the comparison FAKE - ABF revealed: i) a significant decrease ($p < 0.05$) of $\alpha$ power in the right inferior parietal cortex (Brodmann area 40) for the eyes open task; ii) a significant increase ($p <$

* Corresponding author: Lorenzo Chiari, Ph.D., DEIS - Università di Bologna, Viale Risorgimento, 2 I-40136, Bologna - ITALY, ph: (+39) 051 209 3014, fax: (+39) 051 209 3073, e-mail: lorenzo.chiari@unibo.it.

0.05) of γ power in the left temporo-occipital areas in the eyes open task (Brodmann areas 17,18,19, and 30); iii) a significant increase ($p < 0.05$) of γ power in left temporo-parietal areas for the eyes closed task (Brodmann areas 21,37, and 41).

All in all, the findings reported above suggest a completely different usage of the ABF sound by healthy subjects in the EC Task as compared to the EO Task.

It would indeed seem that, in the eyes open task, the spatial information coded in the ABF sound is primarily used by the brain in association with visual information: the significant decrease of α power in the right IPL and the significant increase of γ power in primary and associative visual areas suggest that the ABF sound could i) just modulate the processing of visual information and ii) trigger some specific multi-sensory integration processes in areas associated with multisensory, perceptual integration.

It is obvious that, in the eyes closed task, the brain cannot use the visual information. In the absence of visual information, the perception and the elaboration of the spatial content of the ABF sound would originate, at least partially, by an additional processing workload of the associative cortical auditory areas in the left temporal lobe and in the left temporo-parietal junction. This hypothesis is consistent with the fact that a significant increase of γ power due to ABF was found for the eyes closed task, but not for the eyes open task.

# 1. Introduction

## Mechanisms for Postural Control

The postural control depends on the dynamic integration of multisensory information in the Central Nervous System (CNS). Effective postural control requires peripheral input from the visual, somatosensory and vestibular systems to detect the body's position and movement in space. Each of these senses provides different information based on a different frame of reference (Gurfinkel and Levick 1991). The somatosensory system provide static and dynamic proprioceptive as well as exteroceptive information using the physical surround as the ultimate reference frame. The visual system is designed to give static and dynamic information of the body's position and movement with respect to the visual surround. The vestibulum is essentially a system of accelerometers sensitive to both linear and rotational accelerations in all planes of motion. All types of postural information are continuously processed and integrated at the levels of the brainstem, the cerebellum and the cerebrum in order to monitor ongoing body movements, to compare this movements with the actions planned, to detect movement errors and to correct these errors by adjusting the motor output (Kandel, Schwartz et al. 2000). This mode of balance regulation is often referred to as 'feedback' control of posture.

This CNS process is known as sensory integration. The prevailing theory states that the various sources of sensory information are integrated to form an internal model of the body that the CNS uses to plan and execute motor behaviors . This internal model must be adaptive, to accommodate changes associated with growth and development, aging, and injury (Horak and Macpherson 1996). In fact, basic research has shown that the CNS is able to shift emphasis between somatosensory, visual and vestibular inputs depending on the availability and validity of the sensory information. When one sense is not providing optimal or accurate information about the body's position and movement, the 'weight' given to that sense as a source of orientation is temporarily reduced, while the weight of other, more accurate senses is increased, a phenomenon sometimes referred to as sensory 're-weighting' (Oie, Kiemel et al. 2002). Thus, there is a flexible hierarchy in the CNS between different senses to maintain balance.

## Augmentation of Sensory Information in Postural Control

Sensory loss or abnormal, inadequate sensory information from the vestibular, somatosensory and visual senses can jeopardize the CNS ability to control postural stability. In this case, providing the CNS with substitutive, artificial, sensory information may help restore the ability to control posture. Augmentation of sensory information normally implies the use of an external device able to provide information about body motion through biofeedback, eventually presented in a virtual reality environment.

### *Design of a Biofeedback System*

Three main parts essential for the design of a biofeedback system for postural control are: 1) a sensor or an instrument able to measure some aspect of human motion, 2) a restitution device, able to convey the biofeedback information to the subject (e.g. via the auditory, visual, or tactile sense), and 3) some circuit or a computer able to implement a conversion algorithm which transposes the information sensed by the sensor into a convenient activation of the restitution device.

### *Overview in Biofeedback*

The use of biofeedback for improving control of posture in subjects with motor disorders has been oriented to provide augmented movement information of body segments. Visual-biofeedback of center of pressure displacement has been the most popular biofeedback system design for improving postural stability. In particular, visual-biofeedback has been extensively used for balance rehabilitation of subjects after stroke (Nichols 1997) in order to reduce postural asymmetries. Recently, the interest in biofeedback design is moving from the visual-biofeedback of force plate measurements to audio- and tactile-biofeedback of inertial sensors measurements (Chiari, Dozza et al. 2005; Wall and Kentala 2005). This trend in the design is driven by the intent of producing new cost-effective and portable systems for balance training and rehabilitation. In particular, audio-biofeedback do not rely on expensive and cumbersome monitor, and it is more unobtrusive and comfortable than a tactile one.

Augmentation of sensory information during auditory biofeedback (ABF) of the trunk acceleration, has been shown to improve postural control, as indicated by a reduction of the root mean square (RMS) of the center of pressure displacement and of the trunk acceleration (Dozza, Horak et al. 2007). Such improvement is particularly evident when natural sensory information is limited by environmental conditions or pathology such as in subjects suffering from bilateral vestibular loss (Dozza, Chiari et al. 2005; Dozza, Horak et al. 2007). In (Dozza, Horak et al. 2007), comparison of postural sway under a variety of sensory conditions suggested that patients with profound bilateral loss of vestibular function show larger than normal information redundancy among the remaining senses and ABF of trunk sway. This result supports the hypothesis that the CNS uses augmented sensory information differently depending on both the environment and the individual tendencies to rely on vestibular, somatosensory or visual information to control sway, in proportion to the extent that other sensory information is reduced.

Moreover, it has been shown, through stabilogram diffusion analysis combined with electromyography, that ABF does not simply increase stiffness (and hence co-activation) in leg muscles, but rather helps the brain to actively change to a more feedback-based control activity over standing posture (Dozza, Chiari et al. 2005).

More recently, a pilot study in patients with progressive supranuclear palsy showed the efficacy of an ABF-based physical training in improving posture and dynamic balance as well as psychosocial aspects (Nicolai, Mirelman et al. 2010). Interestingly, the positive effect of the training sustained until 4 weeks after the completion of the training, which argues for possible prolonged effect of the training in these patients cohort.

However, the effects of ABF on the CNS, the neural mechanisms associated with its sensory augmentation and with the integration of such sensory augmentation in feedback-based control mechanisms are still unknown. A better understanding of which are the basic processes in the brain involved in the perception and usage of auditory signals used in ABF is desirable. Moreover, a better knowledge of the neural information processing associated with the ABF exercise would improve our knowledge in understanding how the CNS gathers and interprets time-dependent information from the vast array of sensory stimuli (including artificially augmented channels) and how it turns this into strategies to improve balance or motor performance. This would ultimately support, also, the development of enhanced, tuned, adaptive audio-biofeedback systems to assist motor and balance control, e.g. for older people at risk for falls or in people with postural disabilities.

## 2. How Does ABF Work?

### Current or Recent Research on Cortical Correlates of Postural Control

A number of studies, especially in the recent years, have investigated some central mechanisms involved in postural control through neuroimaging (fMRI, PET) or electro/magnetoencephalography techniques. In particular, (Saitou, Washimi et al. 1996) investigated the cortical potentials preceding postural adjustment followed by voluntary ballistic rising on tiptoe; (Ouchi, Okada et al. 1999) depicted the neural substrates for maintaining different standing postures in humans with a mobile gantry PET system; (Quant, Adkin et al. 2004) investigated the cortical potentials following a balance perturbation; (Quant, Adkin et al. 2004) studied the effect of a concurrent cognitive task on cortical potentials evoked by unpredictable balance perturbations; (Adkin, Quant et al. 2006) contrasted the cortical potentials associated with predictable and unpredictable compensatory balance reactions; (Slobounov, Hallett et al. 2005) showed that the initiation of self-paced postural movement is preceded by slow negative DC shift, similar to movement-related cortical potentials accompanying voluntary limb movement, and that a burst of gamma activity precedes the initiation of compensatory backward postural movement when balance was in danger; (Slobounov, Hallett et al. 2008) specifically examined the modulation of EEG as a function of voluntary postural sway direction. Another important research thread focused on the search for central correlates of the detection of postural instabilities. Slobounov and colleagues showed that: i) power in the EEG $\gamma$ band is influenced by visual recognition of non-stable postures (Slobounov, Tutwiler et al. 2000); ii) parietal and cingulated cortex, cerebellum and basal ganglia activities are modulated by the visual recognition of unstable postures (through fMRI) (Slobounov, Wu et al. 2006); and iii) the cingulate cortex the junction of precuneus and parietal lobe, and the occipital cortex are involved in the recognition of future postural instability in phases immediately preceding falls (Slobounov, Cao et al. 2009).

### The Need for further Investigations on Cortical Correlates of ABF

The effects of ABF on the CNS, the neural mechanisms associated with its sensory augmentation and with the integration of such sensory augmentation in feedback-based control mechanisms are still unknown. A better understanding of which are the basic processes in the brain involved in the perception and usage of auditory signals used in ABF is desirable. A better knowledge of the neural information processing associated with the ABF exercise would in fact improve our knowledge in understanding how the CNS gathers and interprets time-dependent information from the vast array of sensory stimuli (including artificially augmented channels) and how it turns this into strategies to improve balance or motor performance. This would ultimately support, also, the development of enhanced, tuned, adaptive audio-biofeedback systems to assist motor and balance control, e.g. for older people at risk for falls or in people with postural disabilities.

We are not aware of any study previous to (Pirini, Mancini et al. 2011) aimed to investigate the cortical correlates of biofeedback effectiveness for postural control. Indeed, studies investigating the cortical correlates of sensory-guided motor acts / strategies mainly focused on the upper limb, on the hands or fingers movements. Consequently, focused on discrete motor acts (e.g., target reach (Ghilardi, Ghez et al. 2000)) rather than on the modulation of continuously produced motor patterns as during a postural task. Moreover, most of the previous studies exploited the visual channel to instruct the subject about what to do and/or to give feedback about the action being performed (i.e., to return some kind of error measure). Most of them used metabolic neuroimaging techniques (fMRI, PET), that, however, are not suitable for studying ABF in quiet standing tasks due to obvious practical reasons.

For all these reasons, we opted for bringing electroencephalographic (EEG) signals in the routine of ABF-related experiments, EEG being the only technique which is available, at the present time, for a direct, non-invasive investigation of the behavior of the CNS in the present paradigm.

## 3. Insight: Methodological and Interpretative Key Issues in EEG Research

The analysis of the behavior of cortical CNS through high density (19+ channels) EEG is becoming increasingly widespread, both in clinical and in research domains (Niedermeyer and Da Silva 2005). New linear modeling and analysis techniques have been developed in the recent years, allowing researchers to face the poor spatial resolution and the artifact issues related to the EEG signal.

In particular, spatial model-based localization techniques (see the review by (Pascual-Marqui 1999)), like the Standardized Low Resolution Electromagnetic Tomography (sLORETA) make use of spatial models of the skull and head to resolve the inverse localization problem and to localize some specific features at the cortical level (in the time, frequency or time-frequency domains) of the EEG data. In such a context, the EEG can be viewed as a neuroimaging technique, similar to fMRI or PET. The freely available software sLORETA-KEY (http://www.uzh.ch/keyinst/loreta.htm) makes use of a normalized, 3-layer spherical shells model of the head (Montreal Neurological Institute MNI head model, (Fuchs, Kastner et al. 2002; Jurcak, Tsuzuki et al. 2007)), and of the virtually zero-error localization sLORETA algorithm. The solution space of the algorithm is represented by 6735 voxels in the gray matter of the MNI brain (Pascual-Marqui 2002).

Moreover, blind source separation techniques, like Independent Component Analysis (ICA), may allow for a data-driven spatial filtering of data through the search of a set of sources which maximize mutual independency, thus permitting the experimenter to reject non cortical, artefactual ingredients of the signal.

ICA algorithms act as a data-driven spatial separation of the (n-channel) EEG data-set x (Oja and Hyvarinen 2000). They assume that the electrical signals x recorded at the electrodes are the result of a linear, instantaneous combination (summarized by an n by n mixing matrix A) of the activity of a set of n sources s (both cerebral and not), and that such sources are statistically independent:

$$\mathrm{x} = \mathbf{A}\,\mathrm{s} \tag{1}$$

ICA algorithms search for the demixing matrix **W** that will maximize the independence of the estimated set of sources $s_{estim}$:

$$s_{estim} = \mathbf{W}\,x;\ x = \mathbf{W}^{-1}\,s_{estim};\ \mathbf{W}^{-1} \equiv \mathbf{A} \text{ under the assumption (1)} \tag{2}$$

This searching process is mostly done iteratively and involves the calculation of higher order statistics from the dataset (Lee, Girolami et al. 1999). The relevance of the ICA approach in the removal of EEG artifacts stems from the fact that, once a source has been identified as artefactual (i.e., EOG / ECG related), it is possible to virtually remove it by rebuilding a cleaned version of the data set, as a linear combination of the non artefactual sources only (Jung, Makeig et al. 2000).

It has to be remarked here that sLORETA and ICA techniques seek to address quite different issues: the localization (sLORETA) or the separation (ICA) of EEG sources. Their complementary functions can be of great value in understanding different aspects of an EEG-based experiment.

Regarding the interpretation of the EEG signals in the frequency domain (see (Basar, Basar-Eroglu et al. 2001)), we adopted so – far the simplest, but generally valid, interpretative key, stating power in the $\alpha$ band (8-13 Hz) being positively correlated with cortical idling (mainly produced by thalamo-cortical interactions) and power in the $\beta$ and $\gamma$ bands (13-30 Hz, and >30 Hz, respectively) being positively correlated with cortical processing (mediated by intra-cortical interactions).

# 4. Review of Our Recent Research Activity on ABF

We review and complement here the methodology and the results arising from (Pirini, Mancini et al. 2011), a study focused on the search for cortical correlates of postural ABF.

## Aims

In order to reach a better understanding of the mechanisms involved in the task-oriented perception and cognition of auditory signals used in ABF for postural stabilization, the work aimed at localizing the reliable across-subjects loci of the differential cortical activations due to the preliminary exposure to the routine ABF exercise in completely naive healthy subjects and at interpreting the results in the light of the state-of-the-art knowledge about the motor-aimed perceptive integrative mechanisms in the brain. In order to study how the healthy central nervous system uses the auditory ABF information, and if it integrates such information with those arising from other sensory channels, we asked the subjects to perform the ABF exercise with both eyes open and eyes closed. We hypothesized that the ABF-related cortical activations could be different in the presence and in the absence of the visual information, thus showing that the central nervous system would process the auditory information in different ways depending on the availability of the visual channel. Specifically, we hypothesized the activation of cortical areas known to be involved in multisensory integration processes in the presence of visual information.

**Table 1. Subjects information**

| ID | Age | Sex | Right-handed? |
|---|---|---|---|
| #1 | 61 | F | yes |
| #2 | 48 | M | yes |
| #3 | 72 | M | yes |
| #4 | 26 | M | yes |
| #5 | 40 | M | yes |
| #6 | 68 | F | yes |
| #7 | 33 | M | yes |
| #8 | 60 | M | yes |
| #9 | 34 | F | yes |
| #10 | 24 | M | yes |

## Methods

### *Participants*

Ten healthy subjects participated in the study (7 males and 3 females, range 24-72 years). All participants were free from any neurological, orthopedic, or vestibular disorder. Informed consent was obtained from each subject. None of them had been previously exposed to the ABF exercise, nor was previously informed about the syntax of the ABF sound. Inclusion criteria for subject selection were the absence of hearing and cognitive deficits.

### *Apparatus and Procedure*

A wearable system for the delivery of postural ABF was used. The system includes a sensing unit based on a 3D accelerometer (DynaPort MiniMod TriAcc, McRoberts, The Netherlands) which measures trunk acceleration along the anterior-posterior (AP) and the medio-lateral (ML) anatomical axes. Trunk acceleration is then wirelessly transferred (via Bluetooth) to a palmtop which is responsible for real-time signal processing to produce changes (in volume, pitch, and balance) in a stereo sound used to provide the user with an augmented sensory experience about his/her trunk sway. The non-linear equations used to produce the sound, and hardware and software components of the system are described in detail in (Chiari, Dozza et al. 2005) and (Chiari, Farella et al. 2008). The routine procedure for ABF experiments usually involves a repetitive administration of motor and/or postural tasks, the easiest of which is quiet standing, performed under different sensory conditions (eyes open or closed, rigid or foam support, etc.) with and without the ABF (Dozza, Horak et al. 2007; Mirelman, Herman et al. 2009).

In the study, the experimental protocol consisted of the repetition of 90-s long, quiet standing tasks where trials with eyes open (Task: EO) alternated with trials with eyes closed (Task: EC). In both the Tasks, Subjects were asked to keep the upright standing position as still as possible with arms crossed at the chest. We wanted to detect cortical activations which are specifically linked to the interpretation (and usage) of the ABF semantic structure, and not just the effect of the acoustic stimulation. In order to do that, we designed the protocol as follows: 1) two trials (1 EO, 1 EC) without ABF (PRE), 2) two trials (1 EO, 1 EC) with fake ABF (FAKE) in which the sound was not the direct consequence of subjects' actual movements, 3) two trials (1 EO, 1 EC) with ABF (ABF). We measured trunk linear acceleration (at a sampling frequency of 50 Hz) by means of the accelerometer worn on the subject's back (L5 level) through a waist-strap. Only during the ABF condition this signal was used to generate the real-time audio feedback. At the same time, we recorded 19 EEG channels (Neurowave System, Khymeia, Italy) by means of a dedicated cap at a sampling frequency of 256 Hz. Channels positions (Fp1, Fp2, F7, F3, Fz, F4, F8, T3, C3, Cz, C4, T4, T5, P3, Pz, P4, T6, O1, and O2) were set according to the International 10-20 standard system. Reference electrode was positioned at the right earlobe. Electrode impedances were monitored and kept below 10 KΩ during the entire experiment. The ABF and EEG systems were synchronized by a custom-made electronic system.

Subjects were wearing a pair of headsets for the entire experiment. No sound was played during the PRE set of trials. The sound heard during the FAKE trials was obtained by off-line feeding the sound-producing algorithm running on the palmtop with the accelerometric signal recorded during the corresponding (EO or EC) PRE trial. The accelerometric signal recorded during the FAKE trials did not enter into play in any trials. Subjects were instructed about the syntax of the ABF sound just before the first (EO) ABF trial: subjects were instructed on how ABF codes trunk acceleration into sound, and performed some free-movement trials until they felt confident in performing the subsequent experimental sessions. We did not randomize (among the same Task) the FAKE and ABF trials, since it was evident, from previous experiences with ABF, that order matters: a subject already instructed about the ABF syntax tends to intentionally follow an ABF-like sound even if informed that this signal is off-line and not being caused by their own postural accelerations. In order to prevent such a behavior (a confounding factor in the present context), we decided to present a single trial of the FAKE always preceding the actual ABF trial.

It has to be mentioned that the only function of the PRE trials was to provide subject-specific accelerometric data to the sound-production system, in order to have a subject-specific profile of the sound heard by the subject during the FAKE conditions. Therefore, we did not further used the EEG and accelerometric data arising from the PRE trial in any of the investigations.

### *Accelerometric Signal Analysis*

Acceleration signals were transformed to a horizontal-vertical coordinate system and filtered with a 3.5 Hz cut-off, zero-phase, low-pass Butterworth filter. Subsequently, the RMS was calculated from the planar acceleration (Moe-Nilssen 1998; Moe-Nilssen and Helbostad 2002). For each subject and for each Task, the percentage change in RMS ($\Delta$RMS%) between the FAKE and the ABF conditions was calculated as ($RMS_{FAKE}$ - $RMS_{ABF}$) / $RMS_{FAKE}$ * 100. For each Task, a statistical analysis (t test for zero mean) was performed on the vector of $\Delta$RMS% values to reject the null hypothesis $H_0$: mean of $\Delta$RMS% equals to 0.

### *EEG Analysis*

## Power Modulation of Independent Components – Population Wise Analysis

As mentioned previously, the EEG analysis techniques at the scalp level suffer from the volume conduction problem: the electrical activity produced by strong generator of a given rhythm, i.e., the well known occipital $\alpha$ rhythm active when a subject is resting with eyes closed (Berger,1929), could spread also on electrodes far from its source due to volume conduction of the electromagnetic field. Due to that, it could be totally erroneous to interpret $\alpha$ power over frontal electrodes as a frontal $\alpha$ rhythm, and, consequently, its possible modulation due to experimental conditions. Moreover, different $\alpha$ generators modulated by experimental conditions could be masked by the strongest generator. In order to (at least partially) overcome the volume conduction issue, we tested the modulation of the EEG activity not at the electrodes level, but at the IC level. The procedure described below is equivalent to looking at the behavior of the ingredients of the signals, irrespectively of their relative weights.

For each subject the following algorithm was followed:

1) the portions of the EEG recordings clearly contaminated by spurious events (e.g., electrode bad contacts) were manually erased;

2) for each condition (EO, EC), the FAKE and ABF recordings were merged and the resulting trace was passed to a popular ICA algorithm (*runica* - [Lee *et al.*,1999]);
3) the artifactual IC components due to EOG, ECG, and EMG activities were identified and removed – we based such a selection process on the time profile, the power spectrum and the topography of each component;
4) the remaining non-artifactual ICs were considered;
5) for each IC, the temporal signal was epoched (epoch length: 2 s; superposition: 1 s);
6) PSD was estimated for each epoch through a Blackman-Harris modified periodogram estimator;
7) powers in α, β, and γ bands were calculated for each epoch by integration and log10-transformed to gain normality of their distributions;
8) two-tailed t-tests were conducted to test for significant changes of α, β, and γ powers between FAKE and ABF (significance level set at $p = 0.01$ – Bonferroni corrected for multiple tests (correction factor: 19 ICs * 3 bands =57));
9) ICs showing significant differences were assigned, separately for α, β, and γ powers, to a cortical lobe (Frontal, F; Central, C; Parietal, P; Temporal, T; and Occipital, O) according to their topography (the IC was classified as Frontal if its higher weight was on electrode Fp1, Fp2, F7, F3, Fz, F4, or F8; as Central if its higher weight was on electrode C3, Cz, or C4; as Parietal if its higher weight was on electrode P3, Pz, or P4, as Temporal if its higher weight was on electrode T3, T 4, T5, or T6; and as Occipital if and as Occipital if its higher weight was on electrode O1 or O2).

Once identified and spatially classified the significantly modulated ICs on a single-subject basis, an overall, population-wise description was obtained.

## Cortical Localization of Differential Sources - Population-Wise Analysis

In order to move from a scalp level to a more precise identification of cortical sources and to cortically localize the population-wise differences observed for the α, β, and γ powers between FAKE and ABF we used the sLORETA method to post-process our EEG data, separately for EO and EC tasks.

For each subject the following algorithm was employed:

1) once identified and removed by ICA in the previous step the artifactual components due to EOG, ECG, and EMG activities, the cleaned datasets were returned in the portions relative to FAKE and ABF;
2) the cleaned EEG datasets at the scalp level, as derived in the previous step, were considered;
3) the α, β, and γ powers of the current density at each voxel (cortical power maps) were estimated by sLORETA, separately for FAKE and ABF and for EC and EO;
4) a population-wise, paired-samples, non parametric test was performed, separately for the α, β, and γ powers, and for EC and EO. To this aim, the log of ratio of average-across-subject power (log of F-ratio) statistics was calculated for each voxel (statistical nonparametric map), separately for the α, β, and γ powers and for EC and EO, and significance assessment of calculated statistics was performed through a non-parametric permutation procedure (Nichols and Holmes 2002). This statistical

non-parametric mapping methodology corrects for all multiple comparisons across voxels, and at the same time does not require any assumption of Gaussian normality. A subject-based normalization of the cortical power maps was performed before calculating the statistics. Such an operation is common in the field of neuroimaging (Nichols and Holmes 2002).

# Results

## Quantitative Accelerometric Results

Figure 1 shows the single-subject values of the percentage change in RMS acceleration (ΔRMS%) at L5, between FAKE and ABF. Values for the EO and the EC tasks are treated separately. It can be seen that all but two subjects (Subjects #3 and #9) showed a lower RMS value in the ABF trial compared to the FAKE trial, in both the EO and the EC tasks. We excluded Subject #3 from the subsequent statistical analyses since it can be considered as an outlier regarding the accelerometric data (see also Section 4.1 about this subject). Statistical analyses (t test for zero mean) found that the ΔRMS% is significantly (alpha = 0.05) higher than 0 for both Tasks: $p < 0.038$ for the EC Task, and $p < 0.009$ for the EO Task.

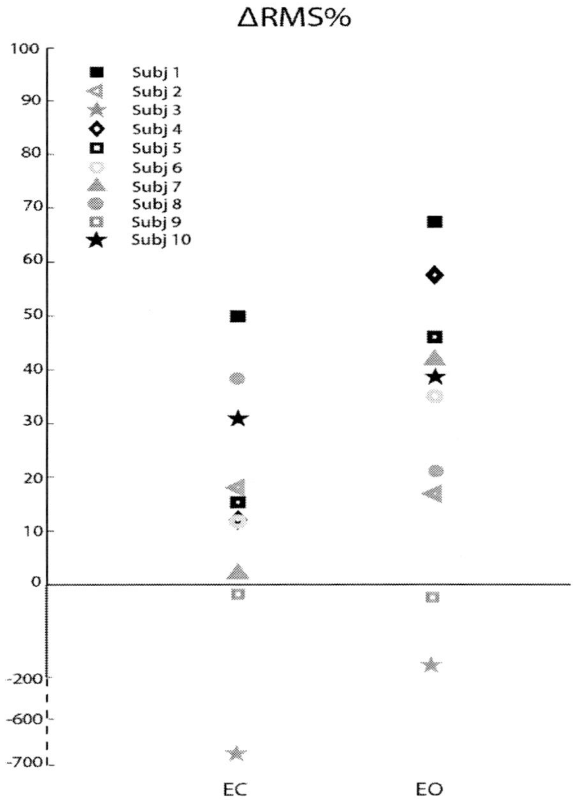


Figure 1. Single-subject ΔRMS% of the accelerometric signal measured at L5, for the eyes open (EO) and the eyes closed (EC) tasks. $\Delta RMS\% = (RMS_{FAKE} - RMS_{ABF}) / RMS_{FAKE} * 100$.

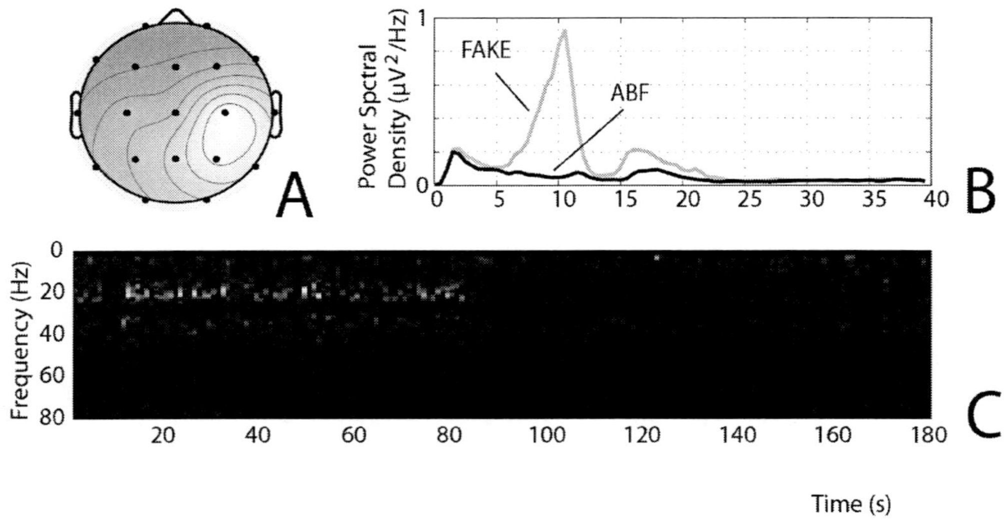


Figure 2. Topography (panel A), spectral power density (panel B - sepatetely shown for the FAKE and the ABF portions), and time-frequency power description (panel C) of an example Indipendent Component (from subject 4). See text for details.

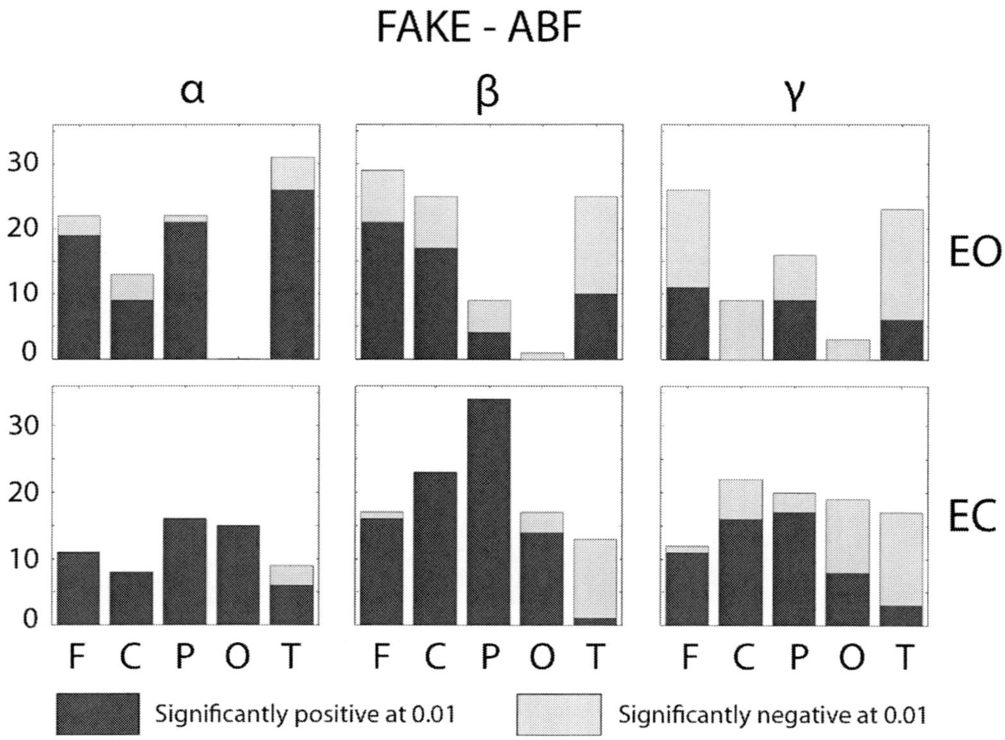


Figure 3. Population-wise representation of the overall ensample of (non artifactual) Indipendent Components showing a statistically ($p < 0.01$) significant difference of power (FAKE Condition - ABF Condition), separately for the α, β, and γ bands and for the EO and EC Tasks. ICs showing a significant negative difference of power are shown in black, while ICs showing a significant positive difference of power are shown in light gray. ICs were classified as Frontal (F), Central (C), Parietal (P), Occipital (O), or Temporal (T). See text for details.

## Power Modulation of Independent Components - Population Wise Analysis

Figure 2 shows, as a way of example, the results of the analysis of a single, non-artifactual Independent Component. The shown IC derived from an ICA of the EEG of the unified FAKE and ABF trials (EC condition) of Subject 4. The total temporal length of the EEG data submitted to the ICA analysis was approximatively 180 s. Figure 3 shows: i) (Panel A) the topography of the IC (a topographical representation of the weights through which the IC propagates on channels, i.e., the corresponding column of the mixing matrix **A**), ii) (Panel B) the estimate of the power spectral density of the IC in the first portion (FAKE) and in the second portion (ABF); and iii) (Panel C) the time-frequency representation of the power spectral density of the IC. The IC is localized in the right central-parietal area (Panel A). It can be seen (Panel B) that ABF heavily modulated the PSD of the IC, by decreasing the power both in the $\alpha$ and in the $\beta$ bands. The decrease was significant at a significance level = 0.05 (not shown here). The modulation depicted in panel B is not due to non-stationary events, but rather due to an abrupt change between two qualitatively stationary regimes (see panel C, showing a clear change of the PSD of the IC at approximatively $t$ = 85 s, i.e., the switching point between FAKE and ABF).

Figure 3 shows the behavior of the whole population-wise cohort of non-artifactual ICs showing a significant (at a significance level = 0.01, Bonferroni-corrected) modulation of power due to ABF, separately for the $\alpha$, $\beta$, and $\gamma$ bands and for the EO and the EC conditions. ICs were reassigned to a cortical lobe, and histograms distinguish between ICs showing a significant increase and decrease in power.

## Cortical Localization of Differential Sources - Population-Wise Analysis

The sLORETA statistical nonparametric maps of the comparison FAKE-ABF, for power in $\alpha$ , $\beta$, and $\gamma$ bands for the EO and the EC tasks, were calculated. sLORETA maps revealed positive values for log-F-ratio statistics of $\alpha$ power and negative values for log-F-ratio statistics of $\beta$ and $\gamma$ power in both the EO and the EC task.

The non-parametric permutation test found: i) significantly positive log-F-ratio regarding the $\alpha$ power for the EO Task (thresh $_{p<0.05}$ = 0.340; maximally significant voxel at 0.370 in the right Inferior Parietal Cortex, Brodmann Area 40) and ii) significantly negative log-F-ratios regarding the $\gamma$ power in some regions for the EC condition (thresh $_{p<0.05}$ = - 0.492; maximally significant voxel at - 0.498) and significantly negative log-F-ratios in some regions for the EO condition (thresh $_{p<0.05}$ = - 0.341; maximally significant voxel at -0.352). The maps for which such statistically significant results were found are shown in Figure 4: areas in red are indicative of positive values of the log-F-ratio statistics (power in FAKE higher than in ABF), while areas in blue are indicative of negative values of the log-F-ratio statistics (power in FAKE lower than in ABF).

Significant effects were not found regarding $\alpha$ power in the EC Task (thresh $_{p<0.05}$ = 0.370; maximally significant voxel at 0.199), nor regarding $\beta$ power for the EO (thresh $_{p<0.05}$ = -0.341; maximally significant voxel at -0.225) and the EC (thresh $_{p<0.05}$ = -0.492; maximally significant voxel at -0.368) s. Tasks.

Table 2 shows the list of regions for which a significant effect at a significance level equal to 0.05 was found.

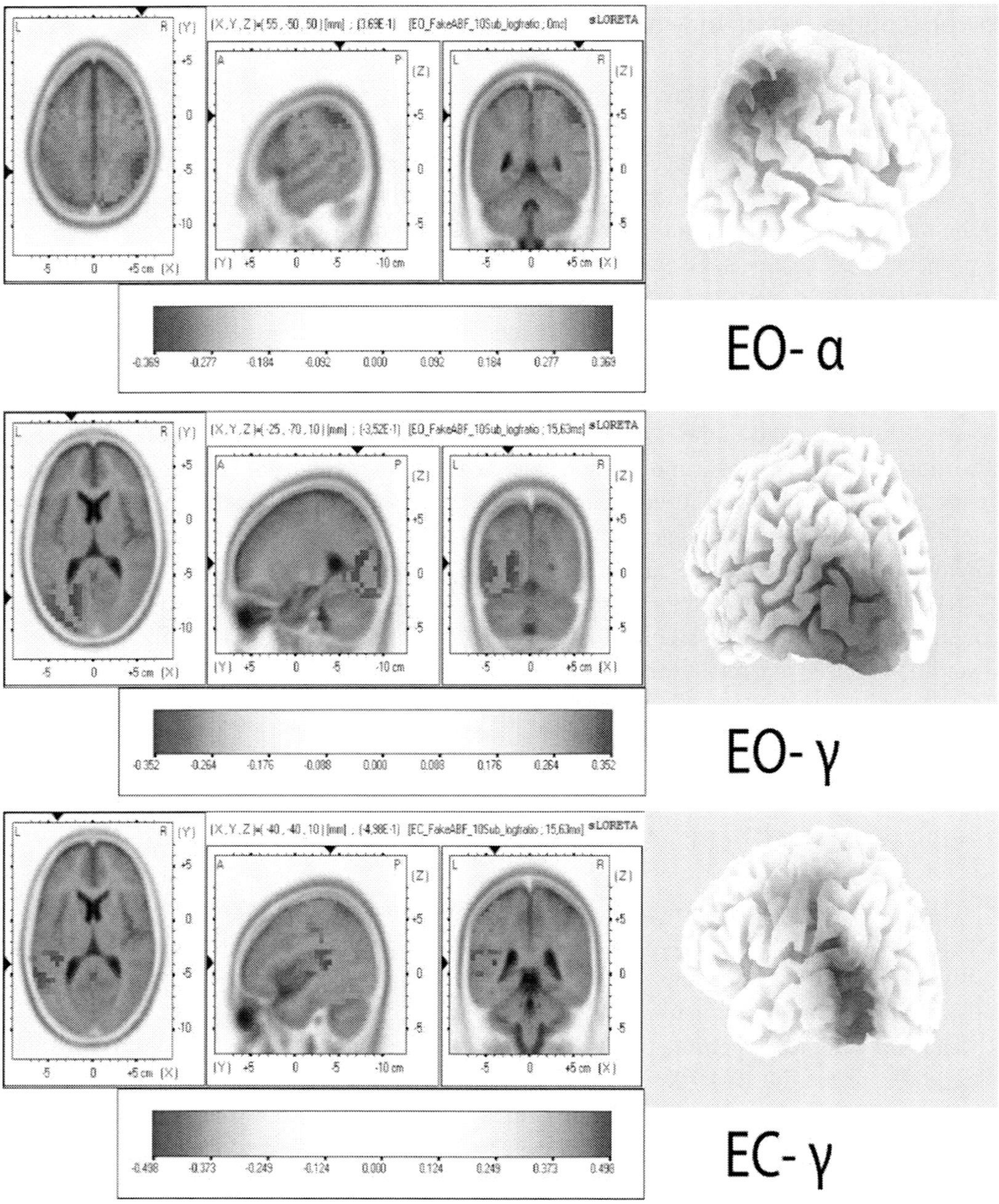


Figure 4. sLORETA maps for which the sLORETA non-parametric permutation test found statistically significant ($p < 0.05$) differences in power (FAKE condition - ABF condition): i) power in the α band for the EO Task (top panel); ii) power in the γ band for the EO Task (central panel); and iii) power in the γ band for the EC Task (bottom panel).

**Table 2. List of brain regions for which the sLORETA non-parametric permutation test found statistically significant ($p < 0.05$) differences in power (FAKE condition - ABF condition) for the α, β, and γ bands and for the eyes open (EO) and the eyes closed (EC) tasks**

| Anatomical regions (Brodmann Areas) |
|---|
| *α power - EO(p<0.05)* |
| Parietal lobe, Inferior Parietal Lobule (Right 40) |
| *β power - EO (p<0.05)* |
| - |
| *γ power – EO(p<0.05)* |
| Occipital Lobe, Cuneus (Left 17, Left 18, Left 30) |
| Occipital Lobe, Lingual Gyrus (Left 19) |
| Limbic Lobe, Posterior Cingulate (Left 18, Left 30) |
| *α power - EC (p<0.05)* |
| - |
| *β power - EC (p<0.05)* |
| - |
| *γ power – EC (p<0.05)* |
| Temporal Lobe, Middle Temporal Gyrus (Left 21, Left 37) |
| Temporal Lobe, Superior Temporal Gyrus (Left 41) |

# Discussion

## The ABF Sound Changed the Postural Behavior of the Subjects

The analysis on the accelerometric signals depicted in Figure 1 clearly showed that the presence of ABF, in both the EO and the EC tasks, helped the subjects reducing their postural oscillations. Such results: i) confirmed previous results about the effects of ABF on trunk sway (see (Dozza, Chiari et al. 2005)), when a decrease in trunk acceleration RMS was observed both in vestibular patients and in healthy subjects even in a minimally challenging task as quiet standing; ii) allowed us to confirm that the subjects clearly understood the ABF exercise, and most importantly, that they actually used the ABF sound to modulate their postural behavior; and, consequently iii) allowed us to treat the whole group of subjects as a homogeneous group for the EEG-related analyses.

It can be seen from Figure 1 that the ΔRMS%, when positive, was higher for the EO than for the EC task in all the subjects but two (Subject #2, for which changes are almost equivalent, and Subject #8, for which the ΔRMS% is higher for the EC than for the EO). It should be remarked, however, that these changes were calculated by comparing the effects of

ABF with a novel condition, never tested before (FAKE), and not with an absence-of-ABF condition, as in (Dozza, Horak et al. 2007).

The subjects who apparently did not understand the exercise and/or did not take advantage of the ABF to reduce their RMS were Subjects #3 and #9. However, the behavior of Subject #3 can be explained as follows. As seen in Figure 1, he *increased* the RMS by several times. From visual observation of his behavior, and from an a-posteriori interview, we argued that the subject modulated his postural behavior not to maintain a clear, stable auditory tone (the target sound, present in a central stable position), but rather tried to reach a perceived absence-of-sound situation. A perceived absence of sound during the ABF exercise could be eventually achieved by swaying backward along the anterior-posterior axis - as the subject did. Indeed, such kind of oscillatory behavior lowers the frequency of the tone, thus giving the sensation that also the loudness of the sound gets lower, due to the non-linear frequency response of the auditory system (see (Fletcher and Munson 1933)). The frequency response decreases as the frequency decreases in the range 150 - 400 Hz, which is in fact the range used to code the backward accelerations in the ABF system. While successfully accomplishing the erroneously-intended task, such oscillatory behavior leads to a much more unstable postural oscillatory regime characterized by a much higher RMS. In any case, even if erroneously, the subject clearly *applied for* an ABF-guided postural exercise, and we considered this behavior as fulfilling the inclusion criteria of our study. Hence we kept also this subject in the subsequent population-wise EEG analyses. A possible modification of the ABF system, in order to equalize the non-linear frequency response of the auditory system (on a single-subject basis, at least partially) and thus to prevent erroneous interpretation of the ABF exercise is under evaluation.

## Discussion of EEG Results

### *Power Modulation of Independent Components - Population Wise Analysis*

Before discussing the present results, we must remind here that such analysis considered all the ICs as equally significant, irrespective of their relative weights in determining the EEG signal, and that it was primarily conduced in order to to get a qualitative picture of the EEG activities modulated by the ABF while limiting at maximum (as far as we know) the "masking effect" that the strongest generators impose when performing simple differential power analysis at the electrode level. We mostly considered such analysis as an intermediate step to be done in order to confirm (or not) our initial working hypothesis regarding the meaning of the power modulations in the different bands, and to get a more conscious picture of data before conducting our “core” sLORETA analysis discussed in the following.

Regarding the ABF modulation in the $\alpha$ band, the great majority of ICs showed a decrease of power due to ABF thus suggesting a come-into-play and/or a release from an idling state of a number of different cortical processes. Notably, it is evident how $\alpha$ - modulated ICs were present in almost all of the tested regions. Interestingly, no significantly modulated occipital ICs were modulated in the $\alpha$ band for the EO Task: such result can be easily interpreted by considering that the opening of the eyes disrupt *per se* the thalamo-cortical idling $\alpha$ activity in the visual occipital areas, with no further effects of the ABF condition. Eventually, the results regarding the $\alpha$ – modulated ICs by ABF were in line with what we expected.

The picture arising from the analysis of the β- and γ -modulated ICs is less straightforward. Differently from what we expected, based on the interpretative framework of EEG power we assumed in the present work, the majority of β-modulated ICs still showed a power decrease, not an increase. It has to be mentioned here that the simple interpretative framework we adopted regarding the power in the different bands could lead itself to erroneous conclusions, due to the fact that often α rhythms are not just "pure" sinusoids; their second and third harmonics fall in the β band (and sometimes also in the γ band), thus further confounding the interpretation of the β (and γ) power modulation by different experimental conditions that modulate also the thalamo-cortical mechanisms responsible for the generation of α rhythms (see (Kozelka and Pedley 1990; Pfurtscheller and Neuper 1997) for a description of this aspect about central sensorimotor α rhythms and (Bianchi, Molteni et al. 2004) for occipital α rhythms). Thus, ICs showing a power decrease in the α band would probably show also a confounding decrease in the β and γ bands (as a partial confirm to this hypothesis, please note that where α-modulated ICs were not found, i.e., the occipital regions in the EO task, no β- and γ-modulated ICS showing a decrease of power were found). Anyway, it should be noted that: i) there is a significant portion of β-modulated ICs showing an increase in power in every region for the EO Task and in the Temporal region for the EC Task); ii) the portion of γ- modulated ICs showing an increase of power further increases when considering the γ band, especially in the Temporal, Central, Frontal, and Occipital regions for the EO Task ands in the Temporal and Occipital regions for the EC Task. As a partial interpretation of results, the increase of β and γ power in Temporal ICs (present both in the EC and in the EO Tasks) could be related to an higher cortical activation of the associative auditory cortex in the temporal lobe, while the additional onset of β and activity in Occipital (present both EC and in the EO Tasks) and Parietal ICs in the EO Task could be due to the well known integrative audio-visual processes that come into play over primary and associative visual areas and in the superior and posterior parietal lobes.

### *Cortical Power Modulation - Population Wise Analysis*

Based on the knowledge of the basic functioning of the healthy CNS (Kandel, Schwartz et al. 2000), it is possible to speculate that the ABF exercise would require several sensory, cognitive, and motor contributions to enter into play. The correct execution of the ABF exercise certainly requires: i) auditory processing, performing a decomposition of the sound into its basic features (pitch, volume, lateralization), surely performed in the primary auditory cortices in the temporal areas; ii) the elaboration of such features guided by the knowledge of the ABF syntax, coded in the working memory, to give rise to a representation of the spatial attributes of the sound; iii) the integration of the information provided by the ABF sound into an internal perceptual spatial representation of the self, that continuously receives information also from other sensory channels (visual, somatosensory, vestibular); iv) the formation of an error signal due to the eventual discrepancy between the perceived position in space and the expected pre-determined target; v) the planning of motor acts to reduce or counterbalance the error (probably performed in the prefrontal cortex); and vi) the execution of such motor acts through specific activations of the primary motor areas. Moreover, the key role of the attentive system(s) (mainly located in the parietal cortices) in promoting and coordinating the whole process should be considered.

We found significant differential cortical activations in the γ band for the EO and the EC Tasks and in the α band for the EO Task. We will try now to read the results of the present study in the light of such hypothesized conceptual framework.

### Modulation of α Power

We found a significant decrease of α power due to ABF for the EO Task in the right Inferior parietal lobule (IPL). The IPL is a functionally and anatomically heterogeneous region that is concerned with multiple aspects of sensory processing and sensorimotor integration. It sustains a wide range of functions related to attention, motion processing, and spatial working memory (Alain, He et al. 2008) and its involvement in auditory and tactile localization has been reported frequently (Clower, West et al. 2001; Holmes and Spence 2005; Alain, He et al. 2008). Among a vast array of corticocortical connections, IPL receives extra-cortical connections primarily from the superior colliculus in the thalamus (one among the most important sub-cortical structures responsible for the multisensory integration functions in the brain), the hippocampus (involved in working memory functions), and the cerebellum, involved in the coordination of voluntary motor activity.

No statistically significant cortical decrease of α power due to ABF was found for the EC tasks.

### Modulation of γ Power

It has been proposed that oscillations in γ band in the EEG reflect multisensory integration through enhanced coherence among the underlying neuronal cortical populations (Kaiser and Lutzenberger 2005; Fries 2009; Kaiser, Lutzenberger et al. 2009).

The areas where we found a statistically significant modulation of γ Power in the EC task (See Table 2) are, interestingly, among the areas previously identified as involved in the preliminary elaboration and perception of speech. In particular, (Hickok and Poeppel 2007) found that the posterior Superior Temporal Gyrus (STG - an auditory association cortex), together with the Superior Temporal Sulcus, is a relevant part of the cortex to construct a perceptual representation of the meaning of auditory inputs, while the Middle Temporal Gyrus (MTG) has been proposed as the substrate for the interface between the phonetic and the lexical content of speech (Indefrey and Levelt 2004; Kiefer, Sim et al. 2008). The left localization of the whole set of structures is not surprising, given that the dominant left hemisphere is specialized for speech perception (Hickok and Poeppel 2007; Kiefer, Sim et al. 2008).

Quite surprisingly, we did not find significant activations of the areas cited above in the EO Task. Instead, in such a Task, we found significant ($p<0.05$) increase of γ power in areas usually thought as primary and associative visual areas (See Table 2). Nevertheless, such activations in the Occipital lobe could be explained considering recent findings in multisensory research. Contrary to the classical idea that multisensory integration of information is performed just after the segregated processing of inputs from different sensory modalities (processed in different sensory cortices), several results recently supported the idea that multisensory integration mechanisms could just enter into play via crosstalk modulations between primary or secondary unisensory cortical areas (see (Holmes and Spence 2005) for a review). In particular (McDonald, Teder-Salejarvi et al. 2003; McDonald, Teder-Salejarvi et al. 2005; Teder-Salejarvi, Di Russo et al. 2005) showed, by Event-Related-Potential-based studies, how spatial congruity between visual and auditory inputs presented simultaneously may trigger cross-modal interactions at the level of the visual processing stream, leading to a higher activation of the ventral occipital cortex and to an enhanced visual perception.

### Interpretation of Results

All in all, the findings reported above suggest a completely different usage of the ABF sound by healthy subjects in the EC Task as compared to the EO Task.

It would indeed seem that, in the EO Task, the spatial information coded in the ABF sound is primarily used by the brain in association with visual information: the significant decrease of $\alpha$ power in the right IPL and the significant increase of $\gamma$ power in primary and associative visual areas suggest the trigger of some specific multi-sensory integration processes, both at the sub-cortical and at the cortical levels.

It is obvious that, in the EC Task, the brain cannot use the visual information. In the absence of visual information, one might argue that the perception and the elaboration of the spatial content of the ABF sound originates, at least partially, by an additional processing workload of the same associative cortical auditory areas in the left temporal lobe and in the left temporo-parietal junction. This hypothesis is consistent with the fact that a significant increase of $\gamma$ power due to ABF was found for the EC Task, but not for the EO Task.

## Limitations of the Work

The aim of the work in (Pirini, Mancini et al. 2011) was not to study the basic physiology of the multisensory integration performed by the Central Nervous System, but rather to study the early EEG modifications due to a *standard* ABF-driven exercise on postural control in completely naive subjects. We wanted to depict the central correlates of a closed-loop process (subject + ABF), rather than to specifically study some open-loop perturbation-related behavior. Therefore, the used protocol, in order to keep the experimental procedure as similar as possible to routine ABF sessions, did not involve the administration of any kind of precisely timed stimulation / request to the subject, thus preventing the use of the well-known event-related analysis techniques (massively used, and much easier to interpret than EEG power changes (Pfurtscheller and Lopes da Silva 1999)).

Surely, a possible source of bias in the population-wise analyses could arise from the fact that in our experimental procedure we did not randomize the EC and the EO tasks across subjects. Indeed, in the present experiment, every subject systematically performed the ABF condition with EO before the ABF condition with EC. Such randomization will be implemented in the next studies regarding ABF.

It was shown how the ΔRMS% values are higher in the EO Task than in the EC Task for most of the subjects. Apparently, this is counter-intuitive, since one might expect that the subjects would gain more benefit from ABF in the EC (a more difficult Task, comparable to a sensory deprivation) than in the EO Task. One may argue that such finding could be a consequence of the lack of randomization cited above; in any case, the effects of the Task over the change in postural parameters induced by ABF surely need to be further investigated in properly re-designed experiments and their consistency checked in order to understand if they change or not with learning (we tested here subjects who were completely naïve to ABF).

In our study, we used the FAKE Condition as a de-facto control condition against which to contrast the ABF Condition. This choice was done since we wanted to detect cortical activations which are specifically linked to the interpretation and usage of the ABF information, and not just the effect of the acoustic stimulation the ABF exercise induces to the subject. However, one may argue that the FAKE condition as a control condition for ABF may not be all together accurate, due to its inherently rich acoustic content. We didn't check if the EEG correlates of normal posture in relative silence or with normal environmental auditory cues available are more like ABF or more like FAKE or something completely different. These data are needed as a foundational piece of information, and future studies should ensure the application of such various controls.

# Conclusion

Depending on the functioning of the natural senses that contribute to balance control, i.e. the vestibular, somatosensory, and visual systems (Day, Guerraz et al. 2002), the biofeedback may be used as a substitute (Dozza, Horak et al. 2007) or as an augmentation (Vuillerme, Pinsault et al. 2008) in the central nervous system's sensorimotor integration. Enhanced effects on movement performance after training with augmented biofeedback may be caused by 'sensory re-weighing' processes, in which the relative dependence of the central nervous system on the different natural senses in integrating sensory information is modified (Horak, Shupert et al. 1989; Peterka and Loughlin 2004).

We have verified that Audio Biofeedback of postural control heavily modulates specific cortical activations in healthy subjects as measured and interpreted by EEG. We believe that such EEG modifications state at least part of the sensory re-weighting processes cited above. In addition, we found completely different ABF-related activations in the EO and EC tasks, stating completely different strategies used by the CNS in using the acoustic ABF information depending on the availability of other sensory information (the visual one). Indeed, it would emerge a multi-level organization of the CNS in allocating resources for the processing of new sensory information for postural control: the re-weighing process (considering here the acoustic and visual input channels) could take part not only at the well-known areas deputed to the multisensory fusion aimed at the creation of the representation of the self in space (e.g., the posterior parietal cortex), but also through inter-sensory, lower-level (in the hierarchy of the sensory information processing) modulations between usually considered unisensory cortical areas. Actually, these findings should not be surprising, due to the recent advances in the multisensory research revealing both hierarchical and parallel organization in the multisensory fusion processes (Lewkowicz and Ghazanfar 2009). Next steps along the present research framework should: i) involve experiments aimed to specifically investigate the influence of ABF over the processing of information for postural control arising from other sensory channels (e.g. the somatosensory one, involving subjects standing on a foam to partially reduce the somatosensory feedback); ii) study if such multisensory fusion processes differ between healthy subjects and elderly and/or in neurological subjects suffering from balance problem (namely in Parkinson's Disease).

## Acknowledgments

The study was co-funded by the European Commission (FP6 project SENSACTION-AAL, IST-045622). We thank Eng. Carlo Tacconi for his help during the experiments with the ABF instrumentation.

## References

Adkin, A. L., Quant, S., Maki, B. E. and McIlroy, W. E. (2006). Cortical responses associated with predictable and unpredictable compensatory balance reactions. *Experimental Brain Research 172 (1)*, 85-93.

Alain, C., He, Y. and Grady, C. (2008). The contribution of the inferior parietal lobe to auditory spatial working memory. *Journal of Cognitive Neuroscience 20 (2)*, 285-295.

Basar, E., Basar-Eroglu, C., Karakas, S. and Schurmann, M. (2001). Gamma, alpha, delta, and theta oscillations govern cognitive processes. *International Journal of Psychophysiology 39 (2-3)*, 241-248.

Bianchi, A., Molteni, S., Panzica, F., Visani, E., Franceschetti, S. and Cerutti, S. (2004). Spectral and bispectral analysis of the EEG rhythms in basal conditions and during photic stimulation. *Conference Proceedings of the 26th Annual International Conference of the IEEE Engineering in Medicine and Biology Society*, San Francisco.

Chiari, L., Dozza, M., Cappello, A., Horak, F. B., Macellari, V. and Giansanti, D. (2005). Audio-biofeedback for balance improvement: an accelerometry-based system. *IEEE Trans. Biomed. Eng. 52 (12)*, 2108-2111.

Chiari, L., Farella, E., Rocchi, L. and Benini, L. (2008). A biofeedback-based portable device to support elderly mobility in the home environment. *Gerontechnology 7 (2)*, 93.

Clower, D., West, R., Lynch, J. and Strick, P. (2001). The inferior parietal lobule is the target of output from the superior colliculus, hippocampus, and cerebellum. *Journal of Neuroscience 21 (16)*, 6283.

Day, B., Guerraz, M. and Cole, J. (2002). Sensory interactions for human balance control revealed by galvanic vestibular stimulation. *Advances in experimental medicine and biology 508*, 129.

Dozza, M., Chiari, L., Chan, B., Rocchi, L., Horak, F. B. and Cappello, A. (2005). Influence of a portable audio-biofeedback device on structural properties of postural sway. *Journal of NeuroEngineering and Rehabilitation 2*, 13-13.

Dozza, M., Chiari, L. and Horak, F. B. (2005). Audio-biofeedback improves balance in patients with bilateral vestibular loss. *Archives of Physical Medicine and Rehabilitation 86 (7)*, 1401-1403.

Dozza, M., Horak, F. and Chiari, L. (2007). Auditory biofeedback substitutes for loss of sensory information in maintaining stance. *Experimental Brain Research 178 (1)*, 37-48.

Fletcher, H. and Munson, W. (1933). Loudness, its definition, measurement and calculation. *Journal of the Acoustical Society of America 5*, 82-108.

Fries, P. (2009). Neuronal gamma-band synchronization as a fundamental process in cortical computation.

Fuchs, M., Kastner, J., Wagner, M., Hawes, S. and Ebersole, J. S. (2002). A standardized boundary element method volume conductor model. *Clinical Neurophysiology 113 (5)*, 702-712.

Ghilardi, M., Ghez, C., Dhawan, V., Moeller, J., Mentis, M., Nakamura, T., Antonini, A. and Eidelberg, D. (2000). Patterns of regional brain activation associated with different forms of motor learning. *Brain Research 871 (1)*, 127-145.

Gurfinkel, V. and Levick, Y. In J. Paillard. *Brain and Space*. Oxford: Oxford Science Publications; 1991; 147-161.

Hickok, G. and Poeppel, D. (2007). The cortical organization of speech processing. *Nature Reviews Neuroscience 8 (5)*, 393-402.

Holmes, N. P. and Spence, C. (2005). Multisensory integration: space, time and superadditivity. *Current Biology 15 (18)*, 762-764.

Horak, F. and Macpherson, J. In S. J. Rowell RB. *Handbook of Physiology: Section 12, Exercise Regulation and Integration of Multiple Systems*. New York: Oxford University Press; 1996; 255-292.

Horak, F., Shupert, C. and Mirka, A. (1989). Components of postural dyscontrol in the elderly: a review. *Neurobiology of Aging 10 (6)*, 727-738.

Indefrey, P. and Levelt, W. J. M. (2004). The spatial and temporal signatures of word production components. *Cognition 92 (1-2)*, 101-144.

Jung, T. P., Makeig, S., Humphries, C., Lee, T. W., McKeown, M. J., Iragui, V. and Sejnowski, T. J. (2000). Removing electroencephalographic artifacts by blind source separation. *Psychophysiology 37 (2)*, 163-178.

Jurcak, V., Tsuzuki, D. and Dan, I. (2007). 10/20, 10/10, and 10/5 systems revisited: their validity as relative head-surface-based positioning systems. *Neuroimage 34 (4)*, 1600-1611.

Kaiser, J. and Lutzenberger, W. (2005). Human gamma-band activity: a window to cognitive processing. *Neuroreport 16 (3)*, 207.

Kaiser, J., Lutzenberger, W., Decker, C., Wibral, M. and Rahm, B. (2009). Task-and performance-related modulation of domain-specific auditory short-term memory representations in the gamma-band. *Neuroimage 46 (4)*, 1127-1136.

Kandel, E., Schwartz, J. and Jessell, T. *Principles of neural science*. 4th Ed. New York: McGraw-Hill; 2000.

Kiefer, M., Sim, E., Herrnberger, B., Grothe, J. and Hoenig, K. (2008). The sound of concepts: four markers for a link between auditory and conceptual brain systems. *Journal of Neuroscience 28 (47)*, 12224.

Kozelka, J. and Pedley, T. (1990). Beta and mu rhythms. *Journal of Clinical Neurophysiology 7 (2)*, 191.

Lee, T. W., Girolami, M. and Sejnowski, T. J. (1999). Independent component analysis using an extended infomax algorithm for mixed subgaussian and supergaussian sources. *Neural Computing 11 (2)*, 417-441.

Lewkowicz, D. and Ghazanfar, A. (2009). The emergence of multisensory systems through perceptual narrowing. *Trends in cognitive sciences 13 (11)*, 470-478.

McDonald, J. J., Teder-Salejarvi, W. A., Di Russo, F. and Hillyard, S. A. (2003). Neural substrates of perceptual enhancement by cross-modal spatial attention. *Journal of Cognitive Neuroscience 15 (1)*, 10-19.

McDonald, J. J., Teder-Salejarvi, W. A., Di Russo, F. and Hillyard, S. A. (2005). Neural basis of auditory-induced shifts in visual time-order perception. *Nature Neuroscience 8 (9)*, 1197-1202.

Mirelman, A., Herman, T., Maidan, I., Chiari, L., Zijlstra, A., Nicolai, S. and Hausdorff, J. (2009). Automated auditory biofeedback training to enhance postural control and mobility in patients with Parkinson's disease: preliminary results from SENSACTION-AAL. *Conference Proceedings of the XIX Conference of the International Society for Posture and Gait Research*, Bologna.

Moe-Nilssen, R. (1998). A new method for evaluating motor control in gait under real-life environmental conditions. Part 1: The instrument. *Clinical Biomechanics 13 (4-5)*, 320-327.

Moe-Nilssen, R. and Helbostad, J. (2002). Trunk accelerometry as a measure of balance control during quiet standing. *Gait and Posture 16 (1)*, 60-68.

Nichols, D. (1997). Balance retraining after stroke using force platform biofeedback. *Physical Therapy 77 (5)*, 553.

Nichols, T. E. and Holmes, A. P. (2002). Nonparametric permutation tests for functional neuroimaging: a primer with examples. *Human Brain Mapping 15 (1)*, 1-25.

Nicolai, S., Mirelman, A., Herman, T., Zijlstra, A., Mancini, M., Becker, C., Lindemann, U., Berg, D. and Maetzler, W. (2010). Improvement of balance after audio-biofeedback. A 6-week intervention study in patients with progressive supranuclear palsy. *Gerontology and Geriatrics Education 43 (4)*, 224-228.

Niedermeyer, E. and Da Silva, F. *Electroencephalography: basic principles, clinical applications, and related fields*. 5th Ed. New York: Lippincott Williams and Wilkins; 2005.

Oie, K., Kiemel, T. and Jeka, J. (2002). Multisensory fusion: simultaneous re-weighting of vision and touch for the control of human posture. *Cognitive Brain Research 14 (1)*, 164-176.

Oja, E. and Hyvarinen, A. (2000). Independent component analysis: algorithms and applications. *Neural Networks 13 (4-5)*, 411-430.

Ouchi, Y., Okada, H., Yoshikawa, E., Nobezawa, S. and Futatsubashi, M. (1999). Brain activation during maintenance of standing postures in humans. *Brain 122 ( Pt 2)*, 329-38.

Pascual-Marqui, R. (1999). Review of methods for solving the EEG inverse problem. *International Journal of Bioelectromagnetism 1 (1)*, 75–86.

Pascual-Marqui, R. (2002). Standardized low-resolution brain electromagnetic tomography (sLORETA): technical details. *Methods and Findings in Experimental and Clinical Pharmacology 24 (Suppl D)*, 5-12.

Peterka, R. and Loughlin, P. (2004). Dynamic regulation of sensorimotor integration in human postural control. *Journal of Neurophysiology 91 (1)*, 410.

Pfurtscheller, G. and Lopes da Silva, F. (1999). Event-related EEG/MEG synchronization and desynchronization: basic principles. *Clinical Neurophysiology 110 (11)*, 1842-1857.

Pfurtscheller, G. and Neuper, C. (1997). Motor imagery activates primary sensorimotor area in humans. *Neuroscience letters 239 (2-3)*, 65-68.

Pirini, M., Mancini, M., Farella, E. and Chiari, L. (2011). EEG correlates of postural audio-biofeedback. *Human Movement Science 30 (2)*, 249-61.

Quant, S., Adkin, A., Staines, W. and McIlroy, W. (2004). Cortical activation following a balance disturbance. *Experimental Brain Research 155 (3)*, 393-400.

Quant, S., Adkin, A. L., Staines, W. R., Maki, B. E. and McIlroy, W. E. (2004). The effect of a concurrent cognitive task on cortical potentials evoked by unpredictable balance perturbations. *BMC Neuroscience 5*, 18.

Saitou, K., Washimi, Y., Koike, Y., Takahashi, A. and Kaneoke, Y. (1996). Slow negative cortical potential preceding the onset of postural adjustment. *Electroencephalogr. Clin. Neurophysiol. 98 (6)*, 449-55.

Slobounov, S., Cao, C., Jaiswal, N. and Newell, K. (2009). Neural basis of postural instability identified by VTC and EEG. *Experimental Brain Research 199 (1)*, 1-16.

Slobounov, S., Hallett, M., Cao, C. and Newell, K. (2008). Modulation of cortical activity as a result of voluntary postural sway direction: An EEG study. *Neuroscience letters 442 (3)*, 309-313.

Slobounov, S., Hallett, M., Stanhope, S. and Shibasaki, H. (2005). Role of cerebral cortex in human postural control: an EEG study. *Clinical Neurophysiology 116 (2)*, 315-23.

Slobounov, S., Tutwiler, R., Slobounova, E., Rearick, M. and Ray, W. (2000). Human oscillatory brain activity within gamma band (30-50 Hz) induced by visual recognition of non-stable postures. *Cognitive Brain Research 9 (2)*, 177-192.

Slobounov, S., Wu, T. and Hallett, M. (2006). Neural basis subserving the detection of postural instability: an fMRI study. *Motor control 10 (1)*, 69.

Teder-Salejarvi, W. A., Di Russo, F., McDonald, J. J. and Hillyard, S. A. (2005). Effects of spatial congruity on audio-visual multimodal integration. *Journal of Cognitive Neuroscience 17 (9)*, 1396-1409.

Vuillerme, N., Pinsault, N., Chenu, O., Demongeot, J., Payan, Y. and Danilov, Y. (2008). Sensory supplementation system based on electrotactile tongue biofeedback of head position for balance control. *Neuroscience letters 431 (3)*, 206-210.

Wall, C. and Kentala, E. (2005). Control of sway using vibrotactile feedback of body tilt in patients with moderate and severe postural control deficits. *Journal of Vestibular Research 15 (5)*, 313-325.

# Index

## E



## F

## G



## H



## I

## N



## O



## P

## Q



## R



## S

## T

## U



## V



## W



## Y